VASCULOGENESIS AND ANGIOGENESIS – FROM EMBRYONIC DEVELOPMENT TO REGENERATIVE MEDICINE

Edited by **Dan T. Simionescu**
and **Agneta Simionescu**

Vasculogenesis and Angiogenesis – From Embryonic Development to Regenerative Medicine
Edited by Dan T. Simionescu and Agneta Simionescu

Published by InTech

Janeza Trdine 9, 51000 Rijeka, Croatia

Publishing Process Manager Marina Jozipovic

Technical Editor Teodora Smiljanic

Cover Designer InTech Design Team

Additional hard copies can be obtained from orders@intechopen.com

Vasculogenesis and Angiogenesis – From Embryonic Development
to Regenerative Medicine, Edited by Dan T. Simionescu and Agneta Simionescu
p. cm.
ISBN 978-953-307-882-3

For EU product safety concerns:
IN TECH d.o.o., Prolaz Marije Krucifikse Kozulić 3, 51000 Rijeka, Croatia,
info@intechopen.com or visit our website at intechopen.com.

Meet the editors

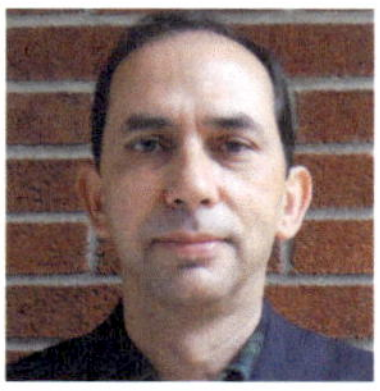

Dr. Dan Simionescu is Director of the Biocompatibility and Tissue Regeneration Laboratories, Department of Bioengineering at Clemson University, Clemson, SC and Director of the Regenerative Medicine Laboratory at Patewood/Clemson University Bioengineering Translational Research Center, Greenville Hospital System, Greenville, SC. He has published 50 papers, invited reviews and book chapters in highly ranked journals such as Circulation, Cardiovascular Pathology, American Journal of Pathology, Tissue Engineering, Biomaterials, Expert Opinions in Biological Therapy, and The Encyclopedia of Biomedical Engineering and has more than 120 peer-reviewed conference proceedings presented worldwide. Dr. Simionescu acts as a grant reviewer for the American Heart Association, Vascular Wall Biology study section and his general research interests include cardiovascular biology, pathology and regeneration using scaffolds and stem cells. His current interest is pre-clinical validation of translational tissue engineering approaches and is being generously funded by NIH, supporting his efforts in the field of regenerative medicine.

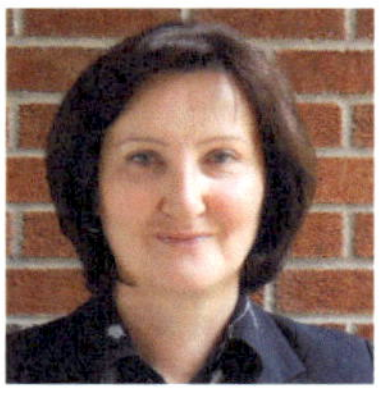

Dr. Agneta Simionescu received her PhD in Biochemistry/Cell Biology for the study of matrix remodeling in cardiovascular diseases. Her research interests include translational tissue engineering, angiogenesis, remodeling and mechanotransduction. She was the first to show that matrix metalloproteinases (MMPs) are involved in degeneration of implanted cardiovascular biomaterials and that matrix-derived degradation products (matrikines) induce pathologic osteogenic activation of cardiovascular cells. She has also shown that stabilization of biomaterials and scaffolds with mild and reversible cross-linking agents might counteract these effects. In recent years she has developed a passion for investigating the effects of diabetes on cardiovascular tissue engineering, including diabetes-related alterations of biomaterials and scaffolds, stem cell differentiation, matrix remodeling and microvascular network formation in vitro and in vivo models of diabetes.

Contents

Preface

The formation, development and persistence of most major organs and tissues depend on adequate vascularization. Blood vessels are among the first functional structures that form during embryonic development. Defects in blood vessel formation frequently lead to congenital malformations which need to be corrected by surgery or by using regenerative medicine approaches. After birth, existing blood vessels grow in size but new blood vessel formation is poorly represented in healthy individuals. This status quo is disturbed in numerous pathological conditions such as wound healing, rheumatoid arthritis, retinopathy, ischemia, and tumor and metastasis. Tumor growth depends greatly on extensive vascularization, and thus cancer research has focused tremendously on agents capable of blocking blood vessel formation.

During aging, blood vessels deteriorate slowly due to lipid and calcium deposition, inflammation, auto-immune reactions, and infections, potentially affecting all major organs and systems. Vascular diseases are a leading cause of morbidity and mortality worldwide and diseased blood vessels require surgical replacement with engineered devices. Tissue engineering and regenerative medicine approaches are diligently working on two main avenues: first, generation of living blood vessels of various calibers to serve as surgical replacements and second, development of vascularized living tissue substitutes with intrinsic 3D blood vessel networks to sustain effective organ perfusion.

New blood vessels may arise by two processes, vasculogenesis and angiogenesis. Endothelial cells are fundamental and common to both processes: however they differ in location, mechanisms of initiation and source of precursor cells. Vasculogenesis is a term describing the general process of de novo blood vessel formation during embryologic development of the cardiovascular system. This refers to two distinct inception scenarios: first, production of new endothelial cells in a developing embryo followed by development of a primordial vascular tree and second, generation of blood vessels in an adult avascular tissue area from precursor cells that migrate and differentiate to endothelial cells as a response to local signals.

Angiogenesis is the process by which new blood vessels form by "sprouting" of endothelial cells from pre-existing blood vessels; after "branching", these new "trees" are then reorganized, "pruned" and remodeled to eventually become 3D networks and also larger diameter vessels. Since this process is graphically similar to the growth and development of trees, there is no wonder that most terms used in angiogenesis are derived from the science of forestry.

Before the discovery of endothelial progenitor cells (EPCs) in the late 90's, the general consensus was that de novo vasculogenesis was restricted to the embryonic development arena and angiogenesis was only limited to growth and remodeling of adult vascular tissue. It is now known that as a response to injury, EPCs that normally reside in the bone marrow are mobilized into the circulation, migrate to avascular areas, differentiate into mature endothelial cells and develop vascular networks. In addition, bone marrow derived stem cells can act as "cytokine factories" and boost remodeling by secreting growth factors that help mature the developing "vascular tree". These cells have now become a central theme around which tissue engineering and regenerative medicine revolves. Vascular tissue engineering using scaffolds and stem cells has made great progress in recent years, highlighted by numerous successful animal experiments and recent clinical trials.

As shown above, basic and applied research in vasculogenesis and angiogenesis has come a long way and has elicited tremendous interest. The study of blood vessel formation is an essential component of embryonic development, congenital malformations, degenerative diseases, and cancer. It is probably almost impossible to contain and review all the research performed in this field in one single book.

The purpose of this book is to highlight novel advances in the field, focusing on four aspects of relevance. Esteemed authors from the USA, Europe and Asia, selected from a variety of fields summarize knowledge in their area of expertise and also contribute with authentic original experimental data to each chapter. The first section focuses on the early stages of human embryogenesis, development of the cardiac vasculature, the fetal lung and a novel signaling marker for vessel formation. This is followed by a section that focuses on regulation of EPCs and their role in diabetic vascular diseases. The role of vasculogenesis and angiogenesis in cancer is highlighted by two chapters that reveal the power of animal models and inhibitors of vasculogenesis and angiogenesis. Finally, looking towards the future, the last chapter highlights use of current knowledge towards regeneration of blood vessels using precursor cells, scaffolds and the proper mechanical cues.

This book is a good source of information for scientists interested in the intricacies of blood vessel formation, maturation, disease and replacement. It is also adequate for graduate students and medical students who wish to acquire basic updated information in the field.

Strolling through it, the reader will appreciate the crucial involvement of various precursor cells, starting with the primordial vascular cells in the embryo, the mesenchymal progenitor cells in healing and pathology and the lessons one can learn from the extraordinary ability of the cancer cells to manipulate blood vessel formation.

We are hoping that this book will help raise interest in the field and will entice new investigators to dwell into the complex and fascinating world of blood vessel formation, from the early days of embryonic development to the prospects of creating blood vessels in vitro for use as surgical replacements.

Dan T. Simionescu
Agneta Simionescu
Clemson University, Clemson, SC,
USA

Part 1

Developmental Biology

1

Human Embryonic Blood Vessels: What Do They Tell Us About Vasculogenesis and Angiogenesis?

Simona Sârb, Marius Raica and Anca Maria Cîmpean
"Victor Babeş" University of Medicine and Pharmacy, Timişoara, România

1. Introduction

The first functioning system during embryonic development is the cardiovascular system; the development of other organs and systems is in strict dependence to the emergence and development of blood vessels. Although the interest in the structure and functioning of the vascular system has existed since antiquity, there are still gaps in knowledge of the vascular system development issues. The process of blood vessel formation plays an important role during prenatal development; in the postnatal life, with few exceptions, this process is, normally, poorly expressed. Usually, an augmentation of postnatal vasculogenesis and angiogenesis is associated with pathological situations: healing wounds, certain degenerative diseases (rheumatoid arthritis, diabetic retinopathy, psoriasis) or malignant growth and metastasis. In this context, it becomes imperative to understand the mechanisms and factors involved in tumor angiogenesis. Mainly, tumor angiogenesis repeats - at least in some aspects - embryonic stages of vascular development. Most studies related to embryonic vascular system development were performed on embryos from other species, and / or cell cultures. Detailed morphogenesis studies, demonstrated the existence of differences between the primitive circulatory system in fish and mammals. In 2004, Ginis and collaborators have conducted a comparative study on cultures of human embryonic versus mice endothelial cells. The authors demonstrated the existence of species-specific differences that are related not only to quantitative aspects, but also to the existence of different signaling pathways. Even when using the same signaling pathways in cells from different species, different members of the same family were involved. Studies on human embryonic tissues, from the points of view stated above, are very rare and controversial; for example, the morphogenesis of embryonic vessels and, the temporal sequence for the onset of smooth muscle actin expression are very well studied and characterized in birds and mice, but not in humans.

2. Material and methods

We investigated the blood vessel morphology, and distribution in human embryos, of different gestational ages. Since the only direct microscopic argument for active angiogenesis is endothelial cell proliferation, we also investigated this parameter, in order to evaluate vasculogenesis versus angiogenesis.

2.1 Materials

This study was conducted on five, seven, and twenty four weeks human embryos; whole embryo specimens were obtained by therapeutic abortions, after signed patient consent, according to the Ethic Comity guidelines, and in compliance with the Helsinki Declaration of Human Rights.

2.2 Methods

The specimens were fixed in buffered formalin and embedded in paraffin according to the usual histological technique. Five-micrometer thick sections were stained with a routine Hematoxylin - Eosin method for morphological diagnosis. Additional sections were prepared for immunohistochemistry, as follows: microwave pH6 citrate buffer antigen retrieval was performed, followed by endogenous peroxidase inhibition with 3% hydrogen peroxide. In pursuing our objectives, first we investigated the morphology of embryo-fetal vessels by double immunostaining: we used as endothelial marker CD34 (clone QBEnd 10, dilution 1:25), and as a perivascular cell marker- smooth muscle actin (SMA, ready to use, clone 1A4 antibody); the cell nuclei were stained with modified Lille's hematoxylin. To assess endothelial cell proliferation, we used another double immunostaining: CD34/Ki-67 (ready to use, clone MIB1 antibody). After incubation with the primary antibody, the LSAB system was applied; the final reaction product was, for the first antibody, visualized in brown, with diaminobenzidine, and, for the second antibody, in red, with aminoethyl carbazole. The entire immunohistochemical technique was performed with DakoCytomation Autostainer. The slides were mounted with an aqueous medium, and examined with a Nikon Eclipse 600 microscope; images were taken, and processed with Lucia G system. On each slide we evaluated the expression/coexpression of the above mentioned markers in embryo-fetal vessels.

3. Results

We assessed embryonic blood vessels in both developing organs, and surrounding mesenchyme; the results varied with the embryo's gestational age, and the staining method.

3.1 Hematoxylin-Eosin staining

As a general remark, this type of staining allowed us to identify with certainty, only vessels with developing/obvious lumen; the vascular islands and vascular cords were less noticeable.

Embryonic tissue examination revealed the presence of blood vessels of different sizes, with different degrees of maturation, in all cases. In five and seven weeks old embryos, the mesenchymal tissue contained small blood vessels with relatively large lumens, thin walls, occasionally surrounded by perivascular cells. In the nervous organs, such small blood vessels were present in the subependymal space, at the boundary between white and gray matter, and in piamater (Fig.1).

In *five weeks embryos*, vessels were extremely rare in the mesenchyme of developing organs, such as esophagus, compared to the peripheral (subperidermal) mesenchyme, and were represented by vascular islands and cords, and small vessels, with thin walls (Fig. 2). Only on rare occasions we found mature vessels, with a well structured wall; some of these vessels had emerging endothelial cords (Fig. 3).

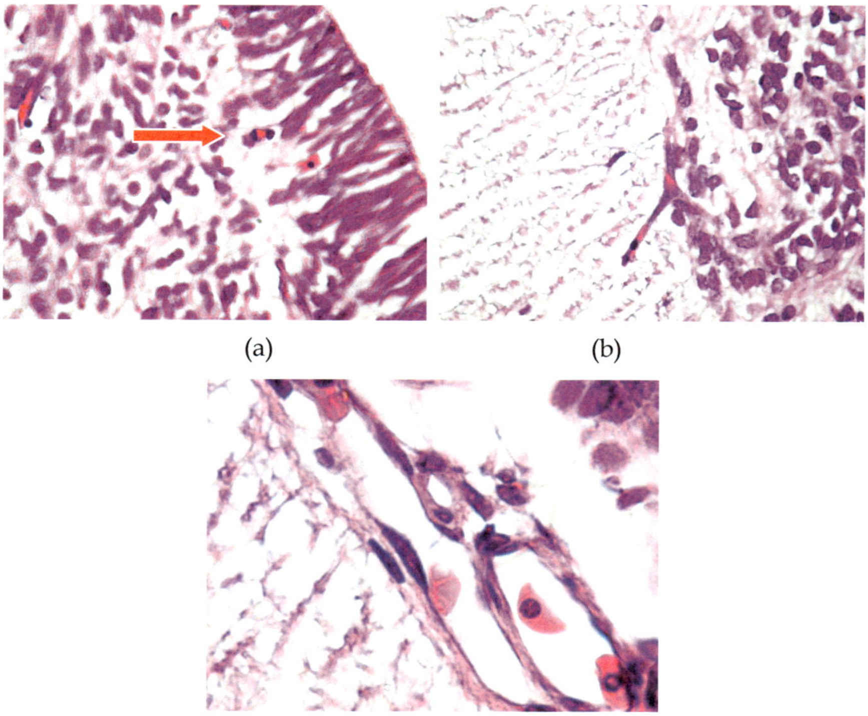

(a) (b)

(c)

Fig. 1. Cross sections of seven weeks embryo spinal cord, HE staining. In the subependymal space there are very small vessels, recognizable by the presence of megalocytes (subfig. a – arrow, X100). If at the white-gray matter border, there are small vessels with/without narrow lumen (subfig.b, X100), in the meningeal membranes there are vessels with larger lumen, that have perivascular cells attached to their endothelial cells (subfig.c, X400).

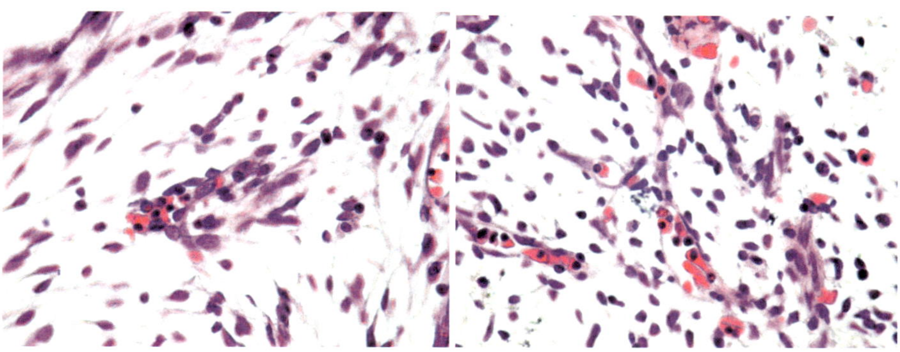

(a) (b)

Fig. 2. Five weeks embryo mesenchyme, HE staining. We frequently identified vascular islands, cords, and vessels with lumen, in the same microscope field (subfig.a, X100); sometimes we found concentrations of branched and anastomozed vessels, that presented budding phenomenon (subfig.b, X100)

In *seven weeks embryos*, the vessels were more numerous in the mesenchyme of the already differentiated organs as the lungs and heart, than in the peripheral mesenchyme. Unlike vessels in other areas of mesenchyme, lung vessels -located close to the bronchi- were characteristically elongated, and their inner tip already presented perivascular cells (Fig.4.a, X200). Again we observed the coexistence, in the same microscope field, of vascular islands, cords, and vessels with large lumen (Fig.4.b, X200).

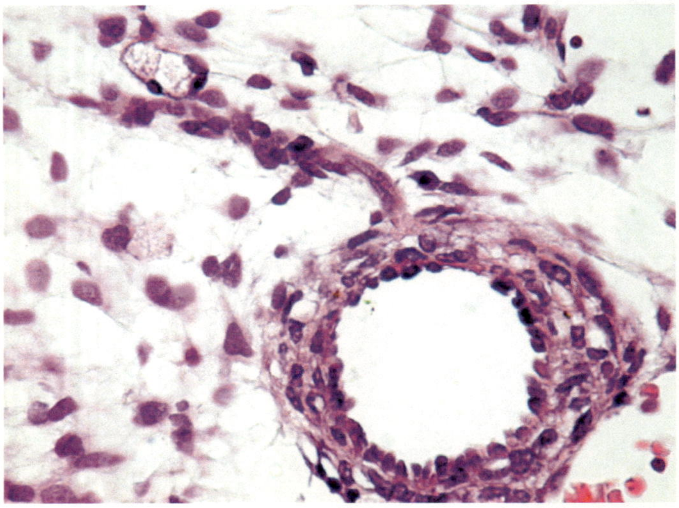

Fig. 3. Blood vessel with arterial morphology, that has in its upper part a cord-like cell proliferation (HE, X400).

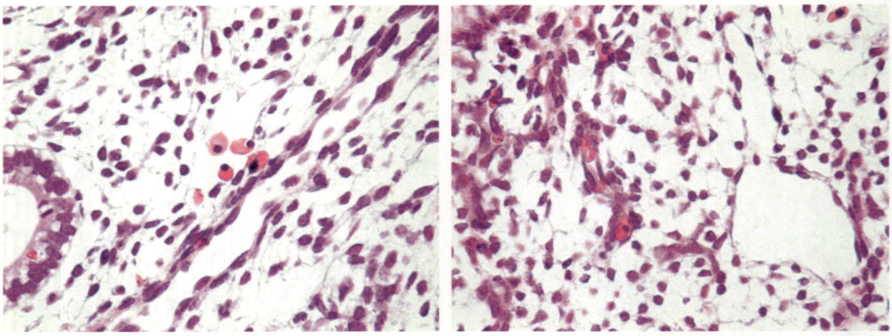

(a) (b)

Fig. 4. Seven weeks embryo lung, HE staining. Next to a bronchus in the canalicular phase of development rests an elongated blood vessel that has perivascular cells (subfig. a, X200). Further from the bronchi, the vascular islands coexist with blood vessels with wide lumen (surfing. b, X200).

3.2 CD34 / SMAct

Blood vessel classification was made according to the criteria described by Gee and his colleagues (2003). We classified as *immature vessels* those items that showed no obvious lumen, and were positive only for CD34; *intermediate vessels* reacted positive for CD34, showed no perivascular cells (negative reaction for SMA), but showed obvious lumen; *mature vessels* showed lumen lined by CD34 positive cells, doubled by SMA positive perivascular cells.

In *five weeks old embryos*, the expression of the two markers depended on the studied area. Thus, in the mesenchyme adjacent to differentiating tissues/organs, the CD34 positive isolated cells, vascular cords (Fig.5) and intermediate CD34 positive/ SMAct negative vessels were predominant. Mature blood vessels positive for both CD34 and SMAct, were detected in the undifferentiated mesenchyme, away from the developing organs; the SMA expression was weak and inconstant (Fig.6).

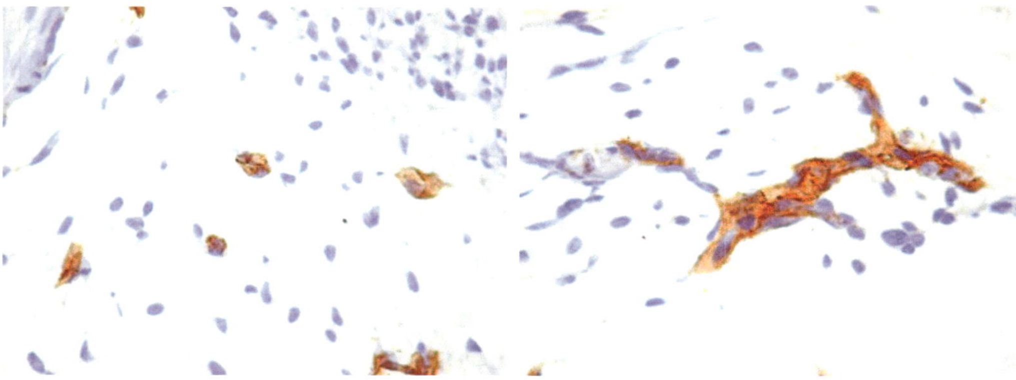

Fig. 5. Isolated CD34 positive cells, and CD34 positive/ SMAct negative vascular cords were the most frequent vascular structures found in the mesenchyme of five weeks old embryos (CD34/SMAct, X400).

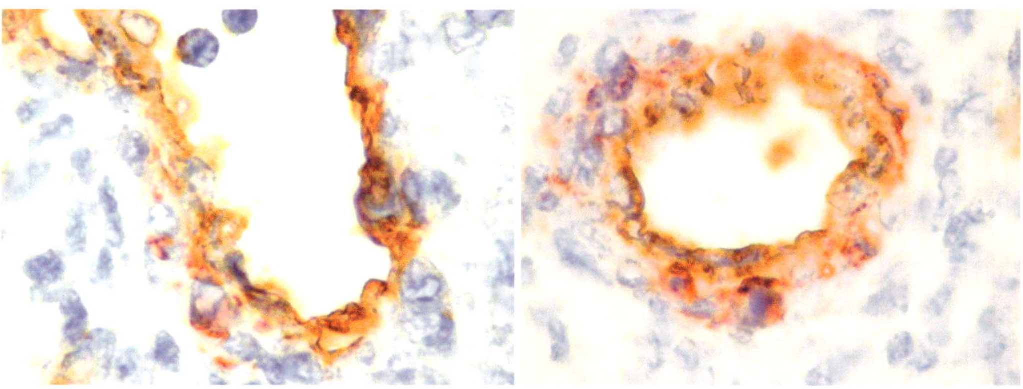

Fig. 6. In five weeks embryos only axial vessels begin to acquire pericytes- positive for SMAct (CD34/ SMAct, X1000).

In *seven weeks old embryos*, the aspects encountered in earlier stages were maintained, with the exception of larger vessels that had an almost complete investment of SMAct positive perivascular cells (Fig.7).

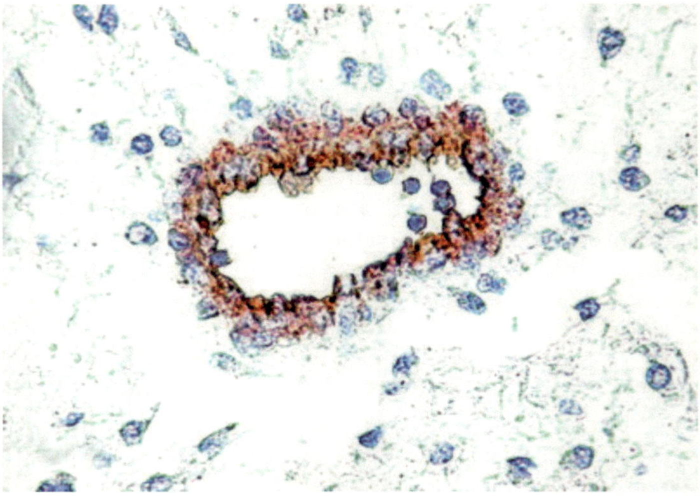

Fig. 7. In the large blood vessel, with a more complex wall structure, the CD34 positive endothelial cells are almost completely surrounded by SMAct positive cells (X400)

In *24 weeks old fetus* we studied the expression of CD34/SMAct in two locations: lungs –as a representative for parenchyma organs-, and esophagus –representative for hollow organs. The lung vessels, from the large ones that accompany the bronchi, to the small, interalveolar capillaries, were all positive for both markers; this means that at 24 weeks, the lung vessels are of mature type (Fig.8). There were some exceptions: at the periphery of the lung parenchyma, immediately under the pleura, we identified cord-like vascular structures positive only for the endothelial marker (immature vessels).

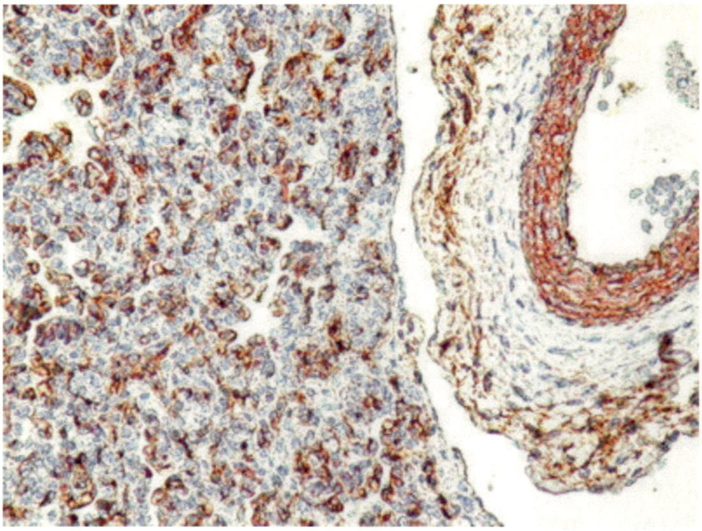

Fig. 8. Large lung blood vessel (right) with CD34 positive endothelium, and a thick SMAct positive muscle layer; note the presence of numerous CD34 positive cells (probably fibroblasts) in the outer adventitia. In the lung parenchyma, the interalveolar capillaries are CD34/ SMAct positive (X200).

In the esophageal wall, the reaction for the two markers was positive in all layers, but with different pattern from one layer to another. In the mucosa of the fetal esophagus immature, CD34 positive /SMAct negative, cord-like vascular structures, and intermediate vessels were observed (Fig.9, subfigure a). The blood vessels of the submucosa had a larger lumen with a more complex wall structure; the proportion of CD34 positive/ SMAct positive vessels versus CD34 positive/ SMA negative ones was approximately equal. Also, the vessels in this layer tended to come in pairs: one immature vessel accompanied by one intermediate/mature vessel (Fig.9, subfigure b). In the connective tissue of the muscular layer, blood vessels were mainly of immature type (CD34 positive /SMA negative), with a marked tendency for branching (Fig.9, subfigure c). In contrast, blood vessels in adventitia were mostly mature vessels, positive for both endothelial and smooth muscle actin markers (Fig.9, subfigure d).

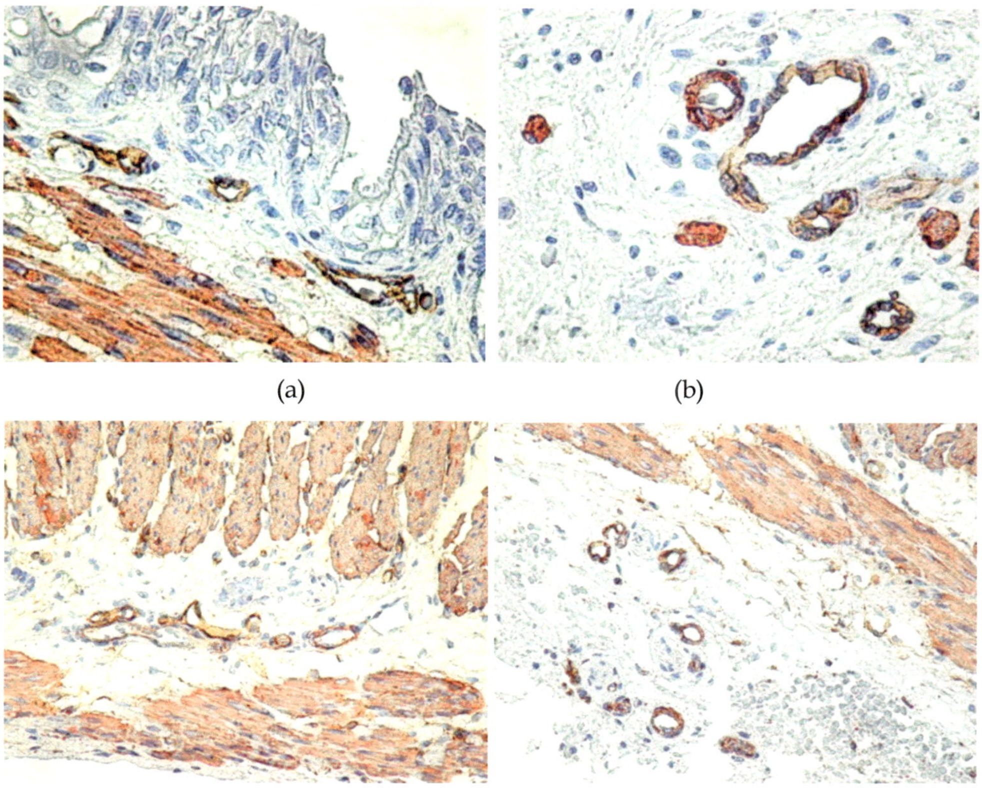

(a) (b)

(c) (d)

Fig. 9. Esophagus of 24 weeks fetus. Subfigure a: vascular cord with the tendency to form lumen, and small CD34 positive/SMAct negative vessels, in the mucosa (X400). Subfigure b: pairs of vessels were the larger one, with a more irregular outline is incompletely surrounded by SMAct positive cells (X400). Subfigure c: blood vessels undergoing remodeling, and as a consequence, the reaction for SMAct is inconstantly positive (X200). Subfigure d: the small blood vessels in the adventitia are completely invested with SMAct positive cells (X200).

3.3 CD34 / Ki67

In the *five weeks old embryos* the reaction for the proliferative marker Ki67 was positive in mesenchymal cells, but negative in all vascular structures identified with CD34 (Fig. 10). In the peripheral mesenchyme of *seven weeks old embryos,* Ki67 was inconstantly positive in the immature and intermediate vessels; only the peripheral cells of the vascular islands were positive for both CD34 and Ki67 (Fig. 11, subfigure a). In larger vessels, on their outer circumferences, we observed cells with an intense positive reaction for Ki67 (Fig.11, subfigure b). These cells were most likely perivascular cells in the process of attaching themselves to the vascular wall. In the vascular structures located in the mesenchyme surrounding developing organs, the endothelial cells lining larger arterial, or venous blood vessels, were CD34 positive/Ki67 negative (Fig. 12). At the same gestational age, even if we found vascular structures both inside, and at the periphery of the developing central nervous system, only those at the periphery were positive for Ki67 (Fig. 13).

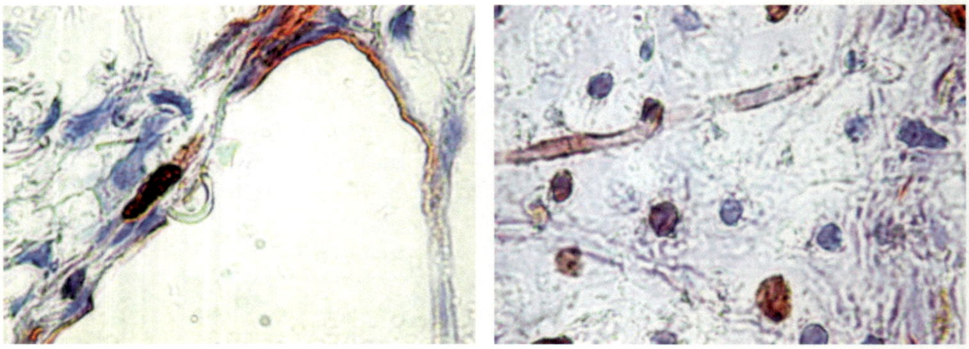

(a) (b)

Fig. 10. In five weeks embryos, endothelial cells nuclei are negative for Ki67; the only positive cells are the mesenchymal cells (subfigure b), and the nuclei of some perivascular cells (CD34/Ki67, X400).

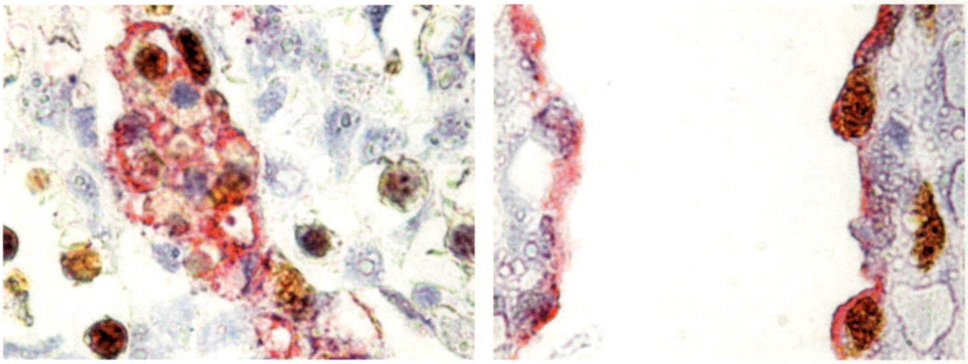

(a) (b)

Fig. 11. Subfigure a: in the central vascular island all cells are positive for CD34, but only those at the periphery are Ki67 positive; the reaction for Ki67 is also positive in some mesenchymal cells. Subfigure b: both endothelial and perivascular cells are positive for Ki67 (X1000).

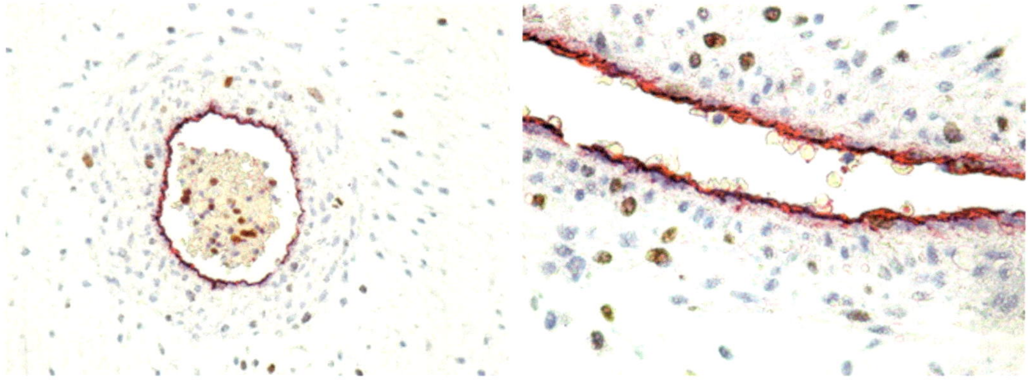

(a) (b)

Fig. 12. Large blood vessels with stabilized wall structure. Only few perivascular cells, and some cells in the mesenchyme are positive for Ki67 (X100, X200).

We also investigated CD34/Ki67 coexpression in the lungs and esophagus of 24 weeks fetuses. In the central zone of the lung parenchyma, in the walls of large blood vessels, occasionally, we encountered endothelial cells that expressed both CD34 and Ki67 (Fig. 14, subfigure a). On the other hand, in the subpleural parenchyma, the reaction for Ki67 was positive in most of the small blood vessels (capillaries) (Fig.14, subfigure b). In the esophagus sections we detected endothelial cell proliferation in the blood vessels of lamina propria and submucosa (Fig.14, subfigure c). A particular aspect was represented by the subepithelial capillaries, whose endothelial cells were negative for Ki67.

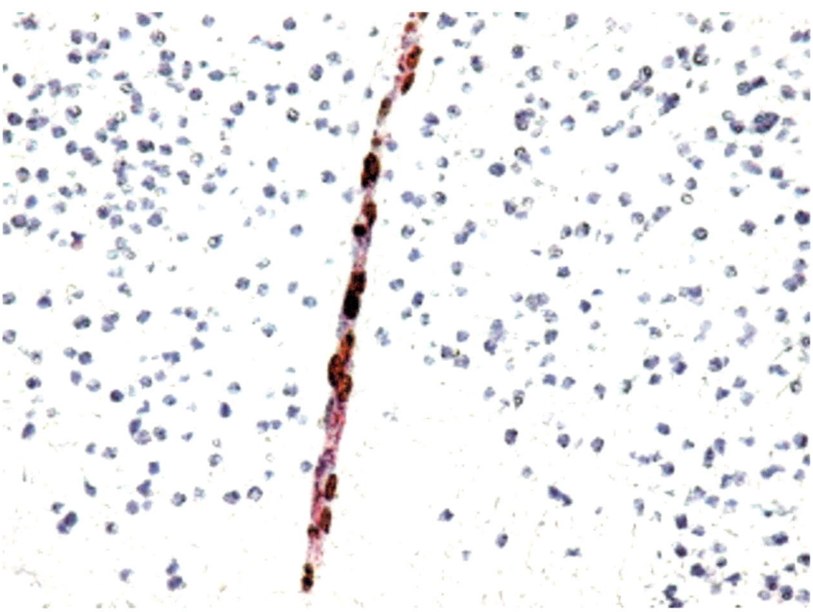

Fig. 13. Vascular cord positive for Ki67 at the periphery of central nervous system in the seven weeks embryos (CD34/Ki67, X200).

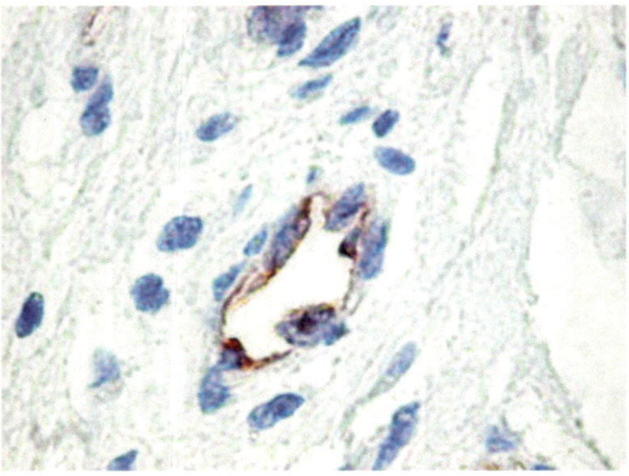

(a)

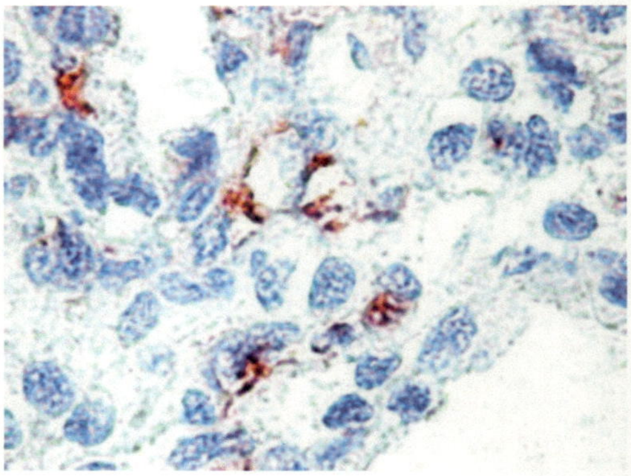

(b)

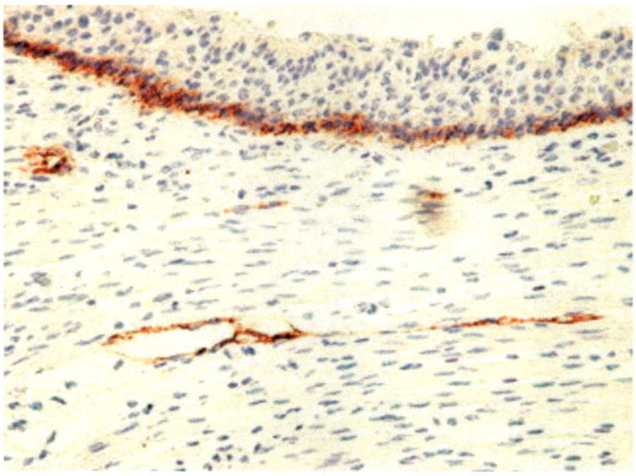

(c)

Fig. 14. Subfigure a, b: Fetus lungs: positive reaction for both CD34 and Ki67 in an isolated endothelial cell of a venous vessel, and in most endothelial cells lining the capillaries (X400). Subfigure c: esophagus wall- Ki67 was positive in the basal layer of the lining epithelium, and in the endothelial cells lining the blood vessels of lamina propria and submucosa.

4. Discussions

In the human species, endothelial cells can be detected in the yolk sac and in the embryo since the 24th day of gestation (Carmeliet, 2000). In the 35 days embryo, in endothelial cells and their precursors, CD34 is uniformly expressed (Tavian et al, 1999). Our results coincided with the literature, for the five weeks embryos; the reaction for CD34 was positive in all immature - isolated cells and vascular cords -, and intermediate vessels. But blood vessel maturation involves, besides endothelial cells, perivascular cells and extracellular matrix. The addition of perivascular cells (pericytes, smooth muscle cells) stabilizes the vascular wall by limiting the proliferation and migration of endothelial cells (Conway et al, 2001). The results that we`ve obtained have varied depending on the gestational age; in embryos aged 5-7 weeks, the response for CD34 was constantly positive in the endothelial cells; the perivascular reaction for SMA was inconstantly positive, with a discontinuous pattern. At this age, next to developing organs, immature and intermediate vessels predominated. Gerecht-Nir (2004) indicates as the time of occurrence of a positive SMA reaction, the gestational age of four weeks, and the presence of mature type arterial vessels - with several layers of SMA positive perivascular cells-, in seven weeks embryos. On our slides we observed the existence of topografic-related differences in the maturation degree of the blood vessels: immature blood vessels next to differentiating organs, and mature ones, even with emerging cords from their walls, in the peripheral mesenchyme. These aspects suggest a more active vasculogenesis in the mesenchyme surrounding developing organs, and the onset of angiogenesis. Blood vessel maturation became more rapid with tissue and organ differentiation. In the fetal mesenchymal tissue, mature vessels were the most numerous; in the developing organs, vascular morphology was organ dependent. The prevalence of vasculogenesis over angiogenesis in five to seven weeks embryos is also supported by our findings regarding the coexpression of CD34 and Ki67; our data showed that there were no proliferating endothelial cells in five weeks embryos, and in seven weeks embryos, proliferation of endothelial cells was inconstant. Our results support also the fact that lung arteries are formed by vasculogenesis while pulmonary capillaries are formed by angiogenesis (Hall et al, 2000).

5. Conclusions

The coexistence of vascular islands, vascular cords, and vessels with lumen, in the same microscopic field, in five to seven weeks human embryos, reflects the dynamic nature of vasculogenesis at this gestational age. The coexistence of budding vessels suggests the early onset of angiogenesis; nevertheless the rarity of this phenomenon indicates the prevalence of vasculogenesis over angiogenesis at this gestational age. Further development of the vascular tree depends on the topographic location, and type of organ.

6. References

Carmeliet, P (2000). Mechanisms of angiogenesis and arteriogenesis. *Nat Med* (2000), No. 6, pp.389- 395.

Conway, EM; Collen, D; Carmeliet, P (2001). Molecular mechanisms of blood vessel growth. *Cardiovasc Res,* (2001), No. 49, pp. 507- 521.

Gee, MS; Procopio, SM; Feldman, MD et al (2003). Tumor vessel Development and Maturation Impose Limits on the Effectiveness of Anti-Vascular Therapy. *Am J Pathol,* No.162 (1), (Jan 2003), 183-93.

Gerecht-Nir, S; Osenberg, S; Nevo, O et al. (2004). Vascular Development in Early Human Embryos and in Teratomas Derived from Human Embryonic Stem Cells. *Biol Reprod,* (2004), No. 71, pp. 2029- 2036.

Ginis, I; Luo, L; Miura, T; et al. (2004). Differences between human and mouse embryonic stem cells. *Dev. Biol.,* No. 269 (2), (May 2004), pp. 360-380.

Hall, SM; Hislop, AA; Pierce, CM; Haworth, SG (2000) - Prenatal Origins of Human Intrapulmonary Arteries. Formation and Smooth Muscle Maturation. *Am J Respir. Cell Mol. Biol.* (2000), No. 23, pp. 194-203.

Tavian, M; Hallais, MF; Peault, B (1999). Emergence of intraembryonic hematopoietic precursors in the pre-liver human embryo. *Development*, (1999), No. 126, pp.793–803

2

Cardiac Vasculature: Development and Pathology

Michiko Watanabe et al.*
Department of Pediatrics, Division of Pediatric Cardiology, Case Western Reserve University School of Medicine, Rainbow Babies and Children's Hospital, Cleveland OH USA

1. Introduction

Coronary vessels are of particular clinical interest to the general public and adult cardiologists because of their propensity in populations of developed countries to get clogged leading to chest pain (angina) and heart attacks (myocardial infarctions; MIs). Coronary artery disease (CAD) is the leading type of heart disease and the leading cause of deaths in the USA in both men and women (representing 51% of all cardiovascular diseases in 2006; American Heart Association Heart Disease and Stroke Statistics 2010 Update-at-a-glance; http://www.americanheart.org/downloadable/heart/1265665152970DS-3241%20HeartStrokeUpdate_2010.pdf; http://www.nlm.nih.gov/medlineplus/coronaryartery disease.html). While the developmental biology of cardiac vessels seems removed from this concern for the adult population, findings from this field may be beneficial and relevant for all age groups. Interest in the development of coronary vessels has increased due to findings that suggest the embryonic epicardium provides components of the coronary vessels and factors that positively influence the myocardium. The possibility has been raised that the epicardium might be sufficiently activated to repair cardiac tissue in the adult in part by promoting coronary vascularization. The aim of this Chapter is to call attention to questions regarding coronary vessels that still require answers and to introduce hypotheses that may lead to answers and strategies for cardiotherapy.

2. The structure of coronary vessels and lymphatics in the four-chambered heart (Allen et al., 2007)

The coronary circulation performs critical functions for the heart as in all organ systems in delivering oxygen and nutrients through the arteries and removing deoxygenated blood

---

* Jamie Wikenheiser[4], Diana Ramirez-Bergeron[3], Saul Flores[1], Amir Dangol[1], Ganga Karunamuni[1], Akshay Thomas[1], Monica Montano[2] and Ravi Ashwath[1]
1 Department of Pediatrics, Division of Pediatric Cardiology, Case Western Reserve University School of Medicine, Rainbow Babies and Children's Hospital, Cleveland OH, USA,
2 Department of Pharmacology, Case Western Reserve University School of Medicine, Cleveland OH, USA,
3 Department of Medicine, Division of Cardiology, Case Western Reserve University School of Medicine, Cleveland OH, USA,
4 Director of Medical Gross Anatomy & Embryology, University of California, Irvine School of Medicine, Department of Anatomy & Neurobiology, Irvine, CA, USA.

and waste through the veins. The lymphatic circulation removes excess fluid within the tissues. In the context of the energy-intensive requirements of the continuously beating heart, the coronary circulation must meet particularly demanding functional requirements that are reflected in its architecture.

The **major vessels** of the heart termed the **coronary arteries** have a very stereotyped architecture (Fig. 1A) that is conserved across individuals within a species and in large part across species (Tomanek et al., 2006b; Sedmera and Watanabe, 2006). With rare exceptions (Frommelt and Frommelt, 2004; Jureidini et al., 1998; Matherne, 2001), the mature four-chambered heart has right and left coronary arteries connected to the aortic lumen by two ostia centrally placed in the right and left sinuses of Valsalva, behind the valvular cusps at the level of the aortic valve. The left main coronary artery (LCA) bifurcates into (1) the circumflex branch of the left coronary artery that wraps around the left atrioventricular groove and (2) the left anterior descending (LAD) coronary artery that courses over the interventricular septum. Other terms for the LAD are anterior interventricular branch of the left coronary artery or anterior descending branch. The right coronary artery (RCA) arises from the right sinus of Valsalva and courses right and posteriorly often with an anterior branch that goes to the sinus node and a posterior branch, the atrioventricular (AV) nodal artery. The main RCA follows the right atrioventricular groove and turns to run along the interventricular sulcus as the posterior descending artery (PDA). In contrast to other tissues that are perfused during systole (end of cardiac contraction when the ventricles are most contracted), the myocardial perfusion of the left ventricle occurs mainly in diastole (when the ventricular lumens are most dilated), while the myocardium of the right ventricle is perfused both during systole and diastole (Epstein et al., 1985; Fulton, 1964; Mosher et al., 1964).

There are rarely variations in the **major coronary arteries**, however there are some variations found in the more distal vessels that have no apparent negative consequences, for example coronary artery dominance. Dominance is determined by what supplies the posterior descending artery (PDA; posterior interventricular artery). In 69% of the population, the right coronary artery is dominant giving rise to the posterior descending coronary artery, which extends to the apex and supplies the posterior part of the ventricular septum, the inferior wall of the left ventricle and the atrioventricular node. In 11% of the population, the left coronary artery is dominant giving rise to the posterior descending coronary artery via the circumflex artery (CF). In 20% of the population it is co-dominant. The dominance has no apparent effect on function under normal circumstances, but is important to note when considering the extent of myocardial damage when a particular artery is occluded or negatively affected. The major coronary arterial system distributes blood to the microcirculation such as capillaries and postcapillary venules which are the main sites of interchange of gas and metabolite molecules between the tissue and blood.

The **major cardiac veins** run along similar avenues as the major arteries. The middle cardiac vein runs within the epicardium from the apex to the base on the posterior surface of the interventricular groove and connects to the coronary sinus. This vein is generally paired with the PDA. Anterior cardiac veins connect to the small cardiac vein that runs posteriorly along the right atrioventricular groove with the right coronary artery and connects to the coronary sinus where the middle cardiac vein also connects. The great cardiac vein courses along the anterior interventricular groove from the apex to the base and wraps around the left atrioventricular groove posteriorly and connects to the coronary sinus. The coronary sinus ultimately drains into the right atrium (Gensini et al., 1965; Gilard et al., 1998).

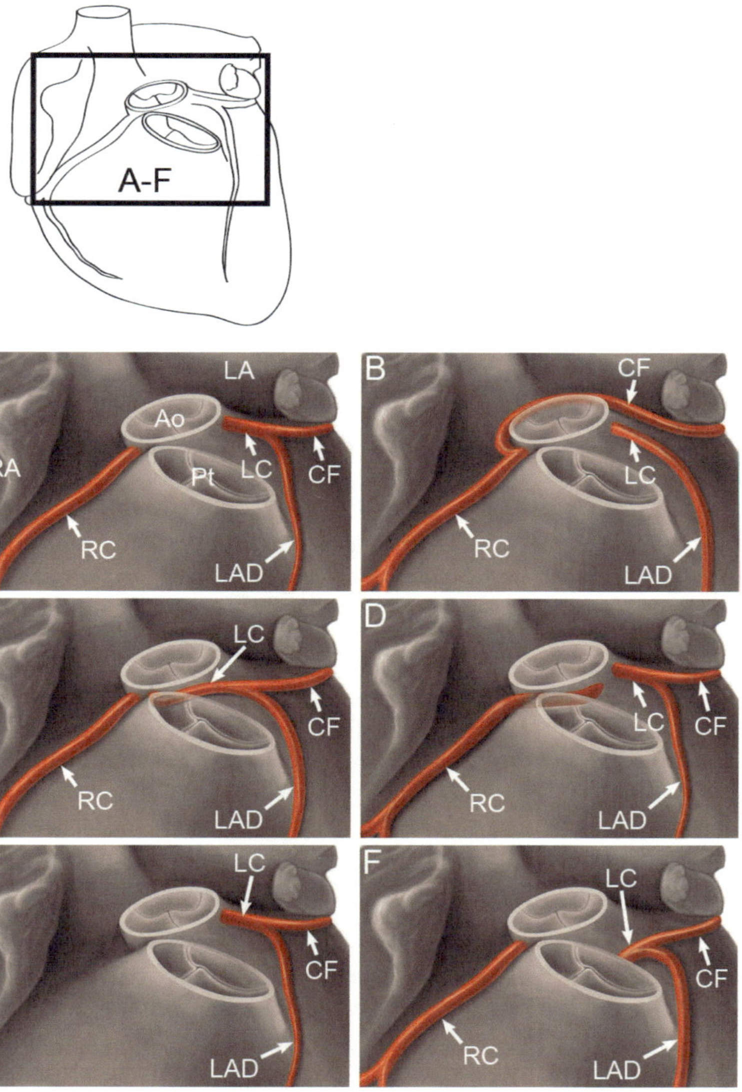

Fig. 1. **Normal morphology and the most frequently seen congenital coronary anomalies.** **A**: Normal coronary artery morphology. **B**: The circumflex artery originating from the right coronary artery near the right sinus of Valsalva. This is the most common coronary artery anomaly (35% of cases). **C**: The left coronary artery originating from the right sinus of Valsalva. This anomaly carries an increased risk of sudden death. **D**: The right coronary artery originating from the left sinus of Valsalva. The frequency of this anomaly is around 30%. **E**: A single coronary artery originating from either the left or right sinus of Valsalva. The frequency of this anomaly is between 5-20%. Note only a single left coronary is shown. **F**: The left coronary artery originating from the pulmonary artery. LA, left atrium; RA, right atrium; Ao, aorta; Pt, pulmonary trunk; RC, right coronary; LC, left coronary; LAD, left anterior descending; CF, circumflex. (Illustrations by Laura M. Bock, BFA).

The cardiac **lymphatic system** (Miller, 1982) also has its larger vessels within the epicardium but their anatomy is not often covered in commonly used textbooks. Surgeons concern themselves with the connection of the largest lymphatics such as the thoracic duct that drains most of the body except the right upper quadrant and usually connects at the junction between the left internal jugular and left subclavian veins. These are not strictly cardiac lymphatics as they are outside the heart. The largest distributing lymphatic vessels within the heart are found in the epicardium running alongside the larger blood vessels. These are connected to a meshwork of lymphatic capillaries that lie within the myocardium mainly in the ventricular walls. While the epicardial lymphatics are documented in several studies, the findings regarding the myocardial lymphatics of the adult heart are controversial and complex and will be discussed separately in a review in preparation (Thomas, A., Watanabe, M. et al., personal communication).

Thus the largest cardiac vessels whether arteries, veins or lymphatics are found embedded within the thick epicardium of the sulcus regions as in the atrioventricular groove and the dorsal and ventral interventricular grooves. This pattern raises several questions. How is this stereotyped pattern of the major named coronaries and veins set up and maintained? Why do the largest coronaries course within the epicardium and do not end up more often within the myocardium as in the cases of myocardial bridging? Why do the left and right coronary arteries normally connect only in two places at the left and right cusps of the aorta and not at the other posterior aortic cusp or at the cusps of the pulmonary artery? What regulates the density of vessels within the epicardium and myocardium and their diameters? The answer to these questions may aid us on intervening in cardiac disease by coaxing collateral growth or enhancing vascular density when myocardial infarctions are a danger or prior to major cardiac surgery. While these fundamental questions have yet to be definitively answered, some hypotheses emerge from studies of the events during coronary vessel development in the embryo and fetus that will be discussed in subsequent sections.

3. Coronary anomalies and consequences. Clinically significant anomalies associated with sudden death and propensity to ischemic heart disease

The major coronary arteries generally follow a specific morphological template (Fig. 1A). Variations from this morphology are rare and may not have clinically significant consequences but are nonetheless important to know about prior to procedures in cardiac surgeries or when inserting leads for pacing for electrophysiological studies. However, specific classes of anomalies have been associated with an increased risk of sudden and exercise related death (Cheitlin and MacGregor, 2009; Eckart et al., 2006a; Frescura, 1999; Haugen and Ellingsen, 2007; Taylor et al., 1992).

Overall, coronary artery anomalies represent a rare and small group of malformations, that are nonetheless important. These anomalies may be isolated or occur as a part of complex congenital heart diseases or associated with hypertrophic cardiomyopathy, dilated cardiomyopathy and sudden cardiac death.

The clinically significant anomalies are near the proximal attachment to the aorta and have been associated with exercise-related deaths. The anomaly in which the left circumflex arises from the right main coronary artery passing posterior to the aorta is the most common coronary anomaly accounting for about 35% of coronary anomaly cases (Fig.1B). There are usually no clinical complications, but compression by the aorta and mitral valve has been reported. In the latter case, implantation of a prosthetic fixation ring could be considered.

This implantation is a series of procedures for the replacement of the mitral valve with an artificial mitral valve and supporting ring (Chiam and Ruiz, 2011).

Another anomaly in which the **left coronary artery arises from the right sinus of Valsalva (ARCA)** and passes between the aorta and the pulmonary artery is rare (3% of cases of coronary anomalies), but has been associated with sudden death (Fig.1C). In this case, it is presumed that during exercise, the abnormal position of the coronary artery running between the aorta and pulmonary trunk causes it to be compressed by the dilated arteries during exercise thus reducing blood flow to a large portion of the heart. There are 4 possible routes for the left main coronary artery (1) posterior to the aorta, (2) anterior to the right ventricular outflow tract, (3) within the ventricular septum under the right ventricular infundibulum, and (4) between the aorta and the right ventricular outflow tract (Fig.1C). Because this last variant carries an increased risk of sudden death, surgical reimplantation may be necessary.

Taylor et al. (Taylor et al., 1992) reviewed the records of 242 patients with isolated coronary artery anomalies and determined that sudden death and exercise related death were most common when the origin of the left main coronary artery came from the right coronary sinus. High risk anatomy involved abnormalities of the initial coronary artery segment or coursing of the anomalous artery between the aorta and pulmonary artery. Frescura et al. (Frescura et al., 1998) analyzed the anatomic collection of 1,200 specimens of individuals with congenital heart disease and anomalous origin of coronary arteries was observed in 27 of these individuals (2.2%). This study concluded that more than half of the postmortem cases with an anomalous origin of the coronary arteries died suddenly. Eckart et al., (Eckart et al., 2006b) reviewed the autopsy reports of sudden cardiac deaths involving U.S. military recruits during basic training from 1977 through 2001. This study found that all sudden cardiac deaths resulting from anomalous coronary origin involved a left main coronary artery originating from the right coronary sinus with a course between the aorta and the right ventricular outflow tract and an otherwise normal distribution of the other major epicardial coronary arteries.

Anomalous origin of right coronary arterial branches from the left sinus of Valsalva occurs in approximately 30% of all major coronary arterial anomalies (Fig.1D). In this condition, the right coronary artery runs between the aorta and the right ventricular outflow tract. Since it carries increased risk for sudden death as does certain cases of ARCA, surgical reimplantation is recommended.

The **anomalous left coronary from the pulmonary artery (ALCAPA;** Bland-White-Garland syndrome; Fig. 1F) results in left ventricular insufficiency or infarction and infants with this condition have a high mortality rate; 65-90% die before age 1 from congestive heart failure (Park, 1988; Pena et al., 2009). This anomaly is usually isolated but can be associated with other congenital heart anomalies such as Tetralogy of Fallot or coarctation of the aorta. It usually presents at birth or shortly after with an increase in myocardial ischemia followed by exhaustion of the coronary vascular reserve. Due to the transition in the neonatal circulation, the pressure in the pulmonary artery remains high. As the pulmonary artery pressure drops, there is more flow from the aorta into the pulmonary artery through the coronary circulation. This results in decreased perfusion of the myocardium and leads to myocardial ischemia. Initially this condition may be transient but with increased exertion, it progresses to infarction of the antero-lateral left ventricle or free wall with dysfunction. Mitral regurgitation can develop secondary to left ventricular delectation and infarction and/or dysfunction of the anterolateral papillary muscle. Diffuse endocardial fibroelastosis of the left ventricle and thickening of the anterior mitral valve leaflet can also occur.

Infants may present with heart failure and the signs of myocardial infarction in the form of irritability with feeding or activity. Older children may be asymptomatic or may have dyspnea, syncope, or angina. Sudden cardiac death after exertion has been known to occur (George and Knowlan, 1959).

The electrocardiogram shows abnormal Q waves in the leads I, aVL and pre-cordial leads V4 to V6. Noninvasive imaging like echocardiography will confirm the diagnosis in most of the cases. If uncertain, angiography or computed tomography (CT) scan with higher resolutions can complement and confirm the diagnosis and also provide insight into the extent of collaterals and help in sorting out which coronary artery is dominant.

About 87% of the patients present in infancy (Neufeld, 1983) and of these 65% to 85% die before one year of age due to congestive heart failure and infarction (Wesselhoeft et al., 1968). It is noted that if the children improve spontaneously (Liebman et al., 1963), it might be from formation of extensive collaterals or there could be ostial stenosis at the entry of the anomalous coronary into the pulmonary artery, thus conferring slight protection. However, they are still at high risk of sudden cardiac death with exercise (Fontana, 1962).

The treatment of such a condition is surgical implantation of the left coronary artery into the aorta (Grace et al., 1977; Huddleston et al., 2001; Jin et al., 1994; Schwartz et al., 1997). An alternative is the Takeauchi procedure, in which an aorto-pulmonary window is created with a tunnel that leads the blood from the aorta to the coronary artery (Takeuchi et al., 1979).

ALCAPA has been separated into the infant type and the adult type (Pena et al., 2009). The infant type is as described earlier in this paragraph. The rare adult type is hypothesized to be the cause of sudden cardiac death that occurs in 80-90% of these individuals. Survival of the adult with ALCAPA is possible because of the development of collaterals between the left and right coronary arteries. In these cases there is likely a pulmonary-coronary steal with a left to right shunt. These account for 15% of ALCAPA patients where the myocardial blood flow can sustain myocardial function at rest or even during exercise allowing these individuals to reach adulthood (Neufeld, 1983).

Even with these collaterals, there is not enough circulation to the left ventricle resulting in ischemia. Surgical repair is usually required and is carried out for the infant by direct reimplantation of the origin of the left coronary artery into the aorta with a "button" (small segment) of pulmonary artery.

Single coronary artery (Fig. 1E): At a frequency of 5-20% of coronary anomalies, a single coronary artery arises from the aorta and then branches to give rise to the right and left coronaries (Ogden, 1970; Shirani and Roberts, 1993). As many as 40% of single coronary artery cases are associated with other congenital cardiac defects such as Tetralogy of Fallot. This anomaly carries a mildly increased risk of sudden death. The branches can pass between the two great arteries, resulting in compression. Of course with only one trunk there is increased vulnerability. For example, atheroma formation (swelling and accumulation of material) at the single trunk can be critical. Surgical repair is considered on a patient to patient basis.

Coronary artery fistulae [reviewed in (Luo et al., 2006; Schamroth, 2009) and (http://emedicine.medscape.com/article/895749-overview)]: Coronary artery fistulae (CAF) are major abnormal connections between a coronary artery and a cardiac chamber (coronary-cameral fistula) or inappropriate vessels and vascular structures (coronary arteriovenous fistula for coronary arterial-venous fistulae; CAVFs) and occur in 50% of coronary vasculature anomalies. For the most part, fistulas are small, have no untoward consequences to hemodynamics, and require no clinical intervention. These are only discovered when echocaradiography or coronary arteriography are performed for other reasons. Larger fistulae may continue to enlarge and eventually cause the "coronary artery steal phenomenon" in

which blood flow to the myocardium is compromised and may cause ischemia during increased activity. These fistula require surgical or percutaneous intervention for their closure. It is proposed that these inappropriate connections are remnants of the primitive coronary network that have failed to remodel and regress appropriately.
The range of **symptoms** associated with coronary artery anomalies can vary based on the specific type of lesion. However, the general concept is based on an imbalance between supply and demand of myocardial perfusion and also due to the steal phenomenon associated with left to right shunting. There are three coronary anomalies associated with myocardial ischemia, infarction, and/or lethal arrhythmias which could then lead to fibrillation or electromechanical dissociation. These are ALCAPA, coronary artery arising from the wrong sinus and coursing between the two great arteries, and large coronary artery fistula.
A history of unexplained syncope (loss of consciousness or fainting) or syncope associated with exercise should raise a diagnostic possibility of an anomalous coronary artery. Initial tests would include an electrocardiogram to rule out arrhythmia, left ventricular hypertrophy or prior evidence of ischemia. An echocardiogram is very helpful in identifying the coronary artery origin and its proximal course should be studied with utmost care. Hypertrophic cardiomyopathy should be ruled out using this method. If the echocardiogram raises the suspicion and is unable to provide enough information, a transesophageal echocardiogram, magnetic resonance imaging and/ or CT scan may be more sensitive and should be considered (Schmitt et al., 2005).
While the association between sudden death and coronary anomalies has been made for certain such anomalies, no treatment has been established for individuals identified with these anomalies but suffering no symptoms.
Classification of coronary artery anomalies: Coronary artery anomalies can be classified as abnormal origin of the coronary arteries from the wrong aortic sinus, anomalous origin of the left or the right coronary artery from the pulmonary artery, absence of a coronary artery, and congenital coronary artery fistulas (See Table 1).

Significant congenital anomalies of the coronary arteries
I. Without congenital heart disease
A. Coronary arteries arising from the wrong sinus
i. without intramural course
ii. with intramural course (within the media of the great vessels)
B. Anomalous origin of the coronary arteries from the pulmonary arteries
i. ALCAPA*
ii. ARCAPA.*
C. Single coronary artery or absence of a coronary artery
D. Coronary artery fistulas
E. Myocardial bridging
II. Coronary artery anomalies associated with congenital heart disease
A. Transposition of the great arteries
B. Tetralogy of Fallot
C. Pulmonary atresia with intact ventricular septum
D. Aortic atresia with mitral atresia/stenosis

*ALCAPA: anomalous origin of the left coronary artery from the pulmonary artery;
*ARCAPA: anomalous origin of the right coronary artery from the pulmonary artery.

Table 1.

Myocardial bridges are another class of coronary anomalies where an artery that normally confines its path within the epicardium dives and travels several millimeters within the myocardium before the terminal branches [Reviewed in (Boktor et al., 2009; Hakeem et al., 2010; Sunnassee et al., 2011; Vales et al., 2010)]. Myocardial bridging has been described as early as 1737 (Rayman, 1737) and have been described since with a wide range of frequencies reported. In one study of 200 adult human hearts collected from autopsies, myocardial bridges were found in 34.5% with a mean length of 31 mm and a mean depth of 12mm (Loukas et al., 2006). The most common site of myocardial bridging was over portions of the left anterior descending coronary artery (LAD). Myocardial bridging usually does not carry a significant increase in risk of sudden death, however ischemia has been reported, in particular when associated with hypertrophic cardiomyopathy. Angiography has identified compression of arteries at the site of myocardial bridging during systolic contraction (Laifer and Weiner, 1991). Surgical repair is considered in select cases to remove the myocardial bridge when there are symptoms such as angina or myocardial infarction. Many patients with myocardial bridges are asymptomatic, but these bridges are hypothesized to lead to a tendency to develop myocardial infarction (MI), ischemia, and other cardiac problems. Long bridges are associated with negative cardiac symptoms (Bourassa et al., 2003). Paradoxically myocardial bridges have been proposed to lead to a decrease or an increase of atherosclerosis. Myocardial bridges correlate with left coronary artery dominance and are thought to be the result of developmental events. Why myocardial bridges and coronary artery dominance would be related is a mystery.

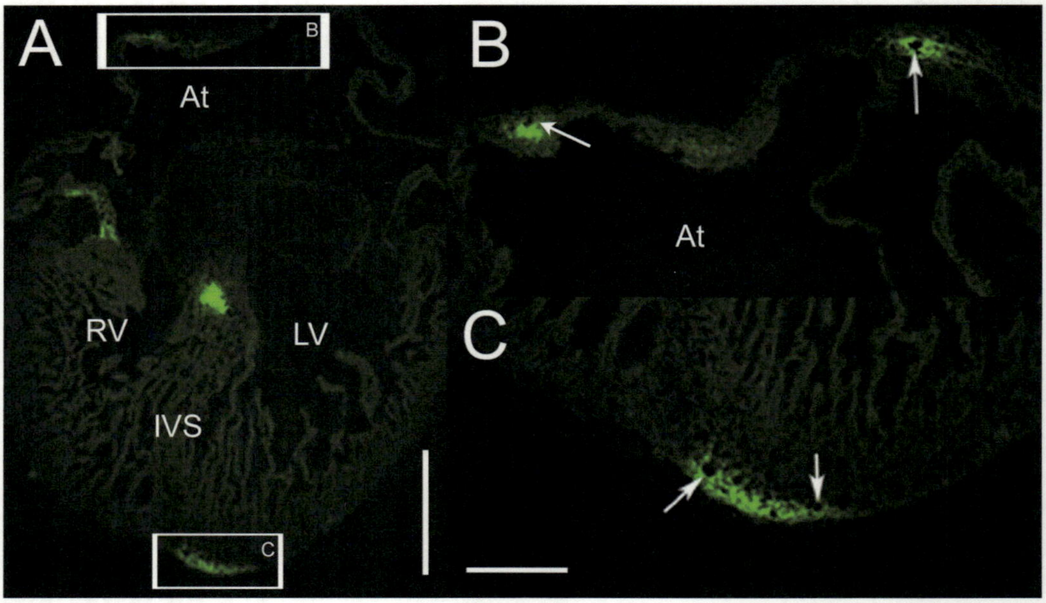

Fig. 2. EF5 at hypoxic regions where major coronary vessels will differentiate. A: EF5 staining in frontal sections of st 30 chicken hearts B: Higher magnification of a region similar to that in the box in A. C: Higher magnification of a region indicated by the box in A. Arrows indicate lumens of small vessels. Scale bar in A = 500 µm and 200 µm in B & C. (Wikenheiser et al., 2006).

Summary: The coronary artery anomalies discussed above are presumed to arise in the embryonic or fetal stages of cardiovascular development from as yet unknown causes. Recent investigations described in Section V, suggest that some coronary anomalies may involve disturbance of a "hypoxic template". Anomalies in the proximal arteries resembling those observed in clinical specimens have been reproduced in avian embryos subjected to conditions that would alter this hypoxic template (Fig 2). ;(Wikenheiser et al., 2009).

Much less attention has been paid to anomalies of the cardiac veins and lymphatics. In one case study, the importance of venography prior to inserting a pacing lead into the coronary sinus was underscored because the contrast agent indicated that the lead may have entered an anomaly of the middle cardiac vein (Yuniadi et al., 2004).

4. Development of coronary vessels

The proepicardial serosa and the embryonic epicardium are known to be sources for the components of the cardiac vessels in the embryo. Recent evidence suggests that the adult epicardium can also be activated to contribute to the vasculature and even the cardiomyocyte population. A number of apparently conflicting interpretations of the data and caveats have been raised that are worth discussing regarding this important cardiac tissue.

The proepicardium and the embryonic epicardium have been the focus of and continue to be the focus of much study [reviewed in (Gittenberger-de Groot et al., 2010; Olivey et al., 2004; Ratajska et al., 2008; Tomanek, 2005; Wessels and Perez-Pomares, 2004)] because it is the source of many cell types critical for the heart including components of the vasculature. The embryonic epicardium arises from the serosal covering of the body wall between the sinus venosus and the future liver. The mesothelial cells at this caudal border of the pericardial cavity form villi and become a small mass appearing as a wrinkled "cauliflower-shaped" structure that is called the proepicardium (PE), proepicardial serosa, or proepicardial organ (PEO) (Manner, 1993). This structure grows up against the atrioventricular groove and migrates to the heart apparently assisted by extracellular matrix fibers that bridge the gap between the myocardium and the proepicardium (Nahirney et al., 2003; Olivey et al., 2004). This structure extends many tissue processes and covers the surface of the naked myocardium of the looped heart in avian species (Hiruma and Hirakow, 1989; Ho and Shimada, 1978; Viragh and Challice, 1981). Bone Morphogenetic Protein (BMP) has been identified as a factor that may be involved in controlling the timing and direction of proepicardial protrusion towards the heart (Ishii et al., 2010). The transcription factor GATA4 has been found to be strongly expressed in the proepicardium and is required for the formation of the epicardium (Watt et al., 2004). When the GATA cofactor FOG-2 is absent in mice, the coronary vasculature does not develop (Tevosian et al., 2000; Tomanek, 2005). The molecular and cellular signals that initiate the growth and coverage of the cardiomyocytes of the embryonic heart are not known. It is likely that proepicardial growth and epicardium coverage would be coordinated closely with the level of hypoxia in cardiac tissues and the contractile function of the heart.

The transition from proepicardium to epicardium is thought to differ between species (Nesbitt et al., 2006). While avians and rats undergo the process as described above, mice and zebrafish may do it a different way. In the mouse, the proepicardial processes appeared to be released as vesicles from the proepicardial serosa that float in the pericardial space and attach to the surface of the myocardium (Viragh and Challice, 1981). Whatever method is used for a particular species, the signal that induces the growth and attachment of the proepicardial processes or vesicles is incompletely understood but likely involves signals from the thickening myocardium and perhaps the endocardium.

Immediately after proepicardial processes or vesicles attach to the surface of the myocardium, an extracellular matrix accumulates between the single layer of mesothelial cells and the myocardium. The epicardial coverage occurs in a stereotyped pattern in the avian heart with the dorsal surface of the atrioventricular junction covered first and radiating out from there, wrapping around the atrioventicular groove, the ventricles and atria and finally the distal portion of the outflow tract (Hiruma and Hirakow, 1989; Ho and Shimada, 1978). This distal portion of the outflow tract has been shown to be covered by epicardial cells from another more cephalic source even when the proepicardial serosa is ablated or impeded (Gittenberger-de Groot et al., 2000). These cells have a different morphology (more cuboidal than squamous), different gene expression, and may also have different capabilities and properties (Perez-Pomares et al., 2003).

The embryonic epicardium consists of a single layer of mesothelial cells, underlying connective tissue, and mesenchymal cells within the connective tissue. These mesenchymal cells arise from epithelial-mesenchymal transition (EMT) of the mesothelium but may also come from the sinus venosus or liver primordia (Perez-Pomares et al., 1997; 1998; Dettman et al., 1998). The cells that undergo EMT are termed epicardial derived cells (EPDCs) and have been tracked into the subepicardium, myocardium and even into the endocardium at sites where valves form (Gittenberger de Groot et al., 1998). Some EPDCs differentiate into the components of the coronary vasculature.

Epicardial EMT is stimulated by vascular endothelial growth factor (VEGF), fibroblast growth factors (FGF-1, FGF-2 and FGF-7) and epidermal growth factor (EGF), but is inhibited by transforming growth factor (TGFb-1-3) (Morabito et al., 2001). The proposed inhibitory role of TGF-β in epicardial EMT is in contrast to its positive role in endocardial EMT and is still seen as controversial (Compton et al., 2006; Olivey et al., 2006). When the myocardium in the embryonic mouse produces an excess of angiopoietin-1 (Ang1), the epicardium fails to develop and that results in an absence of coronary vessels and death (Ward et al., 2004).

The epicardium as a source for cardiac cell types. Lineage studies were conducted using retroviral labeling by injection of engineered virus into the proepicardium (Mikawa and Fischman, 1992). As retroviruses were used for the transfection of reporter genes, the genes integrate into the genome and clonal analysis is possible over many stages of development. In the case of these studies, the reporter gene was the bacterial *lac-z* gene expressing the enzyme beta-galactosidase that can be detected using a dye substrate that turns into a blue precipitate within the cell expressing the reporter gene. The analysis of individual discrete clones of blue cells revealed that there were clones with only endothelial cells or clones with smooth muscle cells and fibroblasts, but no clones were found that included the combination of endothelial cells and smooth muscle cells or endothelial cells and fibroblasts. The findings suggested that there are two populations of precursor cells in the proepicardium, one population that became endothelial cells and a separate population that became smooth muscle cells and fibroblasts. In this study, the virally marked proepicardial cells could have been either the mesothelial cells or the mesenchymal cells of the proepicardium.

Many studies using different approaches confirm that the epicardium can give rise to vascular smooth muscle cells and fibroblasts. However, some lineage tracing approaches do not clearly support that the epicardium serves as a source of endothelial cells. Furthermore, the potential for the epicardium to provide precursors of cardiomyocytes is an exciting idea for cardiac therapy, but has been even more controversial and will be discussed below.

4.1 Where do endothelial cells in the heart come from?

The origin of endothelial cells is still somewhat controversial with several theories being discussed. The theories can be separated into three.

1. The epicardial mesothelial layer undergoes epithelial-mesenchymal transition (EMT) and gives rise to EPDCs (epicardial derived cells) that travel into the epicardium or myocardium and become endothelial cells that form vascular tubes and vessels by vasculogenesis.
2. Endothelial precursors travel within the connective tissue of the epicardium as mesenchymal cells, but do not derive from the epicardial mesothelium. These precursors use the connective tissue of the epicardium as a conduit as do neural crest cells and may originate from outside the heart in the liver primordia.
3. Precursors come from the sinus venosus and veins that transdifferentiate into endothelial cells of the arteries and use the epicardium as a conduit as in (2) (Red-Horse et al., 2010).
4. Endocardial cells differentiate into endothelial cells of the myocardium.

Our findings suggest that lymphatic endothelial precursor cells may travel from outside the heart using the epicardial lining of the outflow tract to travel into the heart (Karunamuni et al., 2010) supporting scheme (2). We also have evidence that lymphatic endothelial cells may also come from precursors within the epicardium.

The Cre-Lox method of lineage tracing has been used widely to trace cell fate and to find evidence for coronary vessel precursors so it is worth discussing the caveats of using this technique. Findings using this method have suggested that cardiomyocytes and few if any endothelial cells arise from the embryonic epicardium. Concerns have been raised regarding the lineage tracing of epicardial cells by this method. The Cre-mice available include, Wt1-Cre, TBX18-Cre and Gata5-Cre, that do appear to allow epicardial specific expression when analyzing limited areas of the heart at certain stages (Cai et al., 2008; Sridurongrit et al., 2008; Zhou et al., 2008). However, these may not be as specific as desired. For example, Wt1-Cre is expressed by cardiac progenitors in the secondary heart field so it may label the lineage prior to their split into myocardial and epicardial lineages. TBX18 is known to be expressed in a subset of cardiomyocytes that are not of epicardial origin (Christoffels 2009). Cre expression can be irreversibly turned on even if the expression of the gene is expressed transiently and in low levels. This expression would be difficult to detect and characterize histologically by immunostaining or in situ hybridization for TBX18 itself.

To address this problem in studies of the role of the epicardium in the adult mouse heart, the Wt1-CreERT2 tamoxifen-inducible reporter constructs have been used (Smart et al., 2011; Zhou et al., 2011). This strategy allowed the investigators to label with a fluorescent reporter (YFP) only those cells expressing Wt1 at the time of tamoxifen injection. Wt1 and YFP expression appeared to be epicardial specific in the adult. However, the same criticism could be invoked for this strategy as for the strategy used to mark the epicardium in the embryo. Thus, transplantation of lineage labeled and explanted epicardial cells was used to support the findings using the Cre-line (Zhou et al., 2011).

Given the uncertainties of the Cre-Lox method of lineage-tracing, several groups have found that the epicardial/mesothelial Cre lineage tracing (Wt1-Cre, TBX18-Cre) rarely if ever provided endothelial cells to the heart or other organs (Cai et al., 2008; Que et al., 2008; Wilm, 2005; Zhou et al., 2008). Other groups including ours found that endothelial cells are indeed part of the Wt1-Cre lineage (personal communication). The staining protocol, background of the mice, and the Cre-construct might be the variables that result in these differences in findings between laboratories.

In summary, multiple avenues for endothelial cells precursors to contribute to the heart have been proposed and at this point, all may be correct.

Coronary vascular development. Several reviews summarize what is known about coronary vascular development (Lie-Venema et al., 2007; Olivey et al., 2004; Olivey and Svensson, 2010; Reese et al., 2002; Tomanek, 2005; Wada, 2003; Wessels and Perez-Pomares, 2004). Precursors of the coronary vasculature are contributed by the embryonic epicardium that arises from the pro-epicardial serosa at a stage when chamber differentiation has begun (Hiruma and Hirakow, 1989; Ho and Shimada, 1978; Viragh and Challice, 1981). The function of the primitive coronary vascular system prior to exhibiting the mature pattern of two arterial connections with the aortic lumen is not known. Are they already moving blood and fluid within the heart? What are the hematopoietic properties of epicardial cells?

Quail endothelial precursors and hemangioblasts are labeled by an antibody Qh-1 (Eralp et al., 2005; Kattan et al., 2004) and appear as individual cells along the back (dorsal surface) of the atrioventricular junction (AVJ), eventually covering the entire heart (Fig. 5). These cells accumulate around the proximal OFT and right ventricular base to form a peritruncal ring of anastomosing capillary-like vessels that surrounds the proximal OFT myocardium and cranial portion of the ventricles in the epicardium (Fig.6). Some vessel precursors enter the myocardium and make multiple connections to the aortic lumen. Subsequent remodeling results in maturation and maintenance of the roots of the right and left coronary arteries connecting to the mature branching vasculature (Tomanek et al., 2006a; Tomanek et al., 2006b; Waldo et al., 1990). Early assembly of coronary vessels occurs by vasculogenesis, the formation of blind-ended tubes that connect with each other to form continuous vessels (Kattan et al., 2004; Mikawa and Fischman, 1992). Once these tubes are connected to each other and to the aortic lumen, angiogenesis, the growth of vessels from preexisting vessels, becomes a prominent mechanism for coronary growth. The signals that promote the formation of the nascent tubes and their eventual connection to each other and to the aortic lumen are incompletely understood. Another equally important issue is the remodeling that eliminates nascent vessels during the transformation of the primitive vascular network into a mature branching vasculature.

To complicate this picture of coronary vessel development, Qh-1 labels not just blood vessel precursors but distinctly labels lymphatic precursors (Parsons-Wingerter et al., 2006) in the chorioallantoic membrane (extraembryonic tissue) and we have recently found that the same is true in the developing epicardium (Karunamuni et al., 2010). Therefore, some of the structures labeled with Qh-1 and identified as nascent blood vessels may be nascent lymphatic vessels.

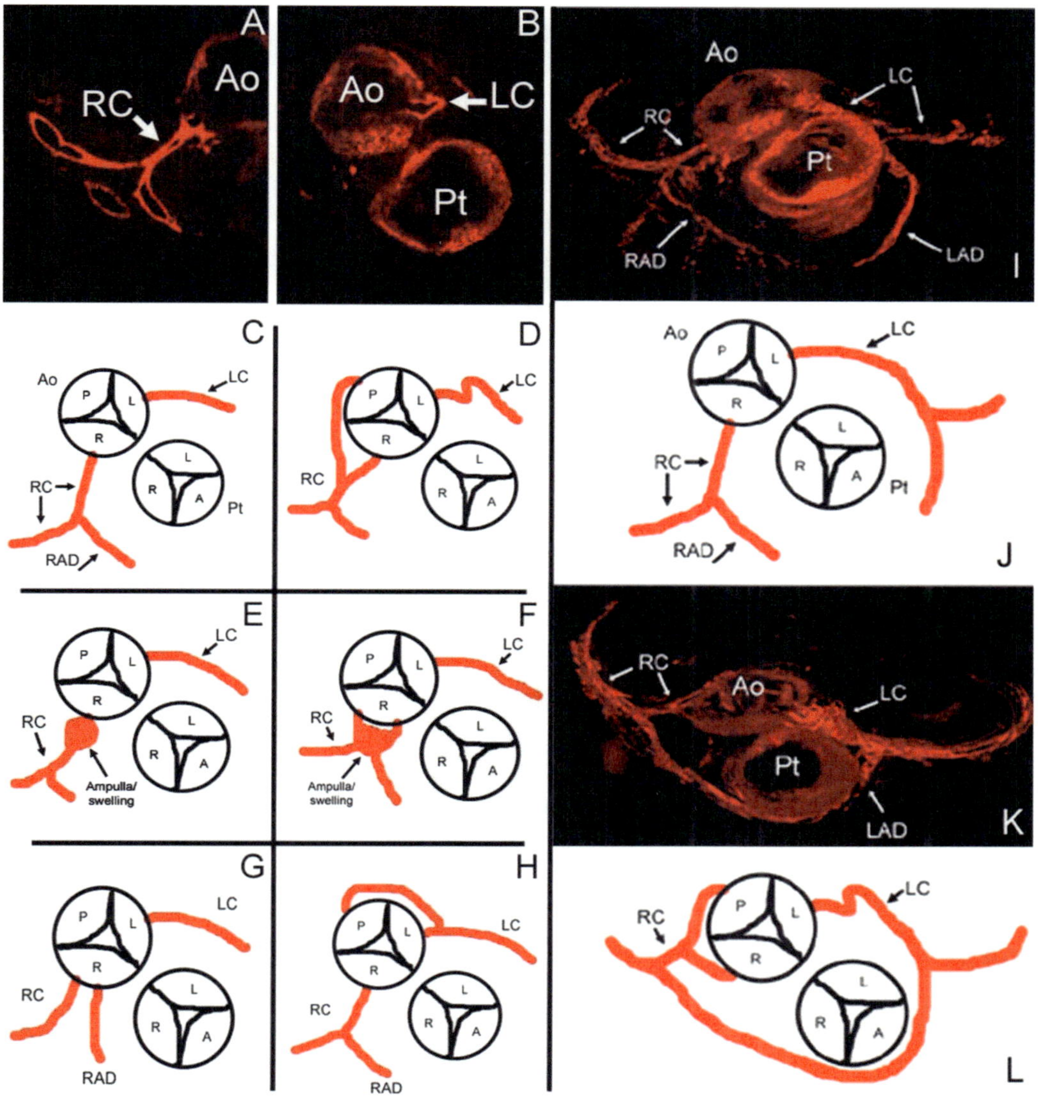

Fig. 3. **Hypoxia-induced defects in coronary vessels.** Transverse sections of stage 35 (ED 9) chicken embryo hearts stained with anti-a-smooth muscle actin-Cy3(A,B). A,B,C were incubated in 20.8% O2 (normoxic) conditions. D-H were incubated in 15% O2 (mildly hypoxic) for 4.5 days. 9 out of 10 embryos had defects that ranged from offset RC's near the posterior cusp (D,H), double RC's (F, G), & swollen RCs (E,F). LC's were tortuous and extended into abnormal positions (D). Ao = aorta, Pt =pulmonary trunk, RC = right coronary, LC = left coronary. [From (Wikenheiser et al., 2009)]

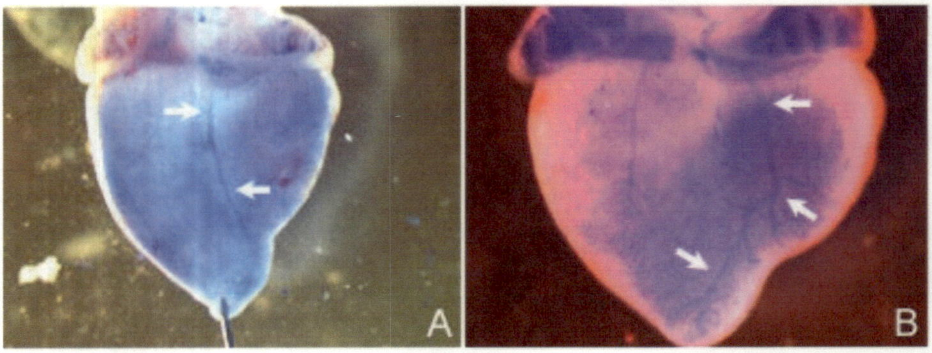

Fig. 4. Abnormal course of the posterior descending branch of the coronary artery after exposure to hypoxic conditions. The coronary vessels were filled by back-injection with blue ink into the aorta. The posterior vessel normally runs straight down the interventricular septum towards the apex (A; white arrows). This hypoxic embryo heart (B) had a vessel that diverged from this pathway along the sulcus before reaching the apex. These embryos were exposed to 15% O2 at stage 24-32, when coronary vessels are differentiating and remodeling, and harvested at stage 38.

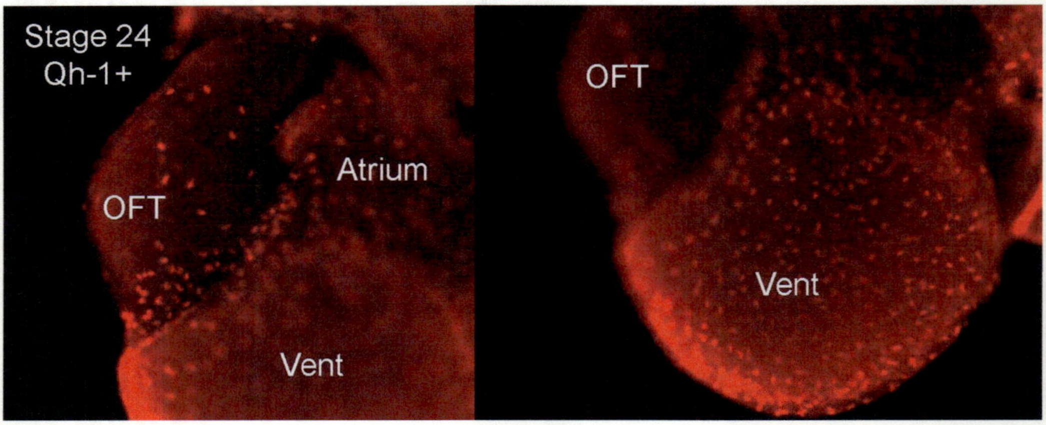

Fig. 5. Qh-1+ staining of vascular precursors cells in the epicardium of the quail heart (stage 24). At a stage prior to the formation of the four cardiac chambers, labeling using the antibody marker Qh-1 for endothelial cells and precursors revealed an evenly spaced set of cells covering the ventricular (Vent) and atrial (Atrium) surfaces and parts of the outflow tract (OFT). Will of these cells become endothelial cells and into which endothelial lineage will they be incorporated, arterial, venous or lymphatic? Why are they so evenly scattered at this stage and why aren't many covering the OFT. Qh-1 labels lymphatic endothelial cells as well as blood vessel endothelial cells and hemangioblasts.

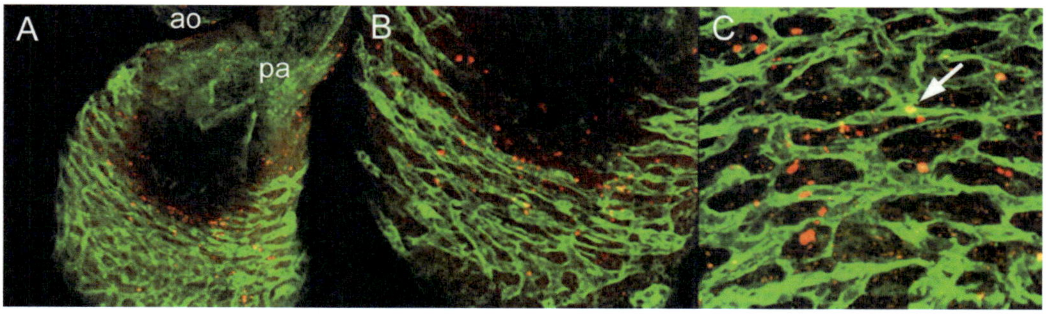

Fig. 6. Confocal microscopy of intact embryonic day E13.5 mouse heart double-labeled with an antibody to an endothelial marker PECAM (green) at the level of the outflow tract. The periarterial anatomoses, the primitive coronary vasculature surrounds the outflow tract. Lysotracker Red staining indicates that most of the apoptotic cells are within the myocardium not in the vasculature. The aorta (ao) and pulmonary artery (pa) are indicated at a low magnification (A, 100x) and higher magnifications are in (B, 200x) and (C, 400x) (Barbosky et al., 2006).

5. Origin of the lymphatics

Much less is known about the development of the lymphatics compared to the blood vessels within the heart. A number of reviews have been recently published regarding lymphangiogenesis (Albrecht and Christofori, 2011; Schulte-Merker, 2011; Witte et al., 2011). Transgenic mice have been created and markers for lymphatics have been identified that have made the study of lymphatic development much more accessible. The markers include antibodies to Prox-1, Lyve-1, Podoplanin, and VEGFR3. Unfortunately, these have limited use when used individually because, they are not exclusive to lymphatic endothelial cells especially in the embryo. They are useful in identifying bona fide lymphatic endothelial cells within the epicardium when used in combination (Karunamuni et al., 2010). It is quite clear that there are lymphatics in the epicardium of the adult heart but it is not known where they come from and exactly how they are distributed within the myocardium and endocardium. In view of their potential importance in cardiac homeostasis and disease, much more work is warranted.

6. Regulation of cardiac blood vessel development

Coronary vessels appear at particular stages of development and particular places within the heart. They can also grow and increase in density within the adult heart. The regulation of coronary vasculature is critical for homeostasis and as a response to stress. An understanding of what regulates these processes would be valuable in cardiotherapy. We expect that cardiac vessels are subject to some of the same regulatory strategies as other vessels in other parts of the body. However, the specific anatomy and demands of the heart suggest that there are likely to be cardiac-specific regulatory mechanisms to investigate.

The emergence of coronary vessels has been documented in quail using the antibody marker Qh1 that detects quail hemangioblasts/angioblasts and endothelial cells (Eralp, 2005; Kattan et al., 2004) and in mouse using PECAM and VEGFR2/Flk1 that detect endothelial cells [e.g.,(Tevosian et al., 2000)]. These early steps also appear to be choreographed such that precursors and endothelial cells assemble within the heart in a reproducible pattern that is similar across species. The resulting mature avian coronary architecture is similar to that found in mammals (Sedmera and Watanabe, 2006; Tomanek et al., 2006a). The mechanisms by which these patterns are established have been speculated to be controlled by (1) the sequence of differentiation of cardiac regions, (2) mechanical factors (shear stress, cyclic stretch and strain), and (3) differential hypoxia.

The location of the largest arteries in the epicardium at the sulcus regions. Why do the largest coronary arteries lie within the epicardium and at the sulcus regions? This can be separated into two questions, why are the sulcus regions preferred and why at the level of the epicardium rather than in the myocardium? We hypothesize that the answer may lie in part in the differential hypoxia at these sites during the earliest stages of coronary vessel development.

Differential Hypoxia. The precursors of endothelial cells are subjected to many environmental influences. An obvious one is hypoxia. The lack of oxygen within cardiac tissues is likely the result of increased proliferation that results in tissues that are too thick for simple tissue diffusion to adequately provide oxygen to the cells. Increased activity of the constantly beating and maturing heart also depletes oxygen from myocardial tissues thus increasing activity would likely increase hypoxia.

We and others (e.g. (Nanka et al., 2008; Naňka et al., 2006; Sugishita et al., 2004c; Tomanek et al., 2003; Wikenheiser et al., 2006)) discovered by the use of hypoxia indicators that there is a pattern of differential hypoxia within the embryonic heart that may explain in part why vessels form or are more concentrated at particular places.

The spatiotemporal pattern of outflow tract (OFT) myocardial hypoxia as measured by the hypoxia indicator EF5 correlates with HIF-1a nuclear localization, cardiomyocyte apoptosis, and morphogenesis of the OFT in both avian and mouse embryos (Sugishita et al., 2004A, B, C; Barbosky et al., 2006; Wikenheiser et al., 2006). Incubation of embryos under hyperoxic conditions reduced tissue hypoxia, HIF-1a nuclear localization and cell death in the OFT myocardium and resulted in abnormal conotruncal morphologies. The expression of hypoxia regulated genes such as VEGFA and VEGFR2 was also affected by hypoxia and hyperoxia in the OFT myocardium. We concluded that relative hypoxia of the chicken embryo OFT at that particular stage was critical to normal morphogenesis. The hypoxia peak also correlated with when coronary vessel precursors accumulated around the proximal OFT in both chicken and mouse (Fig. 6) and when endothelial precursors invade the OFT myocardium (Barbosky et al., 2006; Rothenberg et al., 2002; Wessels and Perez-Pomares, 2004). These findings supported a spatiotemporal correlation between microenivornmental tissue hypoxia, HIF-1a nuclear localization, accumulation of endothelial precursors, and myocardial invasion of endothelial precursors and vessels.

In addition to the OFT, the hypoxia indicator EF5 bound to other cardiac regions that correspond to sites of coronary vessel formation. Using EF5, we determined that the chicken OFT myocardium was one of the most hypoxic cardiac tissues with a peak of EF5 staining intensity at the end of ventricular septation (Sugishita et al., 2004a; Sugishita et al., 2004c). Our subsequent studies (Wikenheiser et al., 2006) revealed additional intensely EF5-positive cardiac regions at intriguing sites that included myocardial regions of the atrial wall, the atrioventricular junction (AVJ), and the interventricular septum (IVS) (Fig 2). These regions were also positive for nuclear-localized HIF-1a suggesting that HIF-1-induced transcriptional regulation may be active at these sites. Many of the intensely EF5+ myocardial regions corresponded to sites where the major vessels of the coronary vasculature will eventually develop. These findings led us to the hypothesis that myocardial hypoxia at specific sites may induce a level of HIF-1a mediated transcriptional activation that regulates gene expression critical to differentiation and organization of the coronary vasculature. The differential hypoxic microenvironments of the heart would provide a template for coronary vessel patterning.

Hypoxia Inducible Factors. An important and well-studied set of hypoxia sensitive transcription factors are the Hypoxia Inducible Factors (HIFs) of which HIF1a has received the most attention. Many cellular responses to hypoxic stress are regulated by the transcription factor HIF-1 (Semenza, 2001) a heterodimeric transcription factor composed of the constitutively expressed HIF-1b (ARNT) and the oxygen-sensitive HIF-1a. Under normoxic conditions, HIF-1a is degraded by ubiquitination. Under hypoxic conditions, HIF-1a escapes degradation, enters the nucleus, becomes a part of the heterdimer HIF-1, and binds to the CBP/p300 co-transactivator to form an active transcription complex that binds to hypoxia responsive elements (HREs) in promoter regions of many genes. In addition to this "canonical" function of HIF1a, this factor may participate in other pathways. For example HIF1a is known to bind to Notch and promote Notch signaling (Gustafsson et al., 2005) that is important in regulating differentiation of various cell types.

HIFs are critical for early development. The HIF-1a knockout mice die at E10.5 with abnormal morphogenesis of cardiac and other structures (Iyer et al., 1998; Ryan et al., 1998). The functional deletion of both HIF-1 and HIF-2 by expressing a dominant negative HIF2a led to embryonic lethality at E11.5. The conditional "knockout" of HIF-1a early in ventricular cardiomyocytes (Krishnan et al., 2008) and HIF-1 and HIF-2 by expression of a dominant negative HIF mutant in endothelial cells also resulted in early death [death by E11.5; (Licht, 2006)]. As coronary vessel development occurs at E10.5-13.5, the early death of these mice precluded determining the role of HIFs in coronary development by the use of these mice. A different strategy was required.

The HIF-1a gene was conditionally knocked out in cardiomyocytes of the left ventricle using the Cre-Lox technique with Cre expression driven by the *MLC2v* promoter (Huang et al., 2004). These mice survived with expected Mendelian frequencies, but with abnormal cardiomyocyte functions and a 15% reduction in vascularity of the left ventricle. These relatively mild effects suggested that HIF-1a is not required in cardiomyocytes for coronary vascular development, but may regulate its extent. However, compensation by HIF-2 (see below) or an alternate pathway is also possible. Another explanation is that the *MLC2v* promoter drives expression primarily in the left ventricle and at a late stage that may not knock out HIF-1a gene expression early and thoroughly enough to interfere with the myocardial paracrine signals for coronary development. These signals may have already been initiated prior to the knockout. Also the promoter may not have disabled the gene in the OFT myocardium or other sulcus regions where signals for early coronary development are likely to be critical. Their finding that smaller, recently developed vessels were more affected than larger vessels supports this idea. Another possibility is that VEGF and other important factors come from another source, the epicardium. Thus, this conditional knockout mouse study supported a role for myocardial HIF-1a on some aspects of coronary vessel organization but it is probably not the only tissue important in this function.

The role of HIFs in the endothelium has been less easily established by conditional knockout studies. Specific deletion of HIF-1a in endothelial cells affected adult tumor angiogenesis but had no detectable effect on embryonic vascular development (Tang et al., 2004). The specific deletion of HIF-2a in endothelial cells has resulted in variable results ranging from no effect on vasculature to yolk sac vascular defects (Compernolle et al., 2002; Duan et al., 2005; Peng, 2000; Scortegagna et al., 2003a; Scortegagna et al., 2003b; Tian et al., 1998). It takes the functional deletion of both HIF-1 and HIF-2 by expressing a dominant negative HIF-2a to see an effect. This deletion as mentioned above caused a embryonic lethality at E11.5. These results support that HIFs can compensate for each other during development and may play a role in other cell types in addition to cardiomyocytes.

A distinguishing feature of the sulcus regions of the heart where the coronary vessels first begin to develop and where the largest coronary arteries end up is a high level of hypoxia and nuclear-localized HIF-1a as well as a high level of expression of HIF downstream genes in both the myocardium and epicardium (Fig. 7). Therefore microenvironmental hypoxia may promote steps in early coronary vessel development in a region-specific pattern by enhancing HIF function in the epicardium as well as the myocardium.

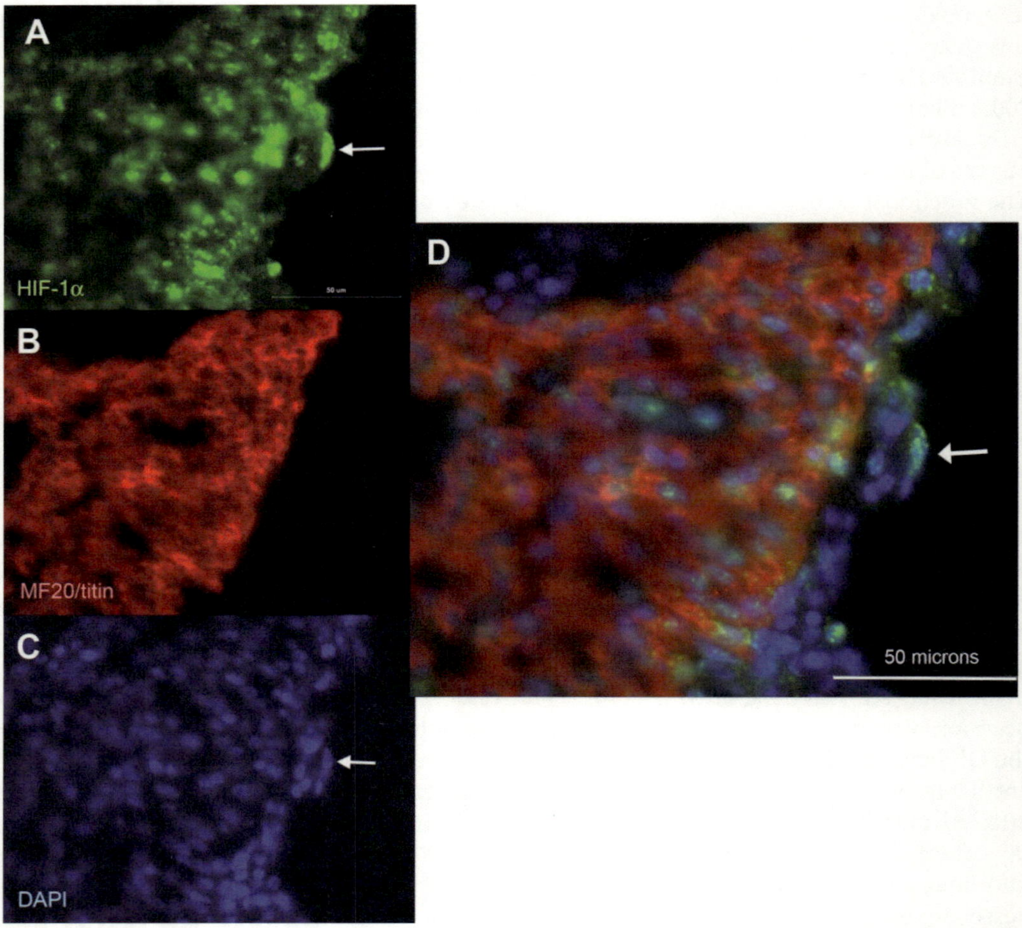

Fig. 7. HIF1a expressed in the epicardium. At the sulcus region of the ventricular apex were epicardial mesothelial cells with nuclear localized HIF1a staining (A, green). The myocardium is delineated using cardiomyocyte markers anti-MF20 and anti-titin (B, red). All nuclei are labeled with DAPI (C, blue). A composite overlay of all three colors (D) indicates an example of where HIF1a is expressed in the nuclei of an epicardial mesothelial cell. The same cell is delineated with a white arrow in A,C,and D.

Molecular factors in early steps of coronary vessel development. Factors that may be important for epicardial EMT and differentiation of these cells have been identified. Explant studies point to FGF (fibroblast growth factor) 2 and 7, VEGF(vascular endothelial growth factor), and EGF (epidermal growth factor) as inducers of EMT with TGFb's (transforming growth factor betas) acting surprisingly as inhibitors of EMT (Morabito et al., 2001). TGFb's act as enhancers of EMT in endocardial cushions. Thus the set of factors that control epicardial EMT resemble the set that control endocardial EMT but differ in their outcomes. These factors are expressed, as detected by immunohistology, within the embryonic epicardium and/or the myocardium. Though some factors involved in EMT and subsequent steps in epicardial cell differentiation have been identified, the mechanism that drives their expression in particular patterns, sites and stages is not fully understood.

Some of the same growth factors also influence the formation of tubes by endothelial precursors. These include VEGF family members and FGFs (Chen et al., 1994; Tomanek, 2006; Tomanek et al., 2008; Tomanek et al., 2002; Tomanek et al., 2006b; Tomanek et al., 2001). A gradient of VEGF expression across the ventricular wall has been observed in embryonic hearts that positively correlates with the level of hypoxia as detected by hypoxia indicators and HIF-1a nuclear localization (Sugishita et al., 2004b; Wikenheiser et al., 2006) and the density of vascular tubes (Tomanek et al., 2001). FGFs are also found in this gradient pattern and ectopic FGF expression caused abnormal coronary patterning within the ventricular wall (Pennisi and Mikawa, 2005). FGF family members are increased in their expression and secreted under hypoxic conditions in other systems (Berger et al., 2003; Moeller et al., 2004). Many factors important in coronary vessel formation are known to be hypoxia inducible and/or controlled directly or indirectly by HIF-1 in other systems.

In summary, a distinguishing feature of the sulcus regions of the heart where the coronary vessels first begin to develop and where the largest coronary arteries end up is a high level of hypoxia and nuclear-localized HIF-1a as well as a high level of expression of HIF downstream genes in both the myocardium and epicardium (Fig. 7).

Abnormally high HIF-1 activity results in abnormal coronary vessel development. If hypoxia via HIFs are an important signal of coronary vessels development, the expectation would be that altering the hypoxic microenvironment would alter coronary vascular development. There is evidence from several studies that this is the case.

Overactive HIF-1 transcriptional activity in the Cited2 knockout mouse results in coronary vascular abnormalities that can be rescued by reducing HIF-1a gene dosage. Cited2, a transcription factor that is regulated by HIF-1 transcriptional activity, down-regulates HIF-1 dependent gene expression in vitro (Bhattacharya et al., 1999)(Bhattacharya et al., 1999). Structural studies (Dames et al., 2002; Freedman et al., 2002; Semenza, 2002) indicated that Cited2 could act as an efficient competitor to HIF-1a binding to CBP/P300 and thus serve as an inhibitor of HIF-1 transcriptional activation. Defects of the Cited2-/- mouse, supported this role for Cited2 in vivo. Cited-/- mice had abnormally high HIF-1 transcriptional activation in the heart and defects in regions that are particularly hypoxic, including the OFT and IVS (Yin et al., 2002). The mRNA levels of HIF-1-regulated genes, VEGF, PGK and Glut-1, were elevated in Cited-/- embryonic hearts. Levels of secreted VEGF were also higher in fibroblast cultures from Cited2-/- as compared to those from Cited+/+ embryos. Vessels in the myocardium of Cited2-/- embryos were larger and leakier resembling vessels developing with VEGF overexpression (Xu et al., 2007). Reducing the gene dosage of HIF-1a in Cited2-/- mice by mating with the HIF-1a knockout line, partially rescued the cardiac defects (Xu et al., 2007). The coronary vasculature and VEGF mRNA transcription were also closer to normal. These results suggested that hypoxia in embryonic heart tissues induces HIF-1 activity to support normal coronary vascular development, but inappropriately high levels of HIF-1 activity have a detrimental effect on coronary vascular and cardiac development. We could not conclude the cell type requirement for HIF-1a and Cited2 using these global Cited2 and HIF-1 knockout mice,

Hypoxic and hyperoxic conditions during embryogenesis alter coronary artery architecture. Regimens of hypoxia (15% O2) and hyperoxia compatible with long-term embryo survival caused coronary artery anomalies in chicken embryos (Wikenheiser et al., 2009)(Fig. 3,4). Regions with relatively high levels of microenvironmental hypoxia within the heart correlated with the expression of HIF-1 nuclear localization and HIF downstream genes at sulcus regions where the epicardium is thickest and where the largest arteries develop. Experimentally increasing the level of hypoxia caused a broadening in the regions of HIF-1a nuclear localized expression within the myocardium and epicardium, abnormal expression of HIF-1 downstream genes, thickening of the epicardium, disruption of the patterns of the early precursors of the coronaries and coronary artery anomalies. The epicardial cells at these sites have a very specific expression of nuclear-localized HIF-1a and N1ICD that indicates that in addition to the paracrine effects of HIFs from the adjacent myocardium, there may be a cell autonomous role for HIF and Notch in the embryonic epicardium (Yang et al., 2009).

Another consideration is the role that normal or abnormal vasculature can play in directing development of other tissues. Vascular development is intimately involved in the growth and development of the liver and pancreas from early inductive events (Bahary and Zon, 2001; Lammert et al., 2001; Lammert et al., 2003; Matsumoto et al., 2001). Evidence also supports the influence of coronary precursors and vessels on myocardial development and function and vice versa (Manner et al., 2001). For example, Purkinje fiber differentiation in avian systems appears to be controlled by factors from the coronary endothelium (Gourdie et al., 1998). *Thus, understanding the factors that regulate normal coronary vascular development is critical to a general understanding of embryonic and adult cardiac diseases and diseases of other tissues.*

7. Regulating the coronary vessels within the adult heart for cardiotherapy

The adult heart can adapt to stress by hypertrophy and vascular growth/remodeling (Bernardo et al., 2010; Weeks KL and McMullen JR, 2011). Physiological or adaptive responses, as in the case of the exercised trained athelete's heart, are characterized by balanced changes in both the cardiomyocytes and the vasculature. Negative consequences arise when these responses are not coordinated, as in the case of prolonged hypertension, and can lead to heart failure, arrhythmia, and death. The physiological and pathological responses overlap in some respects, especially in the early stages of adaptation. However, there are distinct characteristics to the physiological and pathological responses that have been revealed by studies in humans and rodent models (Boström P et al., 2010; Pavlik G et al., 2010; Weeks KL and McMullen JR, 2011). These differences include the degree of vascularization of the myocardium with the physiological response leading to increased vascularization.

Vascular development in the adult heart. Angiogenesis within the myocardium is not limited to developmental stages, but may occur when the mature heart is challenged by enhanced loading conditions or during hypoxia or ischemia. Angiogenesis in the setting of the adult heart can be regulated by hypoxia-induced responses through HIF-1a, that can directly regulate endothelial cell activity and increase capillary density (Pugh CW and Ratcliffe PJ, 2003). Another mechanism is associated with a general stress response following acute hemodynamic overload or hypertrophy induced by exercise or pregnancy (Hilfiker-Kleiner D et al., 2005; Jacobs TB et al., 1984; Sano M et al., 2007; Waters RE et al., 2004). This response would allow the myocardium to coordinate an increase in microvessels with an ensuing hypertrophic response. This load-induced angiogenic response would also protect the heart from developing ischemia, possibly delaying decompensation. That HIF-1α was also activated by mechanical overload (Kim CH et al., 2002) suggests that there is some overlap in the mechanisms.

7.1 Myocardial hypertrophy and angiogenesis

Cardiac hypertrophy is associated with upregulation of VEGF in the myocardium (Izumiya Y et al., 2006). VEGF is required to maintain myocardial capillary density and reductions in the vascular bed are associated with the transition from compensatory hypertrophy to failure (Anversa P et al., 1986; Hudlicka O et al., 1992). In contrast, cardiac growth associated with development, nutritional input, or vigorous exercise is associated with maintained or increased capillary density (Hudlicka O et al., 1992; Shiojima I et al., 2002). Thus, the availability of VEGF may play a role in determining whether the phenotype of the growing heart is "physiological" or "pathological" (Shiojima I et al., 2005). In addition to the VEGF family, bFGF and angiopoietins play major roles in myocardial vascularization (Tomanek RJ et al., 1998; Visconti RP et al., 2002).

It was recently demonstrated that angiogenesis can induce myocardial hypertrophy even in the absence of a hemodynamic stimulus (Tirziu D et al., 2007). In this study an increase in the size of the vascular bed resulted in increased cardiac mass and myocardial hypertrophy paralleled by increased cardiac performance. This points out a complex role played by the endothelium of the heart (and likely other organs) that involves not only participation in a stress response but also regulation of the organ's size. The increase in heart size ceased once the vascular density returned to normal levels (Tirziu D et al., 2007).

Several important transcription factors have been studied for their ability to regulate the coronary vasculature in the adult mouse. These include GATA4 and CEBPb. The coronary vasculature within the myocardium increases in density when GATA4 expression is up-regulated (Heineke et al., 2007), or when CEBPb is down-regulated (Boström P et al., 2010) These vascular changes are also accompanied by improvement in function and survival when mice are subjected to a model of myocardial infarction. While effects on the coronary vasculature are not the only positive changes, this change is probably very important in providing coronary reserve during stresses. These promising preclinical findings suggest that targeting ways to regulate the transcription factors may be important in finding strategies for cardioprotection via increased vascularization.

If it is possible to find the pathways that lead to the morphology, physiology, and gene expression that resemble those of a physiological rather than a pathological response, that knowledge may allow us to coordinate a host of beneficial responses for the heart that would protect it from ischemic insults.

The adult epicardium has recently been shown to act as a paracrine source of factors that increases vessel density and benefits the health of cardiomyocytes (Zhou et al., 2011).

Preclinical studies to develop potential therapies and expected challenges. To prevent or alleviate effects of heart disease including myocardial infarction and heart failure, it would be beneficial to increase the density of the vasculature and therefore perfusion of the myocardium. This increase would have to be controlled and the right mix of vessels would have to be formed in the right place at the right time. This enhancement of the coronary vasculature could be encouraged prior to surgery, or in early stages of coronary artery disease when a coronary occlusion is first noted or when early signs of pathological hypertrophy are identified. In cases of some anomalous coronaries it would be beneficial to encourage collateralization in a controlled way. An ability to promote and nudge coronary vessel development at the right time and place could benefit the outcome of many cardiac diseases.

Gene therapy. Current pharmacologic therapy for ischemic heart disease is limited by several issues including patient compliance and side effects of the medications (Lavu et al., 2011). Also a significant population of patients do not respond to the best medical therapy available. Gene therapy may be a promising alternative that is currently being investigated. Gene therapy with isoforms of growth factors such as Vascular Endothelial Growth Factor A (VEGFA) , Fibroblast Growth Factor (FGF) and Hepatocyte Growth Factor (HGF) induces angiogenesis, decreases apoptosis and leads to protection in the ischemic heart. Stem cell therapy combined with gene therapy promotes myogenesis in animal models of myocardial ischemia. Gene therapy that induces the expression of antioxidants, eNOS, SP, mitogen activated protein kinase and other anti-apoptotic proteins have also been shown to be beneficial in animal models. Clinical trials currently show mixed results and the interpretation of the results are controversial, but some of the therapies appear to be safe.

Vascular endothelial growth factor (VEGF) gene therapy: VEGFA is a highly investigated growth factor that induces angiogenesis in the ischemic heart. Isoforms of VEGFA bind to specific receptors on endothelial cells and play an essential role in angiogenesis (Hao et al., 2007). VEGFA-165 (VEGFA isoform) gene therapy using plasmids in rats (Dong et al., 2009; Yockman et al., 2009) or through non-viral delivery systems in rabbits (Aoki et al., 2000) induces significant neovascularization and improves fractional shortening after modeling myocardial infarction (MI).

Concerns with angiogenic therapies exist because VEGFA is a powerful factor whose expression level must be tightly regulated in isoform expression, timing and location. Deviation from normal levels are known to cause pathology in animal models [e.g. (Autiero et al., 2005; Carmeliet et al., 1996; Flamme et al., 1995; Kaner et al., 2000)]. Novel gene constructs have been created that would allow the gene expression to be responsive to the cellular environments. For example, some constructs allow VEGFA levels to be increased specifically during cardiac ischemia.

(Lee et al., 2003; Su et al., 2002) and the treated animals have reduced infarct size and increased angiogenesis (Dong et al., 2009; Yockman et al., 2009).

Hepatocyte growth factor gene therapy: Human Hepatocyte Growth Factor (hHGF) gene therapy induced angiogenesis in rats and dogs after experimental myocardial infarction (MI) and also improved cardiac function (Ahmet et al., 2002; Ahmet et al., 2003; Cho et al., 2008; Jayasankar et al., 2003; Jin et al., 2004; Li et al., 2003; Taniyama et al., 2002; Yang et al., 2007; Yang et al., 2010). HGF gene therapy combined with a novel gene transfection strategy that looks promising in a rat model of MI (Ahmet et al., 2003) is currently being evaluated in clinical trials.

Fibroblast growth factor gene therapy: Fibroblast growth factors FGF-1 and FGF-2 are known to promote endothelial cell proliferation and formation of tube-like endothelial structures in various pre-clinical models. FGF-2 gene therapy has been shown to improve arteriogenesis and left ventricular (LV) function in a model of chronic ischemia in pigs (Heilmann et al., 2002; Horvath et al., 2002).

Angiogenesis through genetically modified cells: Genetically modified cells can be used to express the transgene of choice and lead to increased levels of the desired proteins in target tissues such as the heart. One obvious potential benefit of this strategy is its ability to activate precursor cells to differentiate into cardiac phenotypes, incorporate into the myocardium and prevent or alleviate harmful cardiac remodeling (Atkins et al., 1999)[29]. Vascular smooth muscle cells (VSMCs) modified to overexpress VEGF, when administered by the intra-coronary route in an intermittent repetitive LAD occlusion model increased collateral circulation in the ischemic heart (Hattan et al., 2004). Fibroblasts, modified to overexpress bFGF gene, when administered by coronary injections in a swine model of chronic ischemia led to improved collateral formation and myocardial contraction as measured by coronary angiography and electromechanical mapping (Ninomiya et al., 2003). Some advantages of mesenchymal stem cells (MSCs) are their ability to be transduced by vectors easily, ability to be delivered systemically and their capacity to home in to damaged tissues. MSCs also possess low immunogenicity and hence can be used allogenically (Ninomiya et al., 2003).

8. Overall summary

There are still many puzzling aspects of cardiac vessel development and anatomy that require further investigation. Fundamental questions regarding lymphangiogenesis in the heart may now be approachable with techniques and reagents currently available and already reveal surprising and puzzling findings. It is still unknown how coronary vessel anomalies develop. Discussions continue on the best way to detect them clinically and how to proceed once detected. Experiments on the developmental biology of coronary vessel development in genetically engineered mice have led to promising leads towards reducing or alleviating the consequences of myocardial infarction and heart disease so as to slow or prevent the progression to heart failure and death. By understanding the mechanisms that control coronary vessel localization and density, it may be possible to increase coronary vasculature with therapies even when exercise is not an option as a preventative measure to reduce or prevent myocardial ischemic damage during surgery or for individuals with a family history of heart disease.

9. Abbreviations

ALCAPA	Anomalous Left Coronary Artery from Pulmonary Artery
ASD	Atrial Septal Defect
AV	Atrioventricular
BMP	Bone Morphogenetic Protein
CAD	Coronary Artery Disease
CF	Circumflex Artery
EGF	Endothelial Growth Factor
EMT	Epithelial Mesenchymal Transition
EPDC	Epicardial Derived Cells
FGF	Fibroblast Growth Factor
FOG	Friend of GATA

HIF	Hypoxia Inducible Factor
HRE	Hypoxia Responsive Elements
LAD	Left Anterior Descending Coronary Artery
MI	Myocardial Infarction
OFT	Outflow Tract
PDA	Posterior Descending Artery
PE	Proepicardium
PEO	Proepicardial Organ
RCA	Right Coronary Artery
TGF	Transforming Growth Factor
VEGF	Vascular Endothelial Growth Factor
VSD	Ventricular Septal Defect

10. Acknowledgements

The authors thank Laura M. Bock, BFA, Medical Illustrator (laurabock.biomed@gmail.com) for artistic contributions, and Dr. Robert J. Tomanek for inspiration, encouragement, and critical discussions. NIH Grant funding (ARRA) from NHLBI HL091171 (M.W.) and AHA Fellowship funding to Ganga Karunamuni

11. References

Ahmet, I., Sawa, Y., Iwata, K., Matsuda, H., 2002. Gene transfection of hepatocyte growth factor attenuates cardiac remodeling in the canine heart: A novel gene therapy for cardiomyopathy. J Thorac Cardiovasc Surg. 124, 957-63.

Ahmet, I., Sawa, Y., Yamaguchi, T., Matsuda, H., 2003. Gene transfer of hepatocyte growth factor improves angiogenesis and function of chronic ischemic myocardium in canine heart. Ann Thorac Surg. 75, 1283-7.

Albrecht, I., Christofori, G., 2011. Molecular mechanisms of lymphangiogenesis in development and cancer. Int J Dev Biol. 55, 483-94.

Allen, H. D. D., D.J.;Shaddy,R.D. RD Shaddy; Feltes,T.F., 2007. Moss and Adams' Heart Disease in Infants, Children, and Adolescents. Lippincott, Williams & Wilkins.

Anversa P, Beghi C, Kikkawa Y, Olivetti G, C. R., 1986. Myocardial infarction in rats. Infarct size, myocyte hypertrophy, and capillary growth. Circ. Res. 58, 26-37.

Aoki, M., Morishita, R., Taniyama, Y., Kida, I., Moriguchi, A., Matsumoto, K., Nakamura, T., Kaneda, Y., Higaki, J., Ogihara, T., 2000. Angiogenesis induced by hepatocyte growth factor in non-infarcted myocardium and infarcted myocardium: up-regulation of essential transcription factor for angiogenesis, ets. Gene Ther. 7, 417-27.

Atkins, B. Z., Hueman, M. T., Meuchel, J., Hutcheson, K. A., Glower, D. D., Taylor, D. A., 1999. Cellular cardiomyoplasty improves diastolic properties of injured heart. J Surg Res. 85, 234-42.

Autiero, M., Desmet, F., Claes, F., Carmeliet, P., 2005. Role of neural guidance signals in blood vessel navigation. Cardiovascular Research. 65, 629-638.

Bahary, N., Zon, L. I., 2001. Development. Endothelium--chicken soup for the endoderm. Science. 294, 530-1.

Barbosky, L., Lawrence, D. K., Karunamuni, G., Wikenheiser, J. C., Doughman, Y. Q., Visconti, R. P., Burch, J. B., Watanabe, M., 2006. Apoptosis in the developing mouse heart. Dev Dyn. 235, 2592-602.

Berger, A. P., Kofler, K., Bektic, J., Rogatsch, H., Steiner, H., Bartsch, G., Klocker, H., 2003. Increased growth factor production in a human prostatic stromal cell culture model caused by hypoxia. Prostate. 57, 57-65.

Bernardo, B. C., Weeks, K. L., Pretorius, L., McMullen, J. R., 2010. Molecular distinction between physiological and pathological cardiac hypertrophy: experimental findings and therapeutic strategies. Pharmacol Ther. 128, 191-227.

Bhattacharya, S., Michels, C. L., Leung, M. K., Arany, Z. P., Kung, A. L., Livingston, D. M., 1999. Functional role of p35srj, a novel p300/CBP binding protein, during transactivation by HIF-1. Genes Dev. 13, 64-75.

Boktor, M., Mansi, I. A., Troxclair, S., Modi, K., 2009. Association of myocardial bridge and Takotsubo cardiomyopathy: a case report and literature review. South Med J. 102, 957-60.

Boström P, Mann N, Wu J, Quintero PA, Plovie ER, Panáková D, Gupta RK, Xiao C, MacRae CA, Rosenzweig A, Spiegelman BM, 2010. C/EBPβ controls exercise-induced cardiac growth and protects against pathological cardiac remodeling. Cell. 143, 1072-1083.

Bourassa, M. G., Butnaru, A., Lesperance, J., Tardif, J. C., 2003. Symptomatic myocardial bridges: overview of ischemic mechanisms and current diagnostic and treatment strategies. J Am Coll Cardiol. 41, 351-9.

Cai, C.-L., Martin, J. C., Sun, Y., Cui, L., Wang, L., Ouyang, K., Yang, L., Bu, L., Liang, X., Zhang, X., Stallcup, W. B., Denton, C. P., McCulloch, A., Chen, J., Evans, S. M., 2008. A myocardial lineage derives from Tbx18 epicardial cells. Nature. 454, 104-108.

Carmeliet, P., Ferreira, V., Breier, G., Pollefeyt, S., Kieckens, L., Gertsenstein, M., Fahrig, M., Vandenhoeck, A., Harpal, K., Eberhardt, C., Declercq, C., Pawling, J., Moons, L., Collen, D., Risau, W., Nagy, A., 1996. Abnormal blood vessel development and lethality in embryos lacking a single VEGF allele. Nature. 380, 435-9.

Cheitlin, M. D., MacGregor, J., 2009. Congenital anomalies of coronary arteries: role in the pathogenesis of sudden cardiac death. Herz. 34, 268-79.

Chen, Y., Torry, R. J., Baumbach, G. L., Tomanek, R. J., 1994. Proportional arteriolar growth accompanies cardiac hypertrophy induced by volume overload. Am J Physiol. 267, H2132-7.

Chiam, P. T., Ruiz, C. E., 2011. Percutaneous transcatheter mitral valve repair: a classification of the technology. JACC Cardiovasc Interv. 4, 1-13.

Cho, K. R., Choi, J. S., Hahn, W., Kim, D. S., Park, J. S., Lee, D. S., Kim, K. B., 2008. Therapeutic angiogenesis using naked DNA expressing two isoforms of the hepatocyte growth factor in a porcine acute myocardial infarction model. Eur J Cardiothorac Surg. 34, 857-63.

Compernolle, V., Brusselmans, K., Acker, T., Hoet, P., Tjwa, M., Beck, H., Plaisance, S., Dor, Y., Keshet, E., Lupu, F., Nemery, B., Dewerchin, M., Van Veldhoven, P., Plate, K., Moons, L., Collen, D., Carmeliet, P., 2002. Loss of HIF-2α and inhibition of VEGF impair fetal lung maturation, whereas treatment with VEGF prevents fatal respiratory distress in premature mice. Nature Medicine.

Compton, L. A., Potash, D. A., Mundell, N. A., Barnett, J. V., 2006. Transforming growth factor-β induces loss of epithelial character and smooth muscle cell differentiation in epicardial cells. Developmental Dynamics. 235, 82-93.

Dames, S. A., Martinez-Yamout, M., De Guzman, R. N., Dyson, H. J., Wright, P. E., 2002. Structural basis for Hif-1 alpha /CBP recognition in the cellular hypoxic response. Proc Natl Acad Sci U S A. 99, 5271-6.

Dong, H., Wang, Q., Zhang, Y., Jiang, B., Xu, X., Zhang, Z., 2009. Angiogenesis induced by hVEGF165 gene controlled by hypoxic response elements in rabbit ischemia myocardium. Exp Biol Med (Maywood). 234, 1417-24.

Duan, L. J., Zhang-Benoit, Y., Fong, G. H., 2005. Endothelium-intrinsic requirement for Hif-2alpha during vascular development. Circulation. 111, 2227-32.

Eckart, R. E., Jones, S. O. t., Shry, E. A., Garrett, P. D., Scoville, S. L., 2006a. Sudden death associated with anomalous coronary origin and obstructive coronary disease in the young. Cardiol Rev. 14, 161-3.

Eckart, R. E., Scoville, S. L., Shry, E. A., Potter, R. N., Tedrow, U., 2006b. Causes of sudden death in young female military recruits. Am J Cardiol. 97, 1756-8.

Epstein, S. E., Cannon, R. O., 3rd, Talbot, T. L., 1985. Hemodynamic principles in the control of coronary blood flow. Am J Cardiol. 56, 4E-10E.

Eralp, I., 2005. Coronary Artery and Orifice Development Is Associated With Proper Timing of Epicardial Outgrowth and Correlated Fas Ligand Associated Apoptosis Patterns. Circulation Research. 96, 526-534.

Eralp, I., Lie-Venema, H., DeRuiter, M. C., van den Akker, N. M., Bogers, A. J., Mentink, M. M., Poelmann, R. E., Gittenberger-de Groot, A. C., 2005. Coronary artery and orifice development is associated with proper timing of epicardial outgrowth and correlated Fas-ligand-associated apoptosis patterns. Circ Res. 96, 526-34.

Flamme, I., von Reutern, M., Drexler, H. C., Syed-Ali, S., Risau, W., 1995. Overexpression of vascular endothelial growth factor in the avian embryo induces hypervascularization and increased vascular permeability without alterations of embryonic pattern formation. Dev Biol. 171, 399-414.

Fontana, R. S., Edwards, J.E., 1962. Congenital Cardiac Disease: A Review of 357 Cases Studied Pathologically. W.B. Saunders, Philadelphia.

Freedman, S. J., Sun, Z. Y., Poy, F., Kung, A. L., Livingston, D. M., Wagner, G., Eck, M. J., 2002. Structural basis for recruitment of CBP/p300 by hypoxia-inducible factor-1 alpha. Proc Natl Acad Sci U S A. 99, 5367-72.

Frescura, C., Basso, C., Thiene, G., Corrado, D., Pennelli, T., Angelini, A., Daliento, L., 1998. Anomalous origin of coronary arteries and risk of sudden death: a study based on an autopsy population of congenital heart disease. Hum Pathol. 29, 689-95.

Frescura, C. B., C.;Thiene, G.;Corrado, D.;Pennelli, T.;Angelini, A.; Daliento, L., 1999. Anomalous origin of coronary arteries and risk of sudden death: a study based on an autopsy population of congenital heart disease. Hum Pathol. 29, 689-695.

Fulton, W. F. M., 1964. Morphology of the myocardial microcirculation. British Heart Journal. 26, 39-50.

Gensini, G. G., Digiorgi, S., Coskun, O., Palacio, A., Kelly, A. E., 1965. Anatomy of the Coronary Circulation in Living Man; Coronary Venography. Circulation. 31, 778-84.

George, J. M., Knowlan, D. M., 1959. Anomalous origin of the left coronary artery from the pulmonary artery in an adult. N Engl J Med. 261, 993-8.

Gilard, M., Mansourati, J., Etienne, Y., Larlet, J. M., Truong, B., Boschat, J., Blanc, J. J., 1998. Angiographic anatomy of the coronary sinus and its tributaries. Pacing Clin Electrophysiol. 21, 2280-4.

Gittenberger-de Groot, A. C., Vrancken Peeters, M. P., Bergwerff, M., Mentink, M. M., Poelmann, R. E., 2000. Epicardial outgrowth inhibition leads to compensatory mesothelial outflow tract collar and abnormal cardiac septation and coronary formation. Circ Res. 87, 969-71.

Gittenberger-de Groot, A. C., Winter, E. M., Poelmann, R. E., 2010. Epicardium-derived cells (EPDCs) in development, cardiac disease and repair of ischemia. J Cell Mol Med. 14, 1056-60.

Gourdie, R. G., Wei, Y., Kim, D., Klatt, S. C., Mikawa, T., 1998. Endothelin-induced conversion of embryonic heart muscle cells into impulse-conducting Purkinje fibers. Proc Natl Acad Sci U S A. 95, 6815-8.

Grace, R. R., Angelini, P., Cooley, D. A., 1977. Aortic implantation of anomalous left coronary artery arising from pulmonary artery. Am J Cardiol. 39, 609-13.

Gustafsson, M. V., Zheng, X., Pereira, T., Gradin, K., Jin, S., Lundkvist, J., Ruas, J. L., Poellinger, L., Lendahl, U., Bondesson, M., 2005. Hypoxia Requires Notch Signaling to Maintain the Undifferentiated Cell State. Developmental Cell. 9, 617-628.

Hakeem, A., Cilingiroglu, M., Leesar, M. A., 2010. Hemodynamic and intravascular ultrasound assessment of myocardial bridging: fractional flow reserve paradox with dobutamine versus adenosine. Catheter Cardiovasc Interv. 75, 229-36.

Hao, X., Mansson-Broberg, A., Grinnemo, K. H., Siddiqui, A. J., Dellgren, G., Brodin, L. A., Sylven, C., 2007. Myocardial angiogenesis after plasmid or adenoviral VEGF-A(165) gene transfer in rat myocardial infarction model. Cardiovasc Res. 73, 481-7.

Hattan, N., Warltier, D., Gu, W., Kolz, C., Chilian, W. M., Weihrauch, D., 2004. Autologous vascular smooth muscle cell-based myocardial gene therapy to induce coronary collateral growth. Am J Physiol Heart Circ Physiol. 287, H488-93.

Haugen, O. A., Ellingsen, C. L., 2007. [Coronary artery anomalies as a cause of sudden death in young people]. Tidsskr Nor Laegeforen. 127, 190-2.

Heilmann, C., von Samson, P., Schlegel, K., Attmann, T., von Specht, B. U., Beyersdorf, F., Lutter, G., 2002. Comparison of protein with DNA therapy for chronic myocardial ischemia using fibroblast growth factor-2. Eur J Cardiothorac Surg. 22, 957-64.

Heineke, J., Auger-Messier, M., Xu, J., Oka, T., Sargent, M. A., York, A., Klevitsky, R., Vaikunth, S., Duncan, S. A., Aronow, B. J., Robbins, J., Cromblehol, T. M., Molkentin, J. D., 2007. Cardiomyocyte GATA4 functions as a stress-responsive regulator of angiogenesis in the murine heart. Journal of Clinical Investigation. 117, 3198-3210.

Hilfiker-Kleiner D, Hilfiker A, Kaminski K, Schaefer A, Park JK, Michel K, Quint A, Yaniv M, Weitzman JB, Drexler H, 2005. Lack of JunD promotes pressure overload-induced apoptosis, hypertrophic growth, and angiogenesis in the heart. . Circulation. 112, 1470-1477.

Hiruma, T., Hirakow, R., 1989. Epicardial formation in embryonic chick heart: computer-aided reconstruction, scanning, and transmission electron microscopic studies. Am J Anat. 184, 129-38.

Ho, E., Shimada, Y., 1978. Formation of the epicardium studied with the scanning electron microscope. Dev Biol. 66, 579-85.

Horvath, K. A., Doukas, J., Lu, C. Y., Belkind, N., Greene, R., Pierce, G. F., Fullerton, D. A., 2002. Myocardial functional recovery after fibroblast growth factor 2 gene therapy as assessed by echocardiography and magnetic resonance imaging. Ann Thorac Surg. 74, 481-6; discussion 487.

Huang, Y., Hickey, R. P., Yeh, J. L., Liu, D., Dadak, A., Young, L. H., Johnson, R. S., Giordano, F. J., 2004. Cardiac myocyte-specific HIF-1alpha deletion alters vascularization, energy availability, calcium flux, and contractility in the normoxic heart. FASEB J. 18, 1138-40.

Huddleston, C. B., Balzer, D. T., Mendeloff, E. N., 2001. Repair of anomalous left main coronary artery arising from the pulmonary artery in infants: long-term impact on the mitral valve. Ann Thorac Surg. 71, 1985-8; discussion 1988-9.

Hudlicka O, Brown M, Egginton S, 1992. Angiogenesis in skeletal and cardiac muscle. Physiol. Rev. 72, 369-417.

Ishii, Y., Garriock, R. J., Navetta, A. M., Coughlin, L. E., Mikawa, T., 2010. BMP signals promote proepicardial protrusion necessary for recruitment of coronary vessel and epicardial progenitors to the heart. Dev Cell. 19, 307-16.

Iyer, N. V., Kotch, L. E., Agani, F., Leung, S. W., Laughner, E., Wenger, R. H., Gassmann, M., Gearhart, J. D., Lawler, A. M., Yu, A. Y., Semenza, G. L., 1998. Cellular and developmental control of O2 homeostasis by hypoxia-inducible factor 1 alpha. Genes Dev. 12, 149-62.

Izumiya Y, Shiojima I, Sato K, Sawyer DB, Colucci WS, Walsh K, 2006. Vascular endothelial growth factor blockade promotes the transition from compensatory cardiac hypertrophy to failure in response to pressure overload. . Hypertension. 47, 887-893.

Jacobs TB, Bell RD, McClements JD, 1984. Exercise, age and the development of the myocardial vasculature. . Growth. 48, 148-157.

Jayasankar, V., Woo, Y. J., Bish, L. T., Pirolli, T. J., Chatterjee, S., Berry, M. F., Burdick, J., Gardner, T. J., Sweeney, H. L., 2003. Gene transfer of hepatocyte growth factor attenuates postinfarction heart failure. Circulation. 108 Suppl 1, II230-6.

Jin, H., Wyss, J. M., Yang, R., Schwall, R., 2004. The therapeutic potential of hepatocyte growth factor for myocardial infarction and heart failure. Curr Pharm Des. 10, 2525-33.

Jin, Z., Berger, F., Uhlemann, F., Schroder, C., Hetzer, R., Alexi-Meskhishvili, V., Weng, Y., Lange, P. E., 1994. Improvement in left ventricular dysfunction after aortic reimplantation in 11 consecutive paediatric patients with anomalous origin of the left coronary artery from the pulmonary artery. Early results of a serial echocardiographic follow-up. Eur Heart J. 15, 1044-9.

Kaner, R. J., Ladetto, J. V., Singh, R., Fukuda, N., Matthay, M. A., Crystal, R. G., 2000. Lung overexpression of the vascular endothelial growth factor gene induces pulmonary edema. Am J Respir Cell Mol Biol. 22, 657-64.

Karunamuni, G., Yang, K., Doughman, Y. Q., Wikenheiser, J., Bader, D., Barnett, J., Austin, A., Parsons-Wingerter, P., Watanabe, M., 2010. Expression of Lymphatic Markers During Avian and Mouse Cardiogenesis. Anat Rec (Hoboken).

Kattan, J., Dettman, R. W., Bristow, J., 2004. Formation and remodeling of the coronary vascular bed in the embryonic avian heart. Dev Dyn. 230, 34-43.

Kim CH, Cho YS, Chun YS, Park JW, Kim MS, 2002. Early expression of myocardial HIF-1alpha in response to mechanical stresses: regulation by stretch-activated channels and the phosphatidylinositol 3-kinase signaling pathway. Circ. Res. 90, E25-E33.

Krishnan, J., Ahuja, P., Bodenmann, S., Knapik, D., Perriard, E., Krek, W., Perriard, J. C., 2008. Essential Role of Developmentally Activated Hypoxia-Inducible Factor 1 for Cardiac Morphogenesis and Function. Circulation Research. 103, 1139-1146.
Laifer, L. I., Weiner, B. H., 1991. Percutaneous transluminal coronary angioplasty of a coronary artery stenosis at the site of myocardial bridging. Cardiology. 79, 245-8.
Lammert, E., Cleaver, O., Melton, D., 2001. Induction of pancreatic differentiation by signals from blood vessels. Science. 294, 564-7.
Lammert, E., Cleaver, O., Melton, D., 2003. Role of endothelial cells in early pancreas and liver development. Mech Dev. 120, 59-64.
Lavu, M., Gundewar, S., Lefer, D. J., 2011. Gene therapy for ischemic heart disease. J Mol Cell Cardiol. 50, 742-50.
Lee, M., Rentz, J., Bikram, M., Han, S., Bull, D. A., Kim, S. W., 2003. Hypoxia-inducible VEGF gene delivery to ischemic myocardium using water-soluble lipopolymer. Gene Ther. 10, 1535-42.
Li, Y., Takemura, G., Kosai, K., Yuge, K., Nagano, S., Esaki, M., Goto, K., Takahashi, T., Hayakawa, K., Koda, M., Kawase, Y., Maruyama, R., Okada, H., Minatoguchi, S., Mizuguchi, H., Fujiwara, T., Fujiwara, H., 2003. Postinfarction treatment with an adenoviral vector expressing hepatocyte growth factor relieves chronic left ventricular remodeling and dysfunction in mice. Circulation. 107, 2499-506.
Licht, A. H., 2006. Inhibition of hypoxia-inducible factor activity in endothelial cells disrupts embryonic cardiovascular development. Blood. 107, 584-590.
Lie-Venema, H., van den Akker, N. M., Bax, N. A., Winter, E. M., Maas, S., Kekarainen, T., Hoeben, R. C., deRuiter, M. C., Poelmann, R. E., Gittenberger-de Groot, A. C., 2007. Origin, fate, and function of epicardium-derived cells (EPDCs) in normal and abnormal cardiac development. ScientificWorldJournal. 7, 1777-98.
Liebman, J., Hellerstein, H. K., Ankeney, J. L., Tucker, A., 1963. The Problem of the Anomalous Left Coronary Artery Arising from the Pulmonary Artery in Older Children. Report of Three Cases. N Engl J Med. 269, 486-94.
Loukas, M., Curry, B., Bowers, M., Louis, R. G., Jr., Bartczak, A., Kiedrowski, M., Kamionek, M., Fudalej, M., Wagner, T., 2006. The relationship of myocardial bridges to coronary artery dominance in the adult human heart. J Anat. 209, 43-50.
Luo, L., Kebede, S., Wu, S., Stouffer, G. A., 2006. Coronary artery fistulae. Am J Med Sci. 332, 79-84.
Manner, J., 1993. Experimental study on the formation of the epicardium in chick embryos. Anat Embryol (Berl). 187, 281-9.
Manner, J., Perez-Pomares, J. M., Macias, D., Munoz-Chapuli, R., 2001. The origin, formation and developmental significance of the epicardium: a review. Cells Tissues Organs. 169, 89-103.
Matsumoto, K., Yoshitomi, H., Rossant, J., Zaret, K. S., 2001. Liver organogenesis promoted by endothelial cells prior to vascular function. Science. 294, 559-63.
Mikawa, T., Fischman, D. A., 1992. Retroviral analysis of cardiac morphogenesis: discontinuous formation of coronary vessels. Proc Natl Acad Sci U S A. 89, 9504-8.
Miller, A. J., 1982. Lymphatics of the Heart. Raven Press, New York.
Moeller, B. J., Cao, Y., Vujaskovic, Z., Li, C. Y., Haroon, Z. A., Dewhirst, M. W., 2004. The relationship between hypoxia and angiogenesis. Semin Radiat Oncol. 14, 215-21.
Morabito, C. J., Dettman, R. W., Kattan, J., Collier, J. M., Bristow, J., 2001. Positive and negative regulation of epicardial-mesenchymal transformation during avian heart development. Dev Biol. 234, 204-15.

Mosher, P., Ross, J., Jr., McFate, P. A., Shaw, R. F., 1964. Control of Coronary Blood Flow by an Autoregulatory Mechanism. Circ Res. 14, 250-9.

Nahirney, P. C., Mikawa, T., Fischman, D. A., 2003. Evidence for an extracellular matrix bridge guiding proepicardial cell migration to the myocardium of chick embryos. Dev Dyn. 227, 511-23.

Nanka, O., Krizova, P., Fikrle, M., Tuma, M., Blaha, M., Grim, M., Sedmera, D., 2008. Abnormal Myocardial and Coronary Vasculature Development in Experimental Hypoxia. The Anatomical Record: Advances in Integrative Anatomy and Evolutionary Biology. 291, 1187-1199.

Naňka, O., Valášek, P., Dvořáková, M., Grim, M., 2006. Experimental hypoxia and embryonic angiogenesis. Developmental Dynamics. 235, 723-733.

Nesbitt, T., Lemley, A., Davis, J., Yost, M. J., Goodwin, R. L., Potts, J. D., 2006. Epicardial development in the rat: a new perspective. Microsc Microanal. 12, 390-8.

Neufeld, H. N., Schneeweiss, A., 1983. Coronary Artery Disease in Infants and Children. Lea & Febiger, Philadelphia.

Ninomiya, M., Koyama, H., Miyata, T., Hamada, H., Miyatake, S., Shigematsu, H., Takamoto, S., 2003. Ex vivo gene transfer of basic fibroblast growth factor improves cardiac function and blood flow in a swine chronic myocardial ischemia model. Gene Ther. 10, 1152-60.

Ogden, J. A., 1970. Congenital anomalies of the coronary arteries. Am J Cardiol. 25, 474-9.

Olivey, H. E., Compton, L. A., Barnett, J. V., 2004. Coronary vessel development: the epicardium delivers. Trends Cardiovasc Med. 14, 247-51.

Olivey, H. E., Mundell, N. A., Austin, A. F., Barnett, J. V., 2006. Transforming growth factor-β stimulates epithelial–mesenchymal transformation in the proepicardium. Developmental Dynamics. 235, 50-59.

Olivey, H. E., Svensson, E. C., 2010. Epicardial-myocardial signaling directing coronary vasculogenesis. Circ Res. 106, 818-32.

Park, M. K., 1988. Pediatric Cardiology for Practitioners. Year Book Medical Publishers, Inc., Boca Raton.

Parsons-Wingerter, P., McKay, T. L., Leontiev, D., Vickerman, M. B., Condrich, T. K., Dicorleto, P. E., 2006. Lymphangiogenesis by blind-ended vessel sprouting is concurrent with hemangiogenesis by vascular splitting. The Anatomical Record Part A: Discoveries in Molecular, Cellular, and Evolutionary Biology. 288A, 233-247.

Pavlik G, Major Z, Varga-Pintér B, Jeserich M, Kneffel Z, 2010. The athlete's heart Part I Acta Physiol. Hung. . 97, 337-353.

Pena, E., Nguyen, E. T., Merchant, N., Dennie, G., 2009. ALCAPA syndrome: not just a pediatric disease. Radiographics. 29, 553-65.

Peng, J., 2000. The transcription factor EPAS-1/hypoxia-inducible factor 2alpha plays an important role in vascular remodeling. Proceedings of the National Academy of Sciences. 97, 8386-8391.

Pennisi, D. J., Mikawa, T., 2005. Normal patterning of the coronary capillary plexus is dependent on the correct transmural gradient of FGF expression in the myocardium. Dev Biol. 279, 378-90.

Perez-Pomares, J. M., Phelps, A., Sedmerova, M., Wessels, A., 2003. Epicardial-like cells on the distal arterial end of the cardiac outflow tract do not derive from the proepicardium but are derivatives of the cephalic pericardium. Dev Dyn. 227, 56-68.

Pugh CW, Ratcliffe PJ, 2003. Regulation of angiogenesis by hypoxia: role of the HIF system. Nat. Med. 9, 677-684.

Que, J., Wilm, B., Hasegawa, H., Wang, F., Bader, D., Hogan, B. L., 2008. Mesothelium contributes to vascular smooth muscle and mesenchyme during lung development. Proc Natl Acad Sci U S A. 105, 16626-30.

Ratajska, A., Czarnowska, E., Ciszek, B., 2008. Embryonic development of the proepicardium and coronary vessels. Int J Dev Biol. 52, 229-36.

Rayman, H. C., 1737. Dissertation de vasis cordis propriis. Haller Bibl Anat. 2, 366.

Red-Horse, K., Ueno, H., Weissman, I. L., Krasnow, M. A., 2010. Coronary arteries form by developmental reprogramming of venous cells. Nature. 464, 549-53.

Reese, D. E., Mikawa, T., Bader, D. M., 2002. Development of the coronary vessel system. Circ Res. 91, 761-8.

Rothenberg, F., Hitomi, M., Fisher, S. A., Watanabe, M., 2002. Initiation of apoptosis in the developing avian outflow tract myocardium. Dev Dyn. 223, 469-82.

Ryan, H. E., Lo, J., Johnson, R. S., 1998. HIF-1 alpha is required for solid tumor formation and embryonic vascularization. EMBO J. 17, 3005-15.

Sano M, Minamino T, Toko H, Miyauchi H, Orimo M, Qin Y, Akazawa H, Tateno K, Kayama Y, Harada M, Shimizu I, Asahara T, Hamada H, Tomita S, Molkentin JD, Zou Y, Komuro I, 2007. p53-induced inhibition of Hif-1 causes cardiac dysfunction during pressure overload. . Nature. 446, 444-448.

Schamroth, C., 2009. Coronary artery fistula. J Am Coll Cardiol. 53, 523.

Schmitt, R., Froehner, S., Brunn, J., Wagner, M., Brunner, H., Cherevatyy, O., Gietzen, F., Christopoulos, G., Kerber, S., Fellner, F., 2005. Congenital anomalies of the coronary arteries: imaging with contrast-enhanced, multidetector computed tomography. Eur Radiol. 15, 1110-21.

Schulte-Merker, S., Sabine, A., Petrova, T.V., 2011. Lymphatic vascular mophogenesis in development, physiology, and disease. Journal Cell Biology. 193, 607-618.

Schwartz, M. L., Jonas, R. A., Colan, S. D., 1997. Anomalous origin of left coronary artery from pulmonary artery: recovery of left ventricular function after dual coronary repair. J Am Coll Cardiol. 30, 547-53.

Scortegagna, M., Ding, K., Oktay, Y., Gaur, A., Thurmond, F., Yan, L. J., Marck, B. T., Matsumoto, A. M., Shelton, J. M., Richardson, J. A., Bennett, M. J., Garcia, J. A., 2003a. Multiple organ pathology, metabolic abnormalities and impaired homeostasis of reactive oxygen species in Epas1(-/-) mice. Nature Genetics. 35, 331-340.

Scortegagna, M., Morris, M. A., Oktay, Y., Bennett, M., Garcia, J. A., 2003b. The HIF family member EPAS1/HIF-2 alpha is required for normal hematopoiesis in mice. Blood. 102, 1634-1640.

Sedmera, D., Watanabe, M., 2006. Growing the coronary tree: the quail saga. Anat Rec A Discov Mol Cell Evol Biol. 288, 933-5.

Semenza, G. L., 2001. HIF-1 and mechanisms of hypoxia sensing. Curr Opin Cell Biol. 13, 167-71.

Semenza, G. L., 2002. Physiology meets biophysics: visualizing the interaction of hypoxia-inducible factor 1 alpha with p300 and CBP. Proc Natl Acad Sci U S A. 99, 11570-2.

Shiojima I, Sato K, Izumiya Y, Schiekofer S, Ito M, Liao R, Colucci WS, Walsh K, 2005. Disruption of coordinated cardiac hypertrophy and angiogenesis contributes to the transition to heart failure. . J. Clin. Invest. 115, 2108-2118.

Shiojima I, Yefremashvili M, Luo Z, Kureishi Y, Takahashi A, Tao J, Rosenzweig A, Kahn CR, Abel ED, 37670–37677, W. K. J. B. C., 2002. Akt signaling mediates postnatal heart growth in response to insulin and nutritional status. J. Biol. Chem. 277.

Shirani, J., Roberts, W. C., 1993. Solitary coronary ostium in the aorta in the absence of other major congenital cardiovascular anomalies. J Am Coll Cardiol. 21, 137-43.

Smart, N., Bollini, S., Dube, K. N., Vieira, J. M., Zhou, B., Davidson, S., Yellon, D., Riegler, J., Price, A. N., Lythgoe, M. F., Pu, W. T., Riley, P. R., 2011. De novo cardiomyocytes from within the activated adult heart after injury. Nature. 474, 640-4.

Sridurongrit, S., Larsson, J., Schwartz, R., Ruiz-Lozano, P., Kaartinen, V., 2008. Signaling via the Tgf-beta type I receptor Alk5 in heart development. Dev Biol. 322, 208-18.

Su, H., Arakawa-Hoyt, J., Kan, Y. W., 2002. Adeno-associated viral vector-mediated hypoxia response element-regulated gene expression in mouse ischemic heart model. Proc Natl Acad Sci U S A. 99, 9480-5.

Sugishita, Y., Leifer, D. W., Agani, F., Watanabe, M., Fisher, S. A., 2004a. Hypoxia-responsive signaling regulates the apoptosis-dependent remodeling of the embryonic avian cardiac outflow tract. Dev Biol. 273, 285-96.

Sugishita, Y., Watanabe, M., Fisher, S. A., 2004b. The development of the embryonic outflow tract provides novel insights into cardiac differentiation and remodeling. Trends Cardiovasc Med. 14, 235-41.

Sugishita, Y., Watanabe, M., Fisher, S. A., 2004c. Role of myocardial hypoxia in the remodeling of the embryonic avian cardiac outflow tract. Dev Biol. 267, 294-308.

Sunnassee, A., Shaohua, Z., Liang, R., Liang, L., 2011. Unexpected death of a young woman: is myocardial bridging significant?--A case report and review of literature. Forensic Sci Med Pathol. 7, 42-6.

Takeuchi, S., Imamura, H., Katsumoto, K., Hayashi, I., Katohgi, T., Yozu, R., Ohkura, M., Inoue, T., 1979. New surgical method for repair of anomalous left coronary artery from pulmonary artery. J Thorac Cardiovasc Surg. 78, 7-11.

Tang, N., Wang, L., Esko, J., Giordano, F. J., Huang, Y., Gerber, H. P., Ferrara, N., Johnson, R. S., 2004. Loss of HIF-1alpha in endothelial cells disrupts a hypoxia-driven VEGF autocrine loop necessary for tumorigenesis. Cancer Cell. 6, 485-95.

Taniyama, Y., Morishita, R., Aoki, M., Hiraoka, K., Yamasaki, K., Hashiya, N., Matsumoto, K., Nakamura, T., Kaneda, Y., Ogihara, T., 2002. Angiogenesis and antifibrotic action by hepatocyte growth factor in cardiomyopathy. Hypertension. 40, 47-53.

Taylor, A. J., Rogan, K. M., Virmani, R., 1992. Sudden cardiac death associated with isolated congenital coronary artery anomalies. J Am Coll Cardiol. 20, 640-7.

Tevosian, S. G., Deconinck, A. E., Tanaka, M., Schinke, M., Litovsky, S. H., Izumo, S., Fujiwara, Y., Orkin, S. H., 2000. FOG-2, a cofactor for GATA transcription factors, is essential for heart morphogenesis and development of coronary vessels from epicardium. Cell. 101, 729-39.

Tian, H., Hammer, R. E., Matsumoto, A. M., Russell, D. W., McKnight, S. L., 1998. The hypoxia-responsive transcription factor EPAS1 is essential for catecholamine homeostasis and protection against heart failure during embryonic development. Genes Dev. 12, 3320-4.

Tirziu D, Chorianopoulos E, Moodie KL, Palac RT, Zhuang ZW, Tjwa M, Roncal C, Eriksson U, Fu Q, Elfenbein A, Hall AE, Carmeliet P, Moons L, Simons M, 2007. Myocardial hypertrophy in the absence of external stimuli is induced by angiogenesis in mice. J. Clin. Invest. 117, 3188-3197.

Tomanek, R. J., 2005. Formation of the coronary vasculature during development. Angiogenesis. 8, 273-84.

Tomanek, R. J., 2006. VEGF Family Members Regulate Myocardial Tubulogenesis and Coronary Artery Formation in the Embryo. Circulation Research. 98, 947-953.

Tomanek RJ, Lotun K, Clark EB, Suvarna PR, Hu N, 1998. VEGF and bFGF stimulate myocardial vascularization in embryonic chick. Am. J. Physiol. 274, H1620-H1626.

Tomanek, R. J., Hansen, H. K., Christensen, L. P., 2008. Temporally expressed PDGF and FGF-2 regulate embryonic coronary artery formation and growth. Arterioscler Thromb Vasc Biol. 28, 1237-43.

Tomanek, R. J., Hansen, H. K., Dedkov, E. I., 2006a. Vascular patterning of the quail coronary system during development. Anat Rec A Discov Mol Cell Evol Biol. 288, 989-99.

Tomanek, R. J., Holifield, J. S., Reiter, R. S., Sandra, A., Lin, J. J., 2002. Role of VEGF family members and receptors in coronary vessel formation. Dev Dyn. 225, 233-40.

Tomanek, R. J., Ishii, Y., Holifield, J. S., Sjogren, C. L., Hansen, H. K., Mikawa, T., 2006b. VEGF family members regulate myocardial tubulogenesis and coronary artery formation in the embryo. Circ Res. 98, 947-53.

Tomanek, R. J., Lund, D. D., Yue, X., 2003. Hypoxic induction of myocardial vascularization during development. Adv Exp Med Biol. 543, 139-49.

Tomanek, R. J., Sandra, A., Zheng, W., Brock, T., Bjercke, R. J., Holifield, J. S., 2001. Vascular endothelial growth factor and basic fibroblast growth factor differentially modulate early postnatal coronary angiogenesis. Circ Res. 88, 1135-41.

Vales, L., Kanei, Y., Fox, J., 2010. Coronary artery occlusion and myocardial infarction caused by vasospasm within a myocardial bridge. J Invasive Cardiol. 22, E67-9.

Viragh, S., Challice, C. E., 1981. The origin of the epicardium and the embryonic myocardial circulation in the mouse. Anat Rec. 201, 157-68.

Visconti RP, Richardson CD, Sato TN, 2002. Orchestration of angiogenesis and arteriovenous contribution by angiopoietins and vascular endothelial growth factor (VEGF). Proc. Natl. Acad. Sci. 11, 8219-8224.

Wada, A. M., 2003. Epicardial/Mesothelial Cell Line Retains Vasculogenic Potential of Embryonic Epicardium. Circulation Research. 92, 525-531.

Waldo, K. L., Willner, W., Kirby, M. L., 1990. Origin of the proximal coronary artery stems and a review of ventricular vascularization in the chick embryo. Am J Anat. 188, 109-20.

Ward, N. L., Van Slyke, P., Sturk, C., Cruz, M., Dumont, D. J., 2004. Angiopoietin 1 expression levels in the myocardium direct coronary vessel development. Developmental Dynamics. 229, 500-509.

Waters RE, Rotevatn S, Li P, Annex BH, Yan Z, 2004. Voluntary running induces fiber type-specific angiogenesis in mouse skeletal muscle. Am. J. Physiol. Cell Physiol. 287, C1342–C1348.

Watt, A. J., Battle, M. A., Li, J., Duncan, S. A., 2004. GATA4 is essential for formation of the proepicardium and regulates cardiogenesis. Proc Natl Acad Sci U S A. 101, 12573-8.

Weeks KL, McMullen JR, 2011. The Athlete's Heart vs. the Failing Heart: Can Signaling Explain the Two Distinct Outcomes? Physiology (Bethesda). 26, 97-105.

Wesselhoeft, H., Fawcett, J. S., Johnson, A. L., 1968. Anomalous origin of the left coronary artery from the pulmonary trunk. Its clinical spectrum, pathology, and pathophysiology, based on a review of 140 cases with seven further cases. Circulation. 38, 403-25.

Wessels, A., Perez-Pomares, J. M., 2004. The epicardium and epicardially derived cells (EPDCs) as cardiac stem cells. The Anatomical Record. 276A, 43-57.

Wikenheiser, J., Doughman, Y. Q., Fisher, S. A., Watanabe, M., 2006. Differential levels of tissue hypoxia in the developing chicken heart. Dev Dyn. 235, 115-23.

Wikenheiser, J., Wolfram, J. A., Gargesha, M., Yang, K., Karunamuni, G., Wilson, D. L., Semenza, G. L., Agani, F., Fisher, S. A., Ward, N., Watanabe, M., 2009. Altered hypoxia-inducible factor-1 alpha expression levels correlate with coronary vessel anomalies. Dev Dyn. 238, 2688-700.

Wilm, B., 2005. The serosal mesothelium is a major source of smooth muscle cells of the gut vasculature. Development. 132, 5317-5328.

Witte, M. H., Dellinger, M. T., McDonald, D. M., Nathanson, S. D., Boccardo, F. M., Campisi, C. C., Sleeman, J. P., Gershenwald, J. E., 2011. Lymphangiogenesis and hemangiogenesis: potential targets for therapy. J Surg Oncol. 103, 489-500.

Xu, B., Doughman, Y., Turakhia, M., Jiang, W., Landsettle, C. E., Agani, F. H., Semenza, G. L., Watanabe, M., Yang, Y. C., 2007. Partial rescue of defects in Cited2-deficient embryos by HIF-1alpha heterozygosity. Dev Biol. 301, 130-40.

Yang, K., Doughman, Y. Q., Karunamuni, G., Gu, S., Yang, Y. C., Bader, D. M., Watanabe, M., 2009. Expression of active Notch1 in avian coronary development. Dev Dyn. 238, 162-70.

Yang, Z., Wang, W., Ma, D., Zhang, Y., Wang, L., Xu, S., Chen, B., Miao, D., Cao, K., Ma, W., 2007. Recruitment of stem cells by hepatocyte growth factor via intracoronary gene transfection in the postinfarction heart failure. Sci China C Life Sci. 50, 748-52.

Yang, Z. J., Chen, B., Sheng, Z., Zhang, D. G., Jia, E. Z., Wang, W., Ma, D. C., Zhu, T. B., Wang, L. S., Li, C. J., Wang, H., Cao, K. J., Ma, W. Z., 2010. Improvement of heart function in postinfarct heart failure swine models after hepatocyte growth factor gene transfer: comparison of low-, medium- and high-dose groups. Mol Biol Rep. 37, 2075-81.

Yin, Z., Haynie, J., Yang, X., Han, B., Kiatchoosakun, S., Restivo, J., Yuan, S., Prabhakar, N. R., Herrup, K., Conlon, R. A., Hoit, B. D., Watanabe, M., Yang, Y. C., 2002. The essential role of Cited2, a negative regulator for HIF-1alpha, in heart development and neurulation. Proc Natl Acad Sci U S A. 99, 10488-93.

Yockman, J. W., Choi, D., Whitten, M. G., Chang, C. W., Kastenmeier, A., Erickson, H., Albanil, A., Lee, M., Kim, S. W., Bull, D. A., 2009. Polymeric gene delivery of ischemia-inducible VEGF significantly attenuates infarct size and apoptosis following myocardial infarct. Gene Ther. 16, 127-35.

Yuniadi, Y., Tai, C. T., Ueng, K. C., Chen, S. A., 2004. Anomaly of the middle cardiac vein? Europace. 6, 451-2.

Zhou, B., Honor, L. B., He, H., Ma, Q., Oh, J. H., Butterfield, C., Lin, R. Z., Melero-Martin, J. M., Dolmatova, E., Duffy, H. S., Gise, A., Zhou, P., Hu, Y. W., Wang, G., Zhang, B., Wang, L., Hall, J. L., Moses, M. A., McGowan, F. X., Pu, W. T., 2011. Adult mouse epicardium modulates myocardial injury by secreting paracrine factors. J Clin Invest. 121, 1894-904.

Zhou, B., Ma, Q., Rajagopal, S., Wu, S. M., Domian, I., Rivera-Feliciano, J., Jiang, D., von Gise, A., Ikeda, S., Chien, K. R., Pu, W. T., 2008. Epicardial progenitors contribute to the cardiomyocyte lineage in the developing heart. Nature. 454, 109-113.

3

Vascular Growth in the Fetal Lung

Stephen C. Land
Centre for Cardiovascular and Diabetic Medicine, Division of Medical Science, Ninewells Hospital and Medical School, University of Dundee, Dundee, Scotland, United Kingdom

1. Introduction

The structure of the lung is truly remarkable. It is primarily composed of three branched tubular networks (the airway, pulmonary artery and vein, bronchial artery and vein) which supply blood and air to the site of gas exchange and which maintain nutrient supply to supporting tissues. This complex interwoven network is packed into a chest cavity with a volume of 6 litres but yet it services a gas-exchange surface area of 130m^2, the floor area of a comfortably sized Mediterranean holiday villa! Weibel (1991) tells us that if this surface area were arranged as a balloon it would possess a radius of 3m and a volume of 113,000 litres, more than 18 thousand times the space available in the chest cavity. The process which drives this exceptional packaging involves repeated cycles of ordered branching to create a fractal network of tubules whose core dimensions decrease at a precise and regular rate with each successive branch. This is a high "gain-of–structure" process. In the airway, 23 generations of branching form a conducting tubular network with 17 million branches and a combined length of more than 7km. This provides convective air flow to 480 million alveoli each of which are located along a path length that is no further than 45cm from the external atmosphere. The pulmonary vasculature forms along side the airway but undergoes an additional five generations of branching to form the capillary network that surrounds each alveolus. If you simply assumed that each alveolus (diameter ~200μm) was serviced by only one blood vessel you would calculate that the alveolar capillary bed alone runs to nearly 100 km in length. Realistic attempts at modelling this structure in three dimensions suggest that it is, in all probability, between 2 and 6 *thousand* km long (Muhlfield et al., 2010), illustrating the impressive capacity of fractal branching processes to package colossal structures into ever smaller spaces.

The airway and pulmonary vasculature interface with one another at the alveolar blood-gas barrier where oxygen and carbon dioxide diffuse along partial pressure gradients. This extremely thin (0.65μm) membrane is composed of cytoplasmic leaflets of type I alveolar epithelial cells and capillary endothelial cells held together with a chicken-wire-like mesh of type IV collagen. Here, a compromise must be met between high surface area, thin-ness and tensile strength to ensure that gas exchange proceeds efficiently from rest-to-work without rupture of the membrane caused by pressure differences across between the alveolar and vascular space. One estimate places the inherent tensile strength of this interface at 0.3MPa (West, 2003) which is close to that of pure type IV collagen

(1MPa) and similar to that of building materials such ceramic fibre boards of the type often used to line an office ceiling.

From here, oxygenated blood traverses the branched venous network to the left atrium of the heart from where it is circulated around the body. The physiological outcome of this interwoven, repeated branching structure is to arrive at a balance between the need for a high gas exchange surface area and a minimal energetic cost of breathing, water and heat loss. Fractal branching achieves this by dissipating resistance to air and blood movement among the exponential rise in tubule number towards the blood-gas barrier, allowing ready passage into the recesses of the lung much like water poured into sand. Similarly, this rise in surface area ensures that inhaled air is rapidly warmed and hydrated as it passes through the upper airways so that ventilating the lung costs little in terms of heat and water loss. Thus, for most healthy people, the act of breathing when at rest or asleep is essentially subconscious and requires almost imperceptible movement of the chest to maintain convective gas exchange over the blood-gas barrier without the need for further anatomical specialisation to maintain core body temperature and hydration. Although the mammalian lung is clearly a complex organ, this is not to imply that it sits at the pinnacle of evolution amongst gas-exchange systems; in fact its structure is derived from imperfect compromise between competing selective forces and the interested reader is referred to several articles for further insight (Sander et al., 2011; West et al., 2007; Perry et al., 2001; Weibel et al., 1998; Weibel, 1984).

To generate this branched, fractal network a molecular system must be in place to programme the duration, bifurcation, orientation and damped repetition of the branching cycle. This chapter reviews the process which controls vascular growth in the lung and, in particular, how its regulation is co-ordinated with the fractal branching pattern of the airways.

2. The pattern of vascular development in the lung

Weibel and Gomez (1962) were among the first to document the fractal branching pattern of the airways noting that the decrease in airway diameter for each new branch declined by a constant factor (0.85 as re-analysed by Maury et al., 2009). The physiological outcome is to dissipate resistance to air flow which, according to Poiseuille's Law, decreases in proportion to the 4th power of tubule diameter. Notably, the rate of decline is slightly shallower than the predicted "optimal" rate (0.79) suggesting that there is an excess of dead space within the airways. Thus, an evolutionary compromise exists between lung volume and branching which accommodates dynamic change in airway diameter caused by exercise, inflammation or disease (Maury et al., 2009).

The pulmonary vasculature closely follows the course of the conducting airways, sharing the same rate of branching and decline in diameter up to the 15th generation. Beyond this, vascular branching diverges at a greater rate proceeding through 28 generations to create the microvasculature surrounding each alveolus (Weibel, 1991). As with the airways, the net outcome is to dissipate resistance to blood flow and achieve a compact, high volume, delivery system capable of sustaining a rate of oxygen diffusion over the blood-gas barrier of 158mlO_2/min/mmHg (Weibel et al., 1993). The way in which this pattern of branching is co-ordinated with the growth of the airways is a question of central importance for understanding how gas exchange occurs between the blind ended airway network and the perfused circuitry of the pulmonary vasculature.

Fetal lung development passes through five distinct stages which (in humans) proceed as: I) embryonic (26 days-6 weeks), II) pseudoglandular (6-16 weeks), III) canalicular (16-24 weeks), IV) saccular (24-36 weeks) and V) alveolar (36 weeks - ~6 years of postnatal life). The canalicular stage is the first point at which the vasculature begins to form a functional interface with the airway epithelium, however, there is clear evidence that the fate of these two structures is intimately linked from the earliest stages of development. During the embryonic stage, the lung develops as a protrusion of foregut endoderm into the surrounding mesoderm tissue then bifurcates to form the left and right lung anlage. The next two rounds of branching establish the primordial lung lobes and, with them, the fundamental structure of the pulmonary vasculature.

Three models have been proposed to explain how the vasculature develops in the lung. The Vasculogenesis Model (Hall et al., 2000) proposes that the pulmonary arteries arise by continuous expansion of endothelial cell precursors (angioblasts) that fuse to form blood filled hematopoietic lakes in the mesenchyme around each airway bud. Fusion of these lakes generates a primitive vasculature which matures as the airway grows forward. This model has the advantage of simplicity as it requires only vasculogenic and fusion signals to co-ordinate its formation with the airway, however, it does not readily explain how ordered vascular patterns might form around each airway branch nor how these primitive vessels form junctions with existing major blood vessels. De Mello et al. (2000) proposed the Central Angiogenesis-Distal Vasculogenesis Model which suggests that the major trunks of the pulmonary artery and vein elongate through the mesenchyme surrounding the right and left lung lobes in response to an angiogenic cue generated behind each branch tip (central angiogenesis). These subsequently fuse with hematopoietic lakes around each branch tip (distal vasculogenesis) to form the basis of the pulmonary vasculature. In this model, three vascular growth cues are necessary: one to induce angiogenic growth of the major vessels along side the developing bud, the second to induce vasculogenesis around the tip of each airway branch and the third to fuse these structures together.

A problem with both of these models is that they fail to adequately explain the presence of red blood cells that appear in the vascular structures around each airway branch (Figure 1). Parera et al. (2005) examined this issue using transgenic mice bearing a vascular reporter gene (lacZ driven by the Tie2 angiopoietin receptor promoter; Tie2-LacZ). They found evidence of a continuous, perfused vascular network consisting of Tie2, PECAM-1 and Fli-1 positive endothelial cells in the mesenchyme tissue that surrounds the left and right airway branches. This network is present from the earliest stages of embryonic lung development and is derived from the heart vasculature making it inter-connected with other more distant structures such as liver and yolk sac. In their Distal Angiogenesis model, they argue that a functional vasculature extends from the heart to the distal tip region of each lung branch and that vascular growth occurs by endothelial sprouting from perfused blood vessels towards an angiogenic cue which is generated from the airway tip (the angiogenic zone; Figure 1B). Endothelial sprouts fuse with each other behind the airway bud tip so generating a perfused vascular network which surrounds each airway bud. Importantly, this occurs in three dimensions so that the angiogenic process is sustained in parallel with airway bud branching (Figure 1C). The growth of the vasculature therefore follows angiogenic cues generated by the airway which ensure that the timing and orientation of branching events is co-ordinated between these two structures at least up to the 15th generation of airway branching.

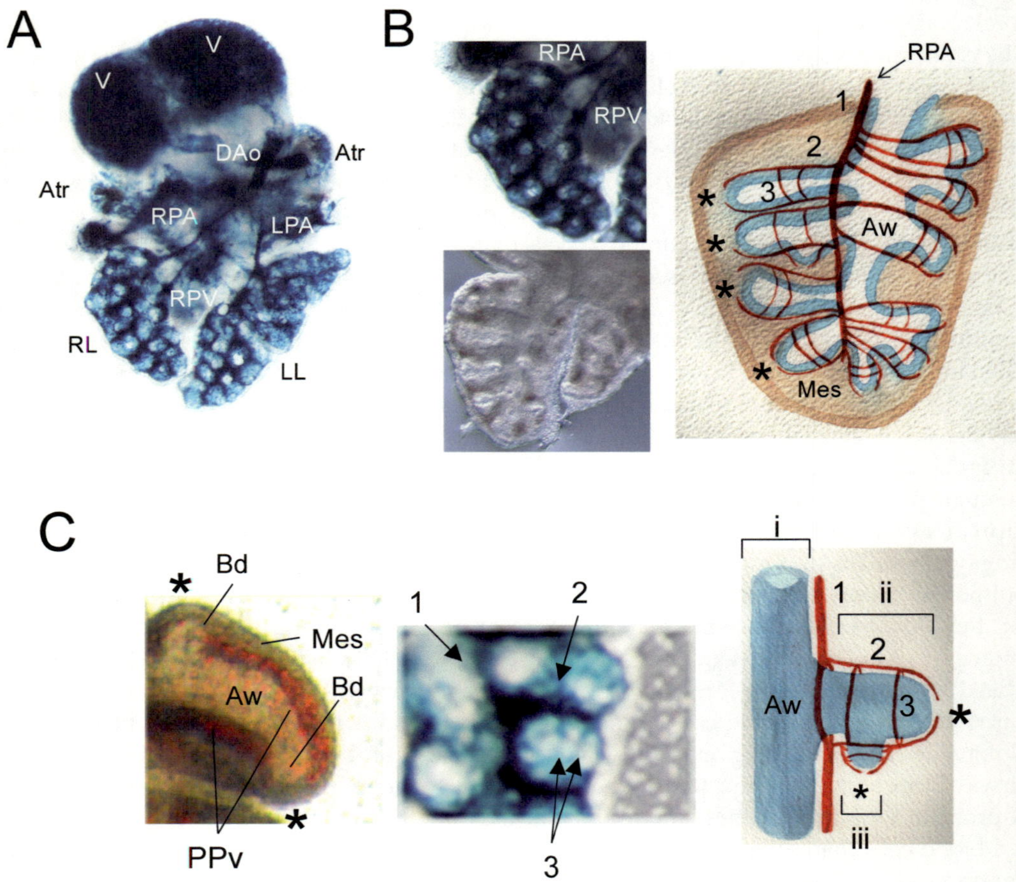

Fig. 1. Vascular growth proceeds by distal angiogenesis in the fetal lung. A. Tie2 expression (blue) in E14 fetal Tie2-LacZ mouse heart and lung. B. Detail showing Tie2 expression surrounding airway branches. Bright field image below shows airway organisation with blood-containing vessels (red hue) in the mesenchyme between each airway branch. Simplified schematic at right indicates angiogenic zone (*) at tip of airway with perfused vessels (3) orthogonal to the axis of the primary (1) and secondary vascular branch (2). C. Detail of vasculature around airway bud tip. *Left panel:* perfused vessels (red hue) can be seen in mesenchyme surrounding airway but are absent from angiogenic zone ahead of each bud tip (*). *Middle panel:* Tie2 positive staining marks primary (1), secondary (2) and tertiary (3) vascular branches around single buds. *Right panel*: Simplified schematic showing parallel branching of airway and vasculature through 3 branch generations (i-iii, airway; 1-3, vasculature). *Abbreviations:* Atr, atrium; Bd, airway bud; Aw, airway; Dao, dorsal aorta; Mes, mesenchyme; PPv, perfused pulmonary vasculature; RL, LL, right and left lung lobes; RPA, LPA, right and left pulmonary arteries; RPV, right pulmonary vein. V, ventricle

3. Airway and vascular growth are inter-dependent processes

Airway outgrowth is induced by secretion of fibroblast growth factor-10 (FGF-10) from discrete regions of the mesenchyme ahead of each new airway branch. As this signal encounters the airway epithelium it activates the tyrosine kinase fibroblast growth factor receptor-2b (FGFR2b) which stimulates airway tube elongation towards the FGF-10 signal (Bellusci et al., 1997). Regulated antagonism of FGF-10 expression and FGFR2b activity determines the duration of the growth stimulus and so regulates the length of each airway tube and entry into branching. A seminal study by Metzger et al. (2008) identified three different types of branching event that generate the three dimensional structure of the conducting airway: *i)* Domain branching, which establishes the overall shape of each lobe, *ii)* Planar bifurcation, which proceeds on the same plane to form branches towards the edge of each lobe and *iii)* Orthogonal bifurcation where branching occurs 90° to the plane of growth. These branching events are governed by four pattern generating events: domain specification (the dimensions of each successive branch generation), branch periodicity generation (rate and number of branching events), bifurcation (spatial separation of branching events) and rotation (angle of branching events relative to the axis of the preceding generations). Precise timing of these events in relation to one another underpins the fractal pattern of tubular branching observed by Weibel & Gomez (1962) for the airway and suggests that airway outgrowth and vascular development are co-ordinated through three types of branching event that is controlled by four pattern generators; but is the growth of these tubular networks inter-dependent and , if so, which regulates which?

3.1 Linking airway and vascular growth cues

Pattern generation in the airways is determined, in the first instance, by factors which control FGF-10 expression and FGFR2b activity. FGFR2b signaling in the airway epithelium is antagonised by Sprouty2 (Spry2) whose genomic expression and activity is induced in response to the FGF-10 signal. Once active, Spry2 suppresses the growth response to FGF-10 by blocking the formation of the protein complex which mediates guanine nucleotide signaling to the extracellular regulated kinase 1&2 (ERK1/2) pathway. The magnitude of this response is governed by the local concentration of FGF-10 around the airway bud and so determines the pattern of growth along the airway tube (Scott et al., 2010; Ramasamy et al., 2007; Tefft et al., 2002). Other ERK1/2 repressors also participate in this process to mediate close control over airway bud growth responses (eg MKP-3, Spred-1). Spry2 is therefore poised to regulate the form and magnitude of downstream signalling in response to FGF-10 and this includes influence over the activity of transcription factors which control vasculogenic signaling (discussed further in Section 4.3).

The duration of FGF-10 expression in the mesenchyme is determined by sonic hedgehog (Shh) whose expression is induced in airway epithelial cells in response to the FGF-10 signal. Secretion of Shh into the surrounding mesenchyme represses FGF-10 expression, forcing lateral movement of this growth inducing cue ahead of regions of low Shh expression. This repression of FGF-10 is locally confined by the transcription factor sine oculis-1 (Six1) and its co-activator, eyes absent-1 (Eya1), which block the expression of the Shh receptor, patched-1 (Ptc1) in the mesenchyme surrounding the airways (El-Hashash et al., 2011a,b). Thus, Six1/Eya1 and Shh form the basis of a regulated feedback loop which determines the spatial expression of FGF-10 in the mesenchyme.

Shh also plays a critical role in patterning the formation of other lung structures such as smooth muscle and connective tissue which develop around the airway tube as it matures (Weaver et al., 2003). It has therefore attracted much attention as a potential link between angiogenic and airway growth. Shh is known to regulate the expression of two families of angiogenic factors, the vascular endothelial growth factor-A isoforms 120, 164 and 188 (VEGF-$A_{120, 164, 188}$) and the vessel maturation factors angiopoietin 1 and 2 (Ang1 and 2). VEGF-A is critical for fetal vascular development and knockout of its splice variant forms or its cognate receptors, VEGFR1 (Fms-related tyrosine kinase 1 (Flt1)) and VEGFR2 (synonyms: mouse: Fetal liver kinase-1 (Flk-1); human: Kinase insert Domain Receptor (KDR)), causes embryonic lethality before lung development occurs (eg Carmeliet et al., 1996; Shalaby et al; 1995; Fong et al., 1995). In the pseudoglandular-stage murine lung, VEGF-A_{120} and VEGF-A_{164} isoforms are expressed in both epithelial and mesenchymal tissue and are necessary for endothelial differentiation and angiogenesis towards the distal tip of the airway (Del Moral et al., 2006; Greenberg et al., 2002). As tubular branching progresses, this angiogenic cue becomes increasingly restricted to the distal lung epithelium where it ultimately establishes the vascular side of the blood-gas barrier throughout the canalicular to alveolar stages of development (Healy et al., 2000). This developmental restriction of VEGF-A_{164} expression is linked to its association with matrix components in the region of the growing bud tip and could be important for delineating different types of vascular growth response by altering the autophosphorylation pattern of VEGFR2. For example, matrix-associated VEGF-A induces distinct phosphorylation of the VEGFR2 tyrosine kinase domain which induces prolonged receptor activation, clustering and association with β1 integrin leading to increased vascular sprouting (Chen et al., 2010; Gerhardt et al., 2003). It is interesting to speculate that this might drive the increased rate of vascular branching that occurs beyond the 15th branch generation to create the alveolar microvasculature. Soluble VEGF-A, on the other hand, stimulates VEGFR2 association with neurolipin-1 and also receptor internalisation which is necessary for vascular maintenance, maturation of the airway epithelium and alveologenesis during the later stages of lung growth (Chen et al., 2010; Voelkel et al., 2006). In fetal lung explants, culture in the presence of soluble VEGF-A_{164} induces vascular growth and endothelial cell differentiation in mesenchyme, whereas inhibition of endogenous VEGF-A_{164} signaling abolishes these effects almost entirely (Zhao et al., 2005; Groenman et al., 2007). Notably, these effects are not solely confined to the vasculature but also alter airway morphogenesis. For example, soluble VEGF-A_{164} augments the rate of tubule branching, however, inhibition of vascular signaling by either VEGFR2 knockdown or blockade leads to fewer branches and extensive dilation of remaining terminal airway buds (Del Moral et al., 2006; Groenman et al., 2007). Thus, VEGF-A signaling is necessary to maintain an appropriate rate of airway tubule elongation and branching but it is not an absolute requirement for airway growth as such.

So what of the role of Shh in this process? Van Tuyl et al (2007) demonstrated that knockout of Shh specifically repressed expression of Ang1, but not VEGF-A_{164} nor VEGFR2 and that this suppressed both airway and vascular morphogenesis. Treatment of fetal lung explants with pro-angiogenic factors such as FGF-2 or Ang1 reinstated vascular growth and this was associated with a partial recovery of tubular branching suggesting that angiogenesis is necessary for airway growth to proceed. A later study showed FGF-9, not FGF-2, to be the physiological ligand which underpins this effect and reported positive synergistic FGF-9/Shh regulation of VEGF-A_{164} expression which controlled the distribution of endothelial cell proliferation in the mesenchyme surrounding the developing airway bud (White et al., 2007). Subsequent vessel maturation is also Shh/Ptc dependent as knockout of either Six1/Eya1 leads to defective smooth muscle actin expression and vessel wall assembly through sustained Shh signaling to the Ptc receptor (El Hayashi et al., 2011a,b). Thus, VEGF-A signaling is critical for co-ordinated vascular and airway development and Shh appears to regulate events associated with vessel maturation as well as endothelial cell proliferation.

Shh could also influence airway growth indirectly by simply regulating the maturation rate of blood vessels. Lazarus et al. (2011) used 3D re-construction coupled with VEGF-A/VEGFR2 genetic ablation to explore perfusion-independent roles of blood vessel formation in airway branching *in vivo*. They demonstrated that the physical absence of blood vessels, rather than the inhibition of VEGF signalling *per se*, has a major influence on airway branching process. They also demonstrated that vessels are required for orthogonal bifurcation events but have no effect on the planar branching process, such that blood vessel ablation leads to an overall "flat" (i.e. planar) lung morphology. This was linked to a disruption of the pattern of FGF-10 expression and de-regulation of the FGF-10/FGFR2b antagonism by Shh and Spry2. Thus, blood vessels appear to control branching patterns which specifically govern the 3-dimensional development of the conducting airways and the factors which control this process are intrinsic to the epithelium-mesenchyme-endothelium interface.

3.2 Does the heart function influence vascular growth of the lung?

Explant studies show that vascular growth occurs in the lung whether or not it is attached to the heart, however, distal angiogenesis ensures that there is a continuously perfused link between heart and lung so changes in heart function might also influence airway and vascular growth. This would be consistent with the role that the heart plays in determining organ placode placement, including trachea and lung, along the primitive foregut (Cardoso & Lü, 2006) and of the vasculature in controlling orthogonal branching later in lung development (Lazarus et al.,2011). We investigated this possibility in intact fetal heart and lung explants from Tie2-LacZ mice using periodic stimulation to slow heart rate for 10 minutes at 30 minute intervals over 6h. Fetal lungs were then allowed to develop without stimulation for a further 24h before fixing and staining for the Tie2 vascular marker (Figure 2).The results show that entrainment of pacemaker activity tends to suppress angiogenesisin the heart (seen as a reduced intensity of the blue stain) but increases airway branching frequency. Lungs grown without the heart attached, but which still received stimulation, showed no such difference in airway and vascular growth. Thus, altering patterns of heart contractility seems to disconnect the relationship between vascular growth and airway morphogenesis suggesting that changes in perfusion rate of the lung, and/or heart-derived growth factors which target airway growth, are important determinants of this relationship. This is likely to have important consequences for understanding how maternal stress and anti-depressant use influences the development of the pulmonary vasculature during pregnancy (Morrison et al., 2002).

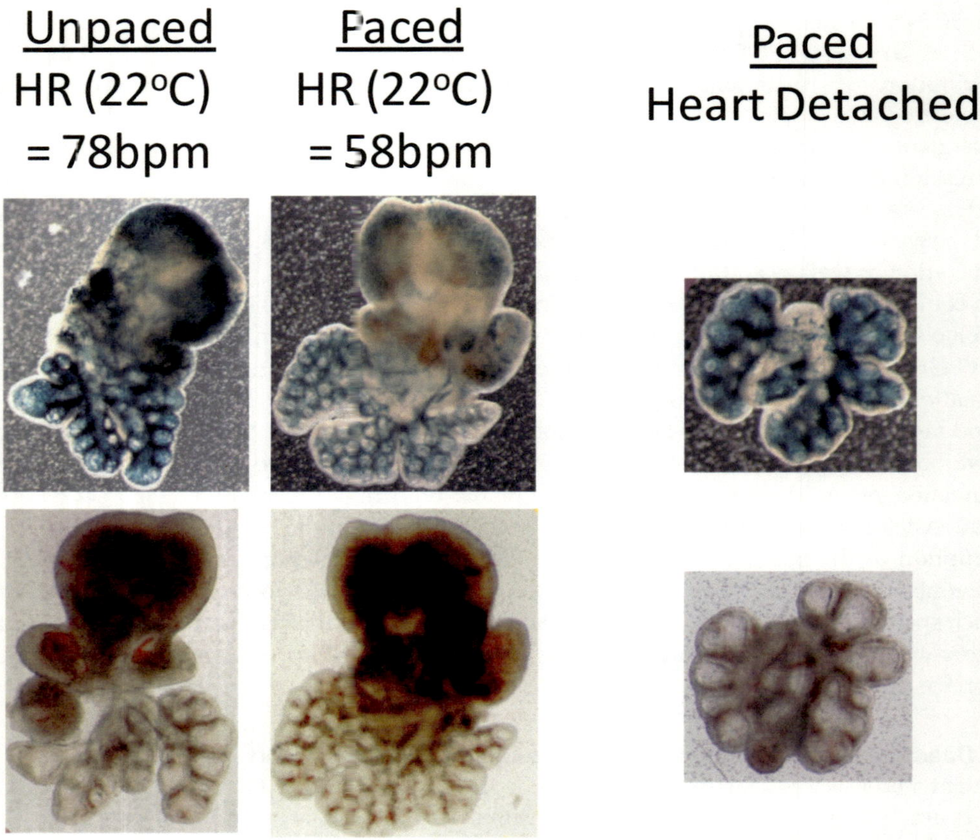

Fig. 2. Altered cardiac pacemaker activity raises airway branching rate and suppresses vascular growth. Heart and lungs from E12 Tie2-LacZ mice were excised with all connections intact and were and placed into organ culture as described by Scott et al. (2010). Pacing was achieved by stimulating preparations (3Hz; 30V) for 10 minute intervals every 30 minutes for 6h after which development was allowed to proceed normally for a further 18h. This produced a sustained suppression of heart rate (measured at 22°C) from 78 to 58bpm. Distribution of Tie2-lacZ expression (blue colour) as a measure of vascular growth was compared to heart-free lung preparation to which the pacing regimen had also been applied. Results shown are representative of 3 independent experiments.

4. Regulation of VEGF-A expression in fetal airway epithelium

Although Lazarus et al. (2011) show that the physical presence of blood vessels is necessary to drive orthogonal branching in the lung, it is clear that VEGF-A expression and secretion from the elongating airway tube is the earliest possible point of cross-talk between factors which regulate airway and vascular growth (Del Moral et al., 2006; Greenberg et al., 2002). VEGF-A gene expression is regulated at multiple levels (transcription factor binding at a

1.2kb (mouse, rat) to 2.362kb (human) 5′ promoter region; mRNA stability through protein interaction with its 3′ untranslated region; mRNA translation via IRES sequences in the 5′ untranslated region) and is intrinsically sensitive to external factors such as oxygen and growth factors (reviewed Pagés & Pouyssegur, 2005). Low oxygen tensions are a persistent feature of the uterine environment, ranging from 0-13mmHg during embryonic implantation to ~30mmHg throughout gestation (reviewed, Land, 2004) and raising oxygen tension beyond this range is known to inhibit vascular growth (van Tuyl et al., 2005). Given the regulated sensitivity of VEGF-A expression to hypoxia, there is therefore an appealing, if teleological, argument to suggest that oxygen availability might direct the growth and development of the gas exchange system that ensures its delivery to the mitochondrial respiratory chain.

4.1 Hypoxia inducible factors direct vascular growth in the lung

Oxygen-sensitive VEGF-A expression is regulated by hypoxia inducible factor (HIF) binding to a HIF consensus site (TACGTGGG) located in the 5′ proximal VEGF-A promoter. HIFs are heterodimeric transcription factors comprising an oxygen regulated α subunit and a nuclear translocating β subunit. In hypoxia, the α subunit is stabilised, dimerises with the β subunit and is translocated to the nucleus by association with the members of the nuclear importer family, importin α1, 3, 5 or 7 (Depping et al., 2008). All three HIFα isoforms are expressed in the developing lung. HIF-1α occurs in the branching airway epithelium and its homozygous knockout in mice causes developmental failure of the vasculature and death by E10.5 (Kotch et al., 1999). HIF-2α occurs in the epithelium and interstitium and its knockout produces vascular defects during alveolar septation (Compernolle et al., 2002). HIF-3α is a truncated isoform that lacks the C-terminal transactivation domain necessary for interaction with p300/CBP and so is thought to act as a competitive repressor of HIF-1α and 2α activity (Bardos & Ashcroft, 2005). Thus, HIF-1α plays the primary role in controlling vascular signalling during lung development, whereas HIF-2α function is predominantly associated with the maturation of vascular structures and the generation of the blood-gas barrier (Groenman et al., 2007). Although growth factors are well known to regulate VEGF-A expression through other transcription factors (eg Sp1, AP2; Pages & Pouyssegur, 2005), it seems that HIF-1α and 2α-dependent regulation of vascular growth and blood vessel maturation is critical for generating the type of vascular growth, reported by Lazarus et al. (2011), that is necessary for three dimensional lung branching to occur.

HIF-1α stability is regulated by O_2-dependent prolyl hydroxylase proteins (PHD1,2,3) and an asparaginyl hydroxylase, factor inhibiting HIF (FIH-1). In normoxia, these enzymes utilise oxygen and the Krebs cycle intermediate, 2-oxoglutarate, to catalyse the hydroxylation of proline residues 402 and 564 in the oxygen-dependent degradation domain of HIFα subunits resulting in ubiquitylation by the von Hippel-Lindau E3 ubiquitin ligase (VHL) (e.g. Flashman et al., 2008). FIH-1 catalyzes the hydroxylation of asparagine 803 and blocks the interaction of the HIF transactivation domain with the CBP/p300 histone acetyltransferase. In hypoxia, the loss of oxygen and a decline in Krebs cycle activity results in PHD substrate limitation, ODD dehydroxylation, diminished VHL binding and rapid HIFα stabilisation and transactivation. PHD substrate limitation may also be associated with the hypoxia-driven degradation of this enzyme by a different E3 ubiquitin ligase, SIAH (seven in absentia homolog) (Qi et al., 2008). PHD proteins critically regulate HIF-1–3α

stability during lung development, as their inhibition augments HIF target gene expression and promotes blood vessel growth and formation of the blood gas barrier (Asikainen et al., 2005, 2006; Groenman et al., 2007). Of the three PHD isoforms, however, PHD2 appears to exert primary regulation of HIF-1α as its knockdown exclusively induces HIF-signaling activity and gene expression in normoxia, whereas knockdown of PHD1 and 3 does not (Berra et al., 2003).

Although airway and vascular development is supported better at fetal rather than postnatal PO_2, and hyperoxia causes severe vascular defects which are associated with silencing of the HIF signaling system, it is unlikely that oxygen gradients direct vascular growth around the airway tip. In the fetal lung, such gradients would be shallow [~15 mmHg (20 μM)]: difference between the PO_2 of the umbilical vein (30 mmHg) and the PO_2 of the amniotic fluid (15mmHg; Land, 2003) and ~10-fold below the Km O_2 of PHD enzymes (230–250 μM; Hirsilä et al., 2003). Moreover, at least in fetal pulmonary vascular smooth muscle cells, HIF-1α protein stability is insensitive to oxygen tension suggesting that other modes of regulation may be more important in fetal tissues (Resnik et al., 2007). It seems more plausible that the low PO_2 of the fetal environment may prime the HIF system by stabilising the α-subunit and that local regulation is mediated by the growth factors which direct airway branching morphogenesis.

4.2 Co-ordinating HIF activity with airway growth regulators

In addition to its regulation by PHD proteins, HIF activity is also influenced by kinases whose signalling is controlled by tyrosine kinase growth factor receptors (Yee Koh et al., 2008) and so it is possible that HIF-directed vascular signaling could be induced from the very first interaction between FGF-10 and FGFR2b in the airway bud tip. FGF-10 activates FGFR2b by promoting receptor subunit homodimerisation which allows autophosphorylation of several tyrosine residues in its intracellular tail region (Figure 3). This promotes the binding and tyrosine phosphorylation of the lipid docking protein, suc-1-associated neurotrophic factor target (FRS2α), to the active receptor complex which then recruits growth factor receptor-binding protein 2 (GRB2) and its partner, son of sevenless (Sos) (Tefft et al., 2002). Simultaneous binding of the protein tyrosine phosphatase, SHP2, to FRS2α potentiates GRB2 recruitment further and establishes the overall magnitude of receptor signalling activity in response to growth factor binding (Hadari et al., 2001; Kouhara et al., 1997). Once this signaling complex is intact, GRB2/Sos catalyses the conversion of GDP to GTP on Ras, enabling the Raf serine/threonine kinase to induce MEK-1 activation of the ERK1/2 signaling pathway.

FRS2α can also recruit alternative adaptor proteins to induce signaling through other pathways. Tyrosine phosphorylation of FRS2α by the active FGF receptor promotes the constitutive binding of GRB2-associated binding protein 1 (GAB1) to the C-terminal SH3 domain of GRB2. This enables tyrosine phosphorylation of GAB1, which is followed by recruitment of phosphoinositide-3- kinase (PI3K) by GAB1 resulting in activation of Akt, inhibition of the tuberous sclerosis complex proteins 1 & 2 (TSC1/2) and subsequent induction of the mammalian target of rapamycin (mTOR) signaling pathway (Eswarakumar et al., 2005). Thus, the intensity of FGF-10 interaction with its receptor can determine the magnitude and duration of signaling through a number of downstream pathways that have the potential to regulate HIF-1α activity and VEGF-A expression from airway epithelium.

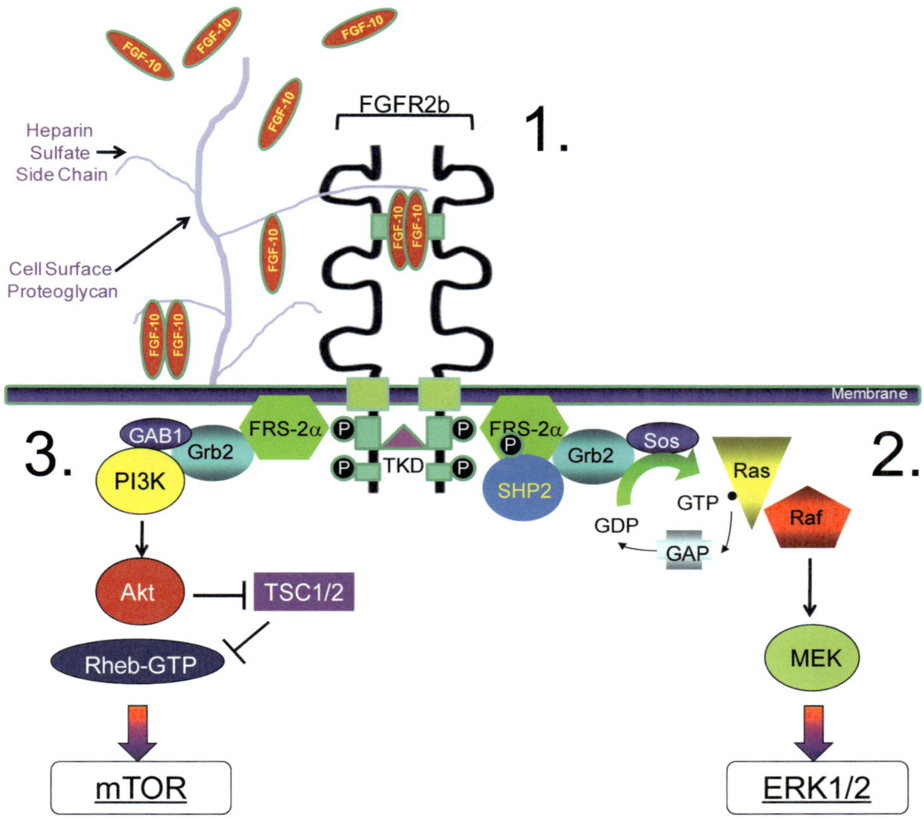

Fig. 3. FGF-10 signal transduction to the mTOR and ERK1/2 pathways. 1. FGF-10, secreted from mesenchyme ahead of the nascent airway bud, binds to heparin sulphate side chains on cell surface proteoglycans and act as a scaffold for FGFR2b homodimerisation. This induces tyrosine autophosphorylation by the active tyrosine kinase domain (TKD) which enables FRS2α to bind specific phosphorylated residues and anchor a signal transduction cascade to the receptor. 2. ERK1/2 signal transduction cascade. 3. mTOR signal transduction cascade. See text for details.

Scott et al., (2010) investigated this by exposing fetal distal lung epithelial cells (FDLE) from pseudoglandular stage rat lungs to FGF-10 concentration gradients at various oxygen tensions. When cultured at alveolar PO_2 (13% O_2), HIF-1α activity and VEGF-A secretion were unresponsive to FGF-10, however, treatment at fetal PO_2 (3% O_2) produced a dose-dependent induction of HIF-1α activity, without change in its stability, and also raised VEGF-A secretion. Both effects were matched by a sustained increase in mTOR activity and were suppressed to the endogenous level (i.e. under fetal oxygen tensions) by the mTOR inhibitor, rapamycin. Moreover, these effects were accompanied by a dose dependent inhibition of ERK1/2 and hypo-phosphorylation of the FGF receptor antagonist, Spry2, causing a band-shift to its lighter (35kDa) active form (Figure 4). Thus, it seems that FGF-10 patterns vascular signalling by favouring mTOR activity over ERK1/2 and that Spry2 may partition signaling between these kinase pathways.

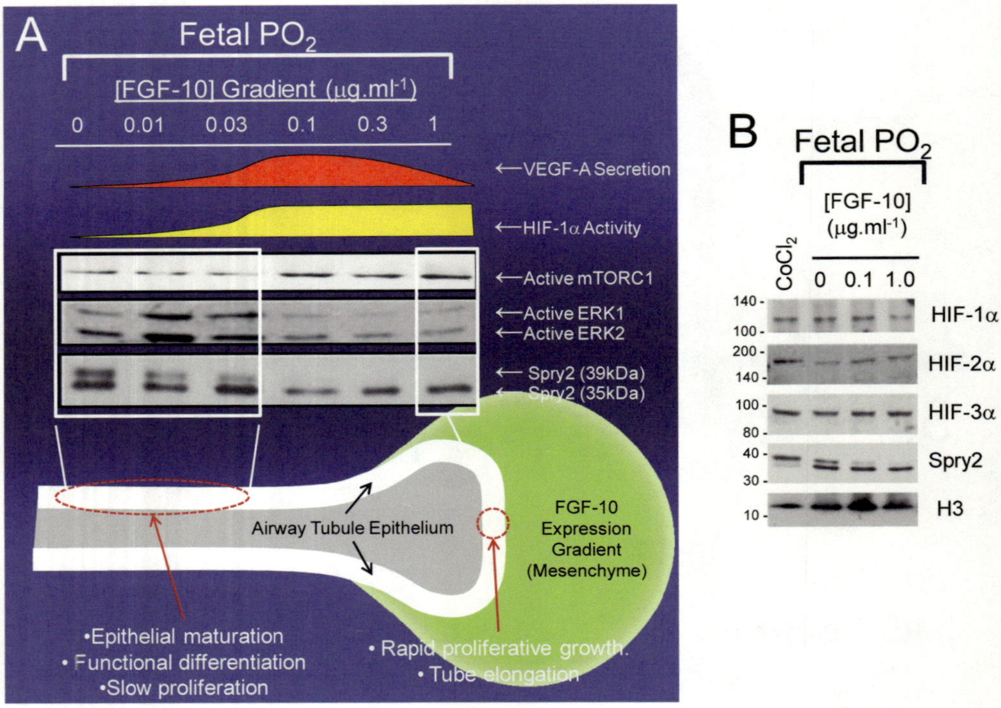

Fig. 4. FGF-10 induces vascular signaling in fetal distal lung epithelial (FDLE) cells. A. FGF-10 induces HIF-1α activity and VEGF-A secretion in hand with altered mTORC-1 (S6K-phospho Thr^{389}), ERK1/2 (Phospho Thr^{202}/Tyr^{204}) and Spry2 activity (see text for details) in FDLE maintained at fetal PO_2. Inferred pattern of signaling within the airway tubule epithelium is shown below; data from Scott et al., (2010) B. FGF-10 does not alter HIF-1,2 or 3α nuclear abundance in FDLE maintained at fetal PO_2.. Positive control, $CoCl_2$ (100μM).

How mTOR regulates HIF-1α activity remains unclear. Although there is some evidence to suggest that this kinase can regulate HIF-1α at the transcriptional level (reviewed Dunlop and Tee, 2006), there remains the exciting possibility that it may also directly interact with the HIF-1α protein to co-ordinate its function with growth factor signals. mTOR forms two distinct multi protein kinase signaling complexes: mTOR complex 1 (mTORC1: mTOR, mammalian LST8/G-protein β-subunit like protein (mLST8/GβL), PRAS40, DEPTOR and a scaffold protein known as regulatory-associated protein of mTOR (RAPTOR)) and mTOR complex 2 (mTORC2: mTOR, GβL, mammalian stress-activated protein kinase interacting protein 1 (mSIN1) and a scaffold protein known as rapamycin-insensitive companion of mTOR (RICTOR)). The arrangement of these complexes partitions mTOR kinase activity amongst different substrates such that mTORC1 generally links nutrient and growth factor cues to the control of translation, whereas mTORC2 links these cues to cytoskeletal proteins which control cell structure (Sarbassov et al., 2004). As mTORC2 is broadly insensitive to rapamycin, the observation that this inhibitor blocks FGF-10-evoked HIF-1α activity and

VEGF-A secretion suggests that mTORC1 drives early vascular signaling in the fetal lung. The scaffold protein RAPTOR binds this complex to its substrates by interacting with conserved penta-peptide sequences known as mTOR signaling (TOS) motifs (FDL/IDL and FEMDI within S6K1 (Schalm & Blenis, 2002) and 4E-BP1 (Schalm et al., 2003), respectively). Mutation of the highly conserved phenylalanine at position 1 of the TOS motif prevents mTOR binding and subsequent phosphorylation of its target residues. We identified a similarly conserved TOS motif located between amino acids 99 and 104 of HIF-1α (FVMVL) which was capable of binding RAPTOR and which was also necessary for growth factor-sensitive regulation of HIF-1α transcriptional activity (Land and Tee, 2007; Scott et al., 2010). Significantly, this interaction specifically promoted the interaction between the stable HIF-1α/β transcription factor and the CBP/p300 histone acetyltransferase resulting in increased efficiency of HIF-regulated gene expression by elevated de-condensation of DNA from its histone complex.

The mTOR pathway plays a critical role in organ development. In mice, its expression arises at E8.5 and its inhibition, by mutation or with rapamycin, results in forebrain defects, loss of somites, poor embryonic rotation and lethality by E12.5 (Hentges et al., 2001). Ontogenic studies of mTOR function in rat fetuses show its activity is high during the early stages of development, declining towards term, but rebounds during the early neonatal period and corresponds with proportionate changes in translation efficiency during gestation and birth (Otulakowski et al, 2009; 2007). In fetal lung *in vivo*, phosphorylation of the mTORC-1 specific substrate, S6 kinase-1 Thr^{389}, is high in the epithelium within the airway bud tip and genomic knockout of its upstream repressor, tuberous sclerosis complex-1 (TSC1), leads to gross vascular defects and widespread expression of VEGF-A in both airway and mesenchymal tissue (Scott et al., 2010). Through its interaction with HIF-1α, mTORC1 therefore links FGF-10/FGFR2b activity to VEGF-A secretion and vascular growth and provides a mechanism by which the growth of the fetal airway epithelium vasculature is linked from the very earliest moment of lung development.

4.3 Linking vascular growth to the FGF-10/FGFR2b/Spry2 airway branching periodicity clock

Although mTORC1 may link the FGF-10 signal to HIF and vascular signaling, it does not explain how branching process might occur. Sprouty proteins direct the duration and magnitude of growth factor receptor signaling and were originally described as repressors of FGF-driven tracheal branching in *Drosophila* (Hacohen et al., 1998). Here, tracheal branching is initiated by the protein product of the Branchless gene (Bnl) whose mammalian equivalent is FGF-10. The receptor for the branchless protein is Breathless (Btl), whose mammalian orthologue is the FGFR family. The duration of signaling between Bnl and Btl (and hence the length of tubule between each branch) is determined by Sprouty whose knockout results in accelerated tracheal branching. Sprouty proteins are therefore evolutionarily conserved, inducible inhibitors of FGF-receptor signalling which control the branching dimensions of the tracheal airway network.

In the developing lung, Sprouty proteins play a similar role to define the dimensions of the airway tree. Four sprouty isoforms (Spry 1-4) are expressed in mammals but it is Spry2 which plays the dominant role in the airway branching process, being expressed at the distal tip of the epithelial tube bud adjacent to sites of FGF-10 expression in the mesenchyme.

Knockdown of Spry2 in fetal lung explants increases epithelial tube branching whereas its over-expression *in vivo* inhibits lung lobation, clefting along the periphery of the lung, failure to septate, mesenchymal thickening and an inhibition of epithelial proliferation (Mailleux et al., 2001; Tefft, et al., 1999). Later work by Metzger et al. (2008) identified Spry2 as an important regulator of airway branching whose knockout increased both branch rate the restriction of airway diameter so that distal branching patterns occurred proximally in the airway. Thus, the FGF-10/FGFR2b/Spry2 feedback loop acts as a timing mechanism which controls airway branching periodicity and so defines the fractal characteristics of the respiratory tree (Metzger et al., 2008; Warburton, 2008).

How might Spry2 co-ordinate airway and vascular branching with one another? Scott et al. (2010) showed that a rise in Spry2 activity (appearance of a hypo-phosphorylated 35kDa form) accompanies the inhibition of ERK1/2 and activation of mTORC1 that occurs in response to FGF-10, therefore, something more than FGFR inhibition must occur to produce this partitioning of kinase activity. Spry2 is well documented as an inhibitor of ERK1/2 signaling following FGF receptor activation (Figure 5). Its structure contains a conserved N-terminal tyrosine residue at position 55 (Y55) whose phosphorylation by FRS2α-activated Src kinase (Li et al., 2004) is necessary for interaction with both protein phosphatase 2A (PP2A) and the ubiquitin ligase, cCbl (reviewed Guy et al., 2009). No single satisfactory explanation exists for what occurs next, however, it is clear that PP2A de-phosphorylates two serine residues in a serine rich region of the protein (Ser^{115} and Ser^{118}) exposing a cryptic proline rich tail that can bind SH3 domain proteins and their interacting partners (Lao et al., 2007). One possibility is that Spry2 therefore acts as an adaptor protein which presents cCbl with substrates for ubiquitylation and degradation. This is supported by the observation that Grb2, a Spry2 interacting SH3 protein, can recruit the cCbl E3 ligase and its associated ubiquitination machinery into a complex with both FRS2α and FGFR1, so repressing signal generation to ERK1/2 (Wong et al., 2002).

In airway epithelium, FGF-10 similarly increases Spry2 tyrosine phosphorylation (presumably at the Y55 residue), promoting its association with the FRS2α/Grb2/Raf signaling complex and disrupting its formation, either by 1) targeting Grb2-associated proteins for proteasomal destruction (Guy et al., 2009; Wong et al., 2002) or 2) inter-calating into the FRS2α/Grb2 signaling complex thereby disrupting downstream activation of ERK1/2 (Tefft et al., 2002). Spry2 activity is repressed by SHP2 which relieves its interaction with the Grb2 complex (possibly by dephosphorylating Y55) and whose inhibition results in sustained ERK1/2 activity (Hanafusa et al., 2004; Jarvis et al., 2006; Tefft et al., 2002). Thus, much like Shh, Spry2 forms the basis of a feedback loop which controls the duration and magnitude of the intracellular signaling response between the FGF receptor and the ERK1/2 pathway and explains the decline in ERK1/2 activity with increasing FGF-10 concentration shown in Figure 4. By implication, ERK1/2 signaling may be more important in the functional maturation of the epithelial tube behind the growing bud tip rather than in the regulation of airway outgrowth towards the FGF-10 signal.

Spry2 regulation of mTORC1 and its role in vascular signaling is less clear. mTORC-1 assembly and activation is held in check by the activity of two interacting protein partners known as Tuberous Sclerosis Complex (TSC) 1 and 2. This acts as a GTPase activating protein (GAP) towards the small G-protein known as ras homolog enriched in brain (Rheb).

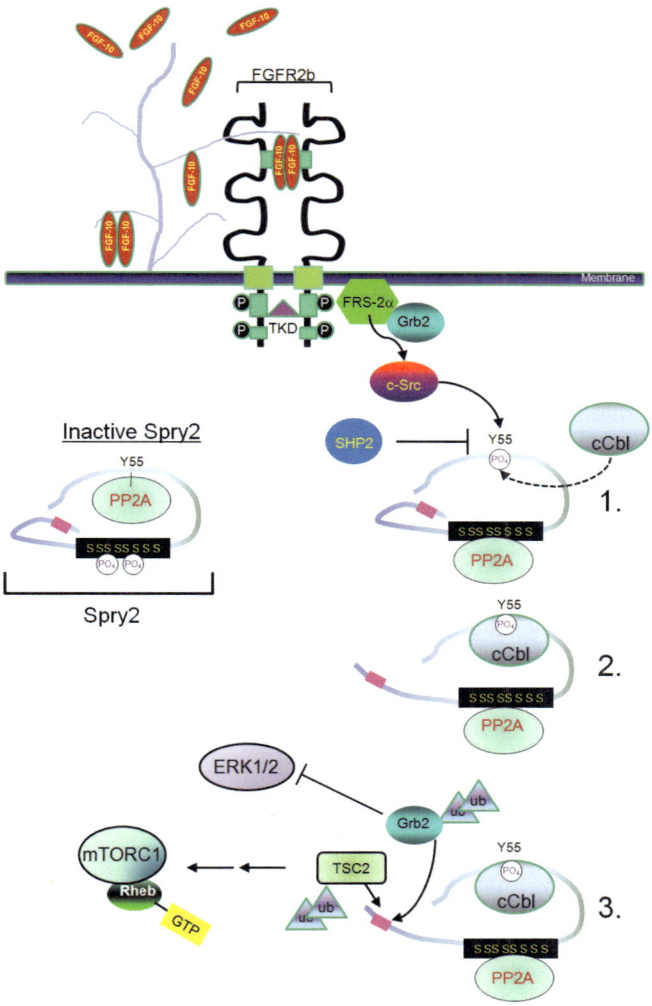

Fig. 5. Activation mechanism of Spry2. In its inactive state, Spry2 binds PP2A and is phosphorylated at serines 115 and 118. The cryptic C-terminal SH3 binding domain (magenta) is hidden within the structure of the protein. FGFR2b autophosphorylation and subsequent FRS2α /Grb2 complex assembly activate Spry2 in three steps: 1. Tyrosine phosphorylation of c-Src kinase phosphorylates the Y55 residue within the tyrosine kinase binding domain of Spry2 (antagonised by the phosphatases, SHP2). This activates protein phosphatase 2A (PP2A) enabling it to bind and dephosphorylate serines 115 and 118 within the serine rich domain (black). Phosphorylated Y55 also enables binding of the cCbl ubiquitin ligase to Spry2. 2. Dephosphorylation of the serine rich domain alters protein conformation to expose the SH3 protein binding region. 3. SH3 domain proteins such as Grb2 and, possibly, TSC2, interact with this region, becoming ubiquitylated and subsequently targeted for proteasomal clearance. Clearance of Grb2 and its associated proteins prevents ERK1/2 signaling whereas TSC2 clearance prevents GAP activity against Rheb, enabling it to bind GTP and activate mTORC1.

When bound to GTP, Rheb potently activates mTORC1 kinase activity and this is suppressed by TSC1/2 which converts Rheb to its GDP-bound state (Zhang et al., 2003). Thus, signaling inputs into TSC1/2 that regulate its GAP activity towards Rheb are critical regulators of mTORC1 activity. Spry2 participates in this process in FGF-10-treated FDLE cells by forming a complex between TSC2 and cCbl which is associated with an increase in Rheb-GTP binding and mTORC1 activation (Figure 5; Scott et al., 2010). Although the mechanism that underpins this interaction is unclear, null mutation of the Spry2 Y55 residue produced an increase in mTORC-1 dependent HIF-1α activity and VEGF-A secretion that was linked to a decline in TSC2 stability and Rheb-GAP activity (Scott et al., 2010).

Thus, Spry2 appears to direct the partitioning of kinase activity within the FGF-10 gradient where pro-vascular mTORC1 activity initiates HIF-1α and VEGF-A secretion from the airway epithelium that is close to the FGF-10 source, whereas ERK1/2 activity is specifically repressed in this region. Whether this partitioning is critical for co-ordinating vascular and airway branching rate is unclear, however, it may be that Spry2-dependent control over mTORC1 governs the duration of proliferative airway and vascular outgrowth around the airway tip and that ERK1/2 activity behind this region limits this process by inducing tubular maturation towards their functionally developed forms. There is precedence for this from the stem cell literature where activation of ERK1/2 drives terminal differentiation of stem cells whereas its inhibition retains cell pleuripotency (Stavridis et al., 2010).

4.4 An epigenetic role for Spry2 in regulating VEGF-A gene expression?

The formation of complex, interwoven, branched tubular networks demands tight control over the timing and placement of gene expression and this is particularly important for VEGF-A where subtle changes in its abundance have major consequences for airway and vascular growth. DNA is packaged around complexes of histone proteins (octamers of histones 2A, 2B, 3 and 4) to form nucleosomes which are further organised into a helical structure to create supercoiled chromatin. Protein tails from each of the histone proteins project outwards from the nucleosome and are modified in different ways (serine phosphorylation, lysine acetylation, lysine SUMOylation, arginine methylation, ubiquitylation) to control DNA organisation. Thus, histone tail modification constitutes an epigenetic code which regulates the association of chromatin modifying proteins with DNA and the formation of active transcriptional complexes. DNA itself is also subject to modification. Methylation of cytosine residues in CG rich promoter regions (CpG islands) leads to gene repression by inhibiting the interaction of transcription complex proteins with the promoter. The three dimensional structure of chromatin enables this effect to act over long distances so that distant hypermethylated CpG domains (CpG shores) are capable of repressing promoter activity located >2kb downstream. The *Vegfa* gene promoter contains a number of CG rich stretches which have been shown to act as binding sites for Sp1 and AP-2 transcription factors (reviewed, Pagès & Pouyssègur, 2005) but probably do not act as CpG methylation islands (Kim et al., 2009). Others have shown that *Vegfa* can be targeted by microRNAs (miR) which either positively or negatively regulate gene expression by altering histone acetylation and the super-ordered structure of the *Vegfa* coding region (Turunen et al., 2009).

Given the central importance of temporal and spatial gene regulation patterns to lung development, it is reasonable to suppose that *Vegfa* is subject to some form of epigenetic regulation that is sensitive to FGF-10 stimulation. In non-fetal cell lines, Spry2 distribution is characteristically endosomal and migrates to the plasma membrane on tyrosine kinase receptor activation by growth factors. In FDLE, however, we have uncovered evidence that

Spry2 also occurs in the nucleus where chromatin immunoprecipitation (ChIP) assays reveal that it interacts with the *Vegfa* promoter (Figure 6). Although the meaning of this interaction is currently unclear, it occurs most strongly in CG-rich regions containing the functional binding sites for Sp1 and its competitive repressor, Sp3. The interaction does not appear to be dependent upon FGF-10, however, this does not preclude FGF-10-sensitive interactions with other protein partners. Clearly, more work is needed here, however, given that Spry2 indirectly promotes the interaction between HIF-1α and the CBP/p300 histone acetyltransferase (HAT), it is interesting to speculate that nuclear Spry2 may fine-tune the epigenetic regulation of the *Vegfa* gene by co-ordinating this effect with the recruitment of other transcriptionally active proteins to CG rich domains of the promoter. Given its role as a regulator of branching periodicity, could nuclear Spry2 act as the "clock" that regulates the timing of gene expression in response to growth factor signals?

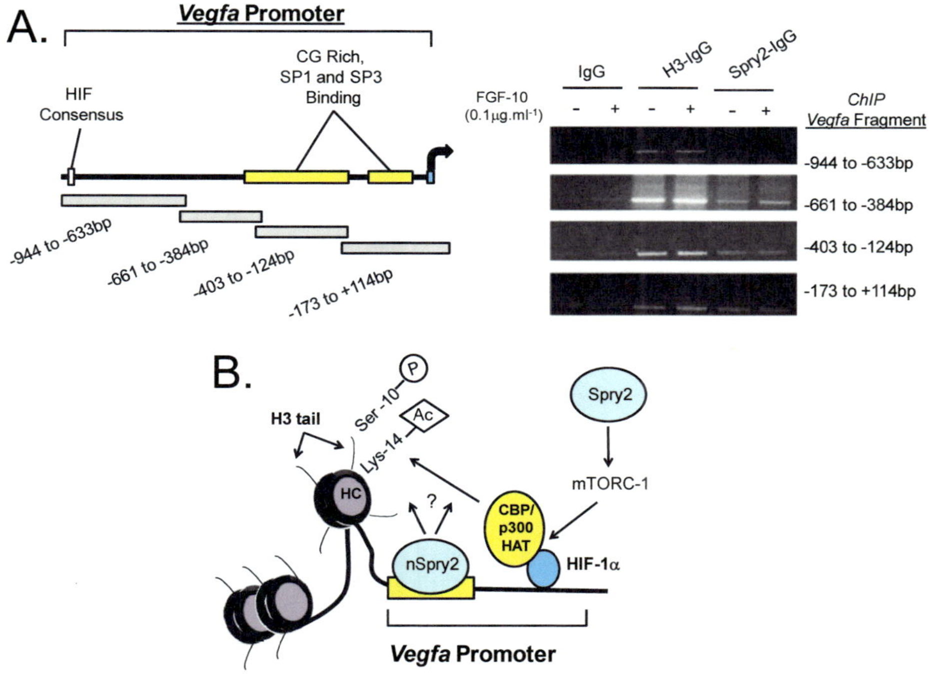

Fig. 6. Spry2 interacts with CG rich regions of the *Vegfa* promoter. A. Location of ChIP assay primers spanning the HIF and Sp1/3 binding sites of the *Vegfa* promoter. Right hand panel shows ChIP assay PCR results which reveal a constitutive interaction between Spry2 and CG-containing regions of the *Vegfa* promoter spanning -661 to -124 bases 5' to the transcription initiation site. IgG and Histone 3 (H3) antibodies are negative and positive control respectively (representative of four independent assays; S.C. Land, Unpubl. Obs). B. Phosphorylation and acetylation of the H3 tail at Ser10 and Lys 14 promotes DNA unwinding from the histone core complex (HC) allowing transcription to proceed. Spry2 promotes this by inducing the recruitment of CBP/p300 to HIF-1α, via mTORC1. The role of nuclear Spry2 (nSpry2) in this process is speculative but may involve recruitment of other transcription factors such as Sp1 or Sp3 to the CG rich region of the *Vegfa* promoter.

5. Conclusion: Towards an integrated model of co-ordinated airway and vascular growth in the fetal lung

The distal angiogenesis model of lung vascular development requires that there is a sustained, localized inductive cue which draws vascular growth along the airway branching path. This may be influenced by fetal heart rate which can alter both rate and intensity of airway and vascular branching. The model presented in Figure 7 suggests that the earliest pro-vascular cue is FGF-10 itself, which induces expression of VEGF-A by amplifying the HIF-1α signaling pathway. This occurs by hypo-phosphorylation of Spry2 and cCbl-dependent inhibition of TSC2 which enables an active mTORC1 complex to interact with the HIF-1α N-terminal TOS motif. HIF-promoted VEGF-A expression occurs by enhanced CBP/p300 histone acetyltransferase activity binding to HIF-1α which, together with Spry2 activity elsewhere in the *Vegfa* promoter, facilitates DNA unwinding and expression of the gene. This initial expression of VEGF-A is accompanied by directional cues which sustain vascular signaling and blood vessel maturation and also ensure that the patterning of the vasculature is confined to appropriate regions of the lung. The precise nature of these cues is unknown, however, it is reasonable to suggest that the FGF-9/Shh interaction performs this role as it does for other lung structures (smooth muscle, for example). Indeed, this interaction could be the basis of the observed need for blood vessels to grow in order to sustain the three dimensional growth of the lung.

Weibel and Gomez's original observation that the branched patterning of the airway and vasculature follows a fractal relationship from one generation to the next implies the presence of a "space and time" precision regulator which controls the rate, location and orientation of each branch process. The tight regulation of airway branching patterns in lung reported by Metzger et al. (2008) suggests that there is a hierarchy of precision regulators which control the "stop", "bifurcate", "re-orientate", "repeat" pattern of branching and that there must be some mechanism to unite these events in time along the entire branch length. The exact identity of these processes remains unknown, however, one possibility is that calcium waves which regulate smooth muscle peristalsis might serve as one periodic orientating cue which co-ordinates these events together on a grand scale (Jesudason et al., 2010). Another, is the repressive role that proteins such as Shh and Spry2 play in determining the spatial patterning and duration of FGF-10 signaling from one branch tip to another. At the molecular end of the scale, epigenetic processes determine the accessibility of RNA polymerases to DNA coding regions and so it is reasonable to expect that the dynamics of histone acetyltransferase and histone deacetylase recruitment to specific gene loci, such as *Vegfa*, determine, when, where and how a developmentally critical gene is expressed. This chapter ends on a speculative, but tantalising, note by suggesting that Spry2 is a good candidate for this role through its interaction with CG rich regions of the *Vegfa* promoter.

In the concluding chapter to his book "The Pathway for Oxygen", Weibel considers whether there is an upper limit to the design of the mammalian respiratory system by examining lung structure in the smallest mammal with the highest energetic demands, the Etruscan shrew. He reveals a lung of truly extraordinary proportions. It is ventilated at a rate of 300 breaths per minute and perfused by a heart that contracts at a rate of 17 beats per *second*. Volume for volume, it has a surface area that is 8-times greater than the human lung and which culminates in a blood-gas barrier which is one third the thickness. Weibel makes the point that this can only occur by taking the dimensions of all lung components to their extreme limit and that, in this organism, the constraints of lung design versus physiological demand cannot be pushed further. This suggests that the molecular regulation of airway and vascular development is an adaptable process that can be tuned, to a finite limit, to generate a lung that can sustain the energetic requirements of the organism. Understanding the molecular regulation of this tuning process in health and disease represents the next major goal in lung developmental biology.

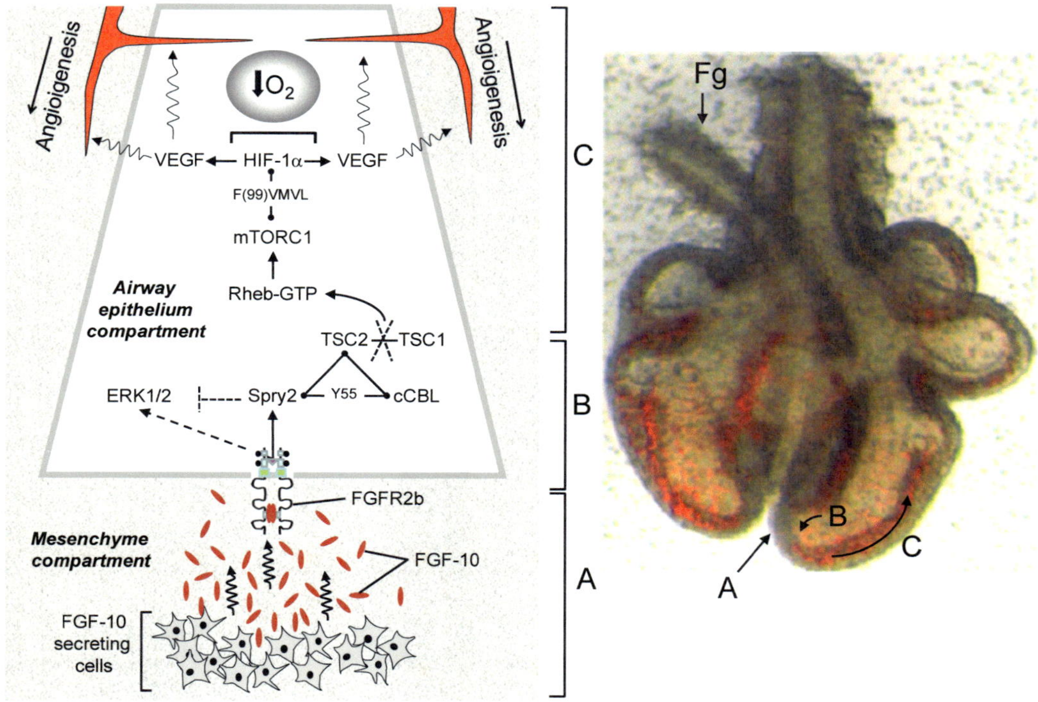

Fig. 7. FGF-10 as a co-ordinator of airway and vascular growth. Right hand panel shows an embryonic stage rat lung where perfused vasculature can be seen within the mesenchyme surrounding the airway branches and proximal to the airway tip (red hue). Foregut (Fg) is shown displaced to left of lung. Signaling in three zones of airway and vascular growth (A-C) are indicated in the left hand panel. **Zone A:** FGF-10 is expressed in the mesenchyme ahead of nascent airway buds and diffuses towards the airway epithelium. **Zone B:** FGF-10 induces FGFR2b autophosphorylation and signaling to Spry2 whose activation inhibits signaling to the ERK1/2 pathway and also induces TSC2 clearance enabling Rheb to bind GTP and activate mTORC1. **Zone C:** mTORC1 promotes transcriptional activity of hypoxia-stabilised HIF-1α by interaction with its FVMVL TOS motif. This augments the expression and secretion of VEGF-A into the surrounding mesenchyme so providing the primary angiogenic cue which sustains vascular growth along with that of the airway. Figure modified from Scott et al. (2010) with permission.

6. Acknowledgements

Work in the author's laboratory is supported by The Wellcome Trust, UK.

7. References

Asikainen TM, Chang LY, Coalson JJ, Schneider BK, Waleh NS, Ikegami M, Shannon JM, Winter VT, Grubb P, Clyman RI, Yoder BA, Crapo JD, White CW. (2006). Improved lung growth and function through hypoxia-inducible factor in primate chronic lung disease of prematurity. *FASEB J* Vol 20: 1698–1700.

Asikainen TM, Schneider BK, Waleh NS, Clyman RI, Ho WB, Flippin LA, Gunzler V, White CW. (2005). Activation of hypoxia-inducible factors in hyperoxia through prolyl 4-hydroxylase blockade in cells and explants of primate lung. *Proc Natl Acad Sci USA* Vol 102: 10212–10217.

Baines DL, Ramminger SJ, Collett A, Haddad J, Best OG, Land SC, Olver RE, Wilson SM. (2001). Oxygen-evoked Na+ transport in rat fetal distal lung epithelial cells. *J Physiol.* Vol 532, No 1: 105-13.

Bardos JI, Ashcroft M. (2005). Negative and positive regulation of HIF-1: a complex network. *Biochim Biophys Acta* Vol 1755: 107–120, 2005.

Bellusci S, Grindley SJ, Emoto H, Itoh N, Hogan BL.(1997). Fibroblast growth factor 10 (FGF10) and branching morphogenesis in the embryonic mouse lung. *Development* Vol 124: 4867–4878.

Berra E, Benizri E, Ginouvès A, Volmat V, Roux D, Pouysségur J. (2003) HIF prolyl-hydroxylase 2 is the key oxygen sensor setting low steady-state levels of HIF-1α in normoxia. *EMBO J* Vol 22. No 16:4082-90.

Cardoso WV, Lü J. (2006) Regulation of early lung morphogenesis: questions, facts and controversies. *Development.* Vol 133, No9:1611-24.

Carmeliet P, Ferreira V, Breier G, Pollefeyt S, Kieckens L, Gertsenstein M, Fahrig M, Vandenhoeck A, Harpal K, Eberhardt C, Declercq C, Pawling J, Moons L, Collen D, Risau W, Nagy A. (1996). Abnormal blood vessel development and lethality in embryos lacking a single VEGF allele. *Nature.* Vol 380, No 6573: 435-9.

Compernolle V, Brusselmans K, Acker T, Hoet P, Tjwa M, Beck H, Plaisance S, Dor Y, Keshet E, Lupu F, Nemery B, Dewerchin M, Van Veldhoven P, Plate K, MoonsL, Collen D, Carmeliet P. (2002) Loss of HIF-2α and inhibition of VEGF impair fetal lung maturation, whereas treatment with VEGF prevents fatal respiratory distress in premature mice. *Nat Med.*Vol 8, No 7: 702-10.

Del Moral, P. M., Sala, F. G., Tefft, D., Shi, W., Keshet, E., Bellusci, S. and Warburton, D. (2006). VEGF-A signaling through Flk-1 is a critical facilitator of early embryonic lung epithelial to endothelial crosstalk and branching morphogenesis. *Dev. Biol.* Vol 290:177 -188.

Depping R, Steinhoff A, Schindler SG, Friedrich B, Fagerlund R, Metzen E, Hartmann E, Köhler M. (2008). Nuclear translocation of hypoxia-inducible factors (HIFs): involvement of the classical importin alpha/beta pathway. *Biochim Biophys Acta.* Vol 1783, No3: 394-404.

Dunlop EA, Tee AR. (2009). Mammalian target of rapamycin complex 1: signalling inputs, substrates and feedback mechanisms. *Cell Signal.* Vol 21, No 6: 827-35.

El-Hashash AH, Al Alam D, Turcatel G, Bellusci S, Warburton D. (2011a). Eyes absent 1 (Eya1) is a critical coordinator of epithelial, mesenchymal and vascular morphogenesis in the mammalian lung. *Dev Biol.* Vol 350. No 1: 112-26.

El-Hashash AH, Al Alam D, Turcatel G, Rogers O, Li X, Bellusci S, Warburton D. (2011b) Six 1 transcription factor is critical for coordination of epithelial, mesenchymal and vascular morphogenesis in the mammalian lung. *Dev Biol.* Vol 353, No 2: 242-58.

Eswarakumar VP, Lax I, Schlessinger J. (2005) Cellular signaling by fibroblast growth factor receptors. *Cytokine Growth Factor Rev.* Vol 16, No 2: 139-49.

Flashman E, Bagg EA, Chowdhury R, Mecinović J, Loenarz C, McDonough MA,Hewitson KS, Schofield CJ. (2008). Kinetic rationale for selectivity toward N- and C-terminal oxygen-dependent degradation domain substrates mediated by a loop region of hypoxia-inducible factor prolyl hydroxylases. *J Biol Chem.* Vol 283, No 7: 3808-15.

Fong, G. H., Rossant, J., Gertsenstein, M. and Breitman, M. L. (1995). Role of the Flt-1 receptor tyrosine kinase in regulating the assembly of vascular endothelium. *Nature* Vol 376: 66 -70.

Greenberg, F.Y. Thompson, S.K. Brooks, J.M. Shannon, K. McCormick-Shannon, J.E. Cameron, B.P. Mallory and A.L. Akeson. (2002). Mesenchymal expression of vascular endothelial growth factors D and A defines vascular patterning in developing lung, *Dev. Dyn.* Vol 224: 144–153.

Groenman F, Rutter M, Caniggia I, Tibboel D, Post M. (2007). Hypoxia-inducible factors in the first trimester human lung. *J Histochem Cytochem.* Vol 55, No 4: 355-63.

Groenman FA, Rutter M, Wang J, Caniggia I, Tibboel D, Post M. (2007). Effect of chemical stabilizers of hypoxia-inducible factors on early lung development. *Am J Physiol Lung Cell Mol Physiol.* Vol 293, No 3:L557-67.

Guy GR, Jackson RA, Yusoff P, Chow SY. (2009). Sprouty proteins: modified modulators, matchmakers or missing links? *J Endocrinol.* Vol 203, No 2: 191-202.Hadari YR, Gotoh N, Kouhara H, Lax I, Schlessinger J. (2001). Critical role for the docking-protein FRS2α in FGF receptor-mediated signal transduction pathways. *Proc Natl Acad Sci U S A.* Vol 98, No 15: 8578-83.

Hanafusa H, Torii S, Yasunaga T, Matsumoto K, Nishida E. (2004) Shp2, and SH2-containing protein-tyrosine phosphatase, positively regulates receptor tyrosine signaling by dephosphorylating and inactivating the inhibitor Sprouty. *J. Bio. Chem.* Vol 279: 22992–22995.

Healy AM, Morgenthau L, Zhu X, Farber HW, Cardoso WV. (2000). VEGF is deposited in the subepithelial matrix at the leading edge of branching airways and stimulates neovascularization in the murine embryonic lung. *Dev Dyn.* 2000 Vol 219 No 3:3 41-52.

Hentges KE, Sirry B, Gingeras AC, Sarbassov D, Sonenberg N, Sabatini D, Peterson AS. (2001). FRAP/mTOR is required for proliferation and patterning during embryonic development in the mouse. *Proc Natl Acad Sci USA* Vol 98: 13796–13801, 2001.

Hirsilä M, Koivunen P, Günzler V, Kivirikko KI, Myllyharju J. (2003). Characterization of the human prolyl 4-hydroxylases that modify the hypoxia-inducible factor. *J Biol Chem* Vol 278: 30772–30780.

Jarvis LA, Toering SJ, Simon MA, Krasnow MA, Smith-Bolton RK. (2006). Sprouty proteins are in vivo targets of Corkscrew/SHP-2 tyrosine phosphatases. *Development* Vol 133: 1133–1142.

Jesudason EC, Keshet E, Warburton D. (2010). Entrained pulmonary clocks: epithelium and vasculature keeping pace. Am J Physiol Lung Cell Mol Physiol. Vol 299, No 4: L453-4.

Kim JY, Hwang JH, Zhou W, Shin J, Noh SM, Song IS, Kim JY, Lee SH, Kim J. (2009). The expression of VEGF receptor genes is concurrently influenced by epigenetic gene silencing of the genes and VEGF activation. *Epigenetics.* Vol 4 No 5: 13-21.

Kouhara H, Hadari YR, Spivak-Kroizman T, Schilling J, Bar-Sagi D, Lax I, Schlessinger J. (1997). A lipid-anchored Grb2-binding protein that links FGF-receptor activation to the Ras/MAPK signaling pathway. *Cell.* Vol 89, No 5: 693-702.

Land, SC.(2004). Hochachka's "Hypoxia Defense Strategies" and the development of the pathway for oxygen. *Comp Biochem. Physiol. B* Vol 139: 415-433.

Land SC. (2003). Oxygen-sensing pathways and the development of mammalian gas exchange. *Redox Report* Vol 8: 326–340.

Land SC, Collett A.(2001) Detection of Cl^- flux in the apical microenvironment of cultured foetal distal lung epithelial cells. *J Exp Biol.* Vol 204, No 4: 785-95.

Lao DH, Yusoff P, Chandramouli S, Philp RJ, Fong CW, Jackson RA, Saw TY, Yu CY & Guy GR (2007) Direct binding of PP2A to Sprouty2 and phosphorylation changes are a prerequisite for ERK inhibition downstream of fibroblast growth factor receptor stimulation. *J. Biol Chem.* Vol 282: 9117–9126.

Lazarus A, Del-Moral PM, Ilovich O, Mishani E, Warburton D, Keshet E. (2011). A perfusion-independent role of blood vessels in determining branching stereotypy of lung airways. *Development.* Vol 138 No 11: 2359-68.

Li X, Brunton VG, Burgar HR, Wheldon LM, Heath JK. (2004). FRS2-dependent Src activation is required for fibroblast growth factor receptor-induced phosphorylation of Sprouty and Suppression of ERK activity. *J. Cell Sci* Vol 117: 6007–6017.

Mailleux AA, Tefft D, Ndiaye D, Itoh N, Thiery JP, Warburton D, Bellusci S. (2001). Evidence that SPROUTY2 functions as an inhibitor of mouse embryonic lung growth and morphogenesis. Mech Dev. Vol102, Nos 1-2: 81-94.

Mauroy B, Filoche M, Weibel ER, Sapoval B. (2004). An optimal bronchial tree may be dangerous. *Nature.* Vol 427 :633-6.

Metzger RJ, Klein OD, Martin GR, Krasnow MA. (2008). The branching programme of mouse lung development. *Nature.* Vol 453:745-50.

Morrison JL, Chien C, Riggs KW, Gruber N, Rurak D. (2002). Effect of maternal fluoxetine administration on uterine blood flow, fetal blood gas status, and growth. *Pediatr Res.* Vol 51 No4: 433-42.

Mühlfeld C, Weibel ER, Hahn U, Kummer W, Nyengaard JR, Ochs M. (2010). Is length an appropriate estimator to characterize pulmonary alveolar capillaries? A critical evaluation in the human lung. *Anat Rec (Hoboken).* Vol 293 No 7: 1270-5.

Ng YS, R. Rohan, M.E. Sunday, D.E. Demello and P.A. D'Amore (2001) Differential expression of VEGF isoforms in mouse during development and in the adult, *Dev. Dyn.* Vol 220: 112–121.

Otulakowski G, Duan W, O'Brodovich H.(2009). Global and gene-specific translational regulation in rat lung development. *Am J Respir Cell Mol Biol* Vol 40: 555–567.

Otulakowski G, Duan W, Gandhi S, O'brodovich H.(2007). Steroid and oxygen effects on eIF4F complex, mTOR, and ENaC translation in fetal lung epithelia. *Am J Respir Cell Mol Biol.* Vol 37, No 4: 457-66.

Pagès G, Pouysségur J. (2005).Transcriptional regulation of the Vascular Endothelial Growth Factor gene-a concert of activating factors. *Cardiovasc Res.* Vol 65 No3: 564-73.

Perry SF, Wilson RJ, Straus C, Harris MB, Remmers JE. (2001). Which came first, the lung or the breath? *Comp Biochem Physiol A Mol Integr Physiol.* Vol 129 No 1: 37-47.

Qi J, Nakayama K, Gaitonde S, Goydos JS, Krajewski S, Eroshkin A, Bar-Sagi D, Bowtell D, Ronai Z. (2008). The ubiquitin ligase Siah2 regulates tumorigenesis and metastasis by HIF-dependent and -independent pathways. *Proc Natl Acad Sci USA* Vol 105: 16713–16718.

Ramasamy SK, Mailleux AA, Gupte VV, Mata F, Sala FG, Veltmaat JM, Del Moral PM, De Langhe S, Parsa S, Kelly LK, Kelly R, Shia W, Keshet E, Minoo P, Warburton D, Bellusci S. (2007). Fgf10 dosage is critical for the amplification of epithelial cell progenitors and for the formation of multiple mesenchymal lineages durin g lung development. *Dev Biol.* Vol 307, No 2: 237-47.

Resnik ER, Herron JM, Lyu SC, Cornfield DN. (2007). Developmental regulation of hypoxia-inducible factor 1 and prolyl-hydroxylases in pulmonary vascular smooth muscle cells. *Proc Natl Acad Sci U S A.* Vol 104 No 47: 18789-94.

Sander PM, Christian A, Clauss M, Fechner R, Gee CT, Griebeler EM, Gunga HC,Hummel J, Mallison H, Perry SF, Preuschoft H, Rauhut OW, Remes K, Tütken T, Wings O, Witzel U. (2011) Biology of the sauropod dinosaurs: the evolution of gigantism. *Biol Rev Camb Philos Soc.* Vol 86 No 1: 117-55.

Sarbassov D, Ali S, Kim D, Guertin D, Latek R, Erdjument-Bromage H, Tempst P, Sabatini D (2004). Rictor, a novel binding partner of mTOR, defines a rapamycin-insensitive and raptor-independent pathway that regulates the cytoskeleton. *Curr Biol* Vol 14, No 14 : 1296–302.

Schalm SS, Blenis J. (2002). Identification of a conserved motif required for mTOR signaling. *Curr Biol.* Vol 12, No 8: 632-9.

Schalm SS, Fingar DC, Sabatini DM, Blenis J. (2003). TOS motif-mediated raptor binding regulates 4E-BP1 multisite phosphorylation and function. *Curr Biol.* Vol 13, No 10: 797-806.

Scott CL, Walker DJ, Cwiklinski E, Tait C, Tee AR, Land SC. (2010). Control of HIF-1α and vascular signaling in fetal lung involves cross talk between mTORC1 and the FGF-10/FGFR2b/Spry2 airway branching periodicity clock. *Am J Physiol Lung Cell Mol Physiol.* Vol 299 No 4: L455-71.

Shalaby, F., Rossant, J., Yamaguchi, T. P., Gertsenstein, M., Wu, X. F., Breitman, M. L. and Schuh, A. C. (1995). Failure of blood-island formation and vasculogenesis in Flk-1-deficient mice. *Nature* Vol 376: 62 -66.

Stavridis MP, Collins BJ, Storey KG. (2010). Retinoic acid orchestrates fibroblast growth factor signalling to drive embryonic stem cell differentiation. *Development* Vol 137: 881–890.

Tefft D, Lee M, Smith S, Crowe DL, Bellusci S, Warburton D. (2002) mSprouty2 inhibits FGF10-activated MAP kinase by differentially binding to upstream target proteins. *Am J Physiol Lung Cell Mol Physiol* Vol 283: L700–L706.

Tefft D, Lee M, Smith S, Leinwand M, Zhao J, Bringas P Jr, Crowe DL, Warburton D (1999). Conserved function of mSpry-2, a murine homolog of Drosophila sprouty, which negatively modulates respiratory organogenesis. *Curr Biol.* Vol 9. No 4 :219-22.

Turunen MP, Lehtola T, Heinonen SE, Assefa GS, Korpisalo P, Girnary R, Glass CK, Väisänen S, Ylä-Herttuala S. (2009). Efficient regulation of VEGF expression by promoter-targeted lentiviral shRNAs based on epigenetic mechanism: a novel example of epigenetherapy. *Circ Res.* Vol 105 No 6: 604-9.

van Tuyl M, Groenman F, Wang J, Kuliszewski M, Liu J, Tibboel D, Post M. (2007). Angiogenic factors stimulate tubular branching morphogenesis of sonic hedgehog-deficient lungs. *Dev Biol.* Vol 303, No 2 :514-26.

van Tuyl M, Liu J, Wang J, Kuliszewski M, Tibboel D, Post M. (2005). Role of oxygen and vascular development in epithelial branching morphogenesis of the developing mouse lung. *Am J Physiol Lung Cell Mol Physiol* Vol 288: L167–L178.

Warburton D. (2008). Developmental biology: order in the lung. *Nature* Vol 453: 733-735.

Weaver M, Batts L, Hogan BL. (2003). Tissue interactions pattern the mesenchyme of the embryonic mouse lung. *Dev Biol.* Vol 258, No 1 :169-84.

Weibel ER, Taylor, CR and L Bolis. (1998). Principles of Animal Design, Cambridge University Press, 315pp.

Weibel ER, Federspiel WJ, Fryder-Doffey F, Hsia CCW, König M, Stalder-Navarro V, Vock R. (1993). Morphometric model for pulmonary diffusing capacity. I. Membrane diffusing capacity. *Respir Physiol.* Vol 93: 125–49.

Weibel ER. (1991). Fractal Geometry: a design principle for living organisms. *Am. J. Physiol. Lung Cell Mol. Physiol.* Vol 261 No. 5: L361-L369.

Weibel ER (1984). The Pathway for Oxygen. Harvard University Press, 425pp

Weibel ER, and Gomez DM. (1962). Architecture of the human lung. Use of quantitative methods establishes fundamental relations between size and number of lung structures. *Science* Vol 137: 577-585.

West BJ, Bhargava V, and Goldberger AL. (1986). Beyond the principle of similitude: renormalization in the bronchial tree. *J Appl Physiol* Vol 60: 1089-1097.

West JB, Watson RR, Fu Z. (2007). The human lung: did evolution get it wrong? *Eur Respir J.* Vol 29 No 1: 11-7.

West JB. (2003). Thoughts on the pulmonary blood-gas barrier. *Am J Physiol Lung Cell Mol Physiol.* Vol 285 No 3: L501-13.

White AC, Lavine KJ, Ornitz DM. (2007). FGF9 and SHH regulate mesenchymal Vegfa expression and development of the pulmonary capillary network. *Development.* Vol 134, No 20: 3743-52.

Wong A, Lamothe B, Lee A, Schlessinger J & Lax I (2002) FRS2α attenuates FGF receptor signaling by Grb2-mediated recruitment of the ubiquitin ligase Cbl. *Proc Natl. Acad. Sci. USA* Vol 99: 6684–6689.

Yee Koh M, Spivak-Kroizman TR, Powis G. (2008). HIF-1 regulation: not so easy come, easy go. *Trends Biochem Sci.* Vol 33, No 11: 526-34.

Zhang Y, Gao X, Saucedo LJ, Ru B, Edgar BA, Pan D. (2003). Rheb is a direct target of the tuberous sclerosis tumour suppressor proteins. *Nat Cell Biol.* Vol 5 No 6: 578-81.

Zhao, L., Wang, K., Ferrara, N. and Vu, T. H. (2005). Vascular endothelial growth factor co-ordinates proper development of lung epithelium and vasculature. *Mech. Dev.* Vol 122: 877 -886.

4

Apelin Signalling: Lineage Marker and Functional Actor of Blood Vessel Formation

Yves Audigier
Research Center of Cancerology of Toulouse,
UMR 1037 INSERM - Universite Toulouse III,
France

1. Introduction

G protein-coupled receptors (GPCR) represent a large family of proteins that share a unique membrane topology made of seven transmembrane segments. These receptors are an evolutionary success as they constitute more than 1% of the genoma. In addition, the same structural archetype has been selected to recognize a large variety of ligands and to activate multiple intracellular cascades via the coupling to different G proteins. Accordingly, G protein-coupled receptors participate in a wide range of physiological functions. The corollary of this physiological importance is that many pathologies are linked to a dysfunction of these signalling pathways. Indeed, half of the pharmacological drugs used to treat human diseases corresponds to molecules which interact with this family of receptors.
In this context, the discovery of new receptors not only has an evident physiological interest, but also represents a therapeutic potential by the development of new pharmacological agents. The discovery and history of apelin signalling provides the best example of the close relationship between basic research and its pharmacoclinical implications.

2. Discovery of apelin signalling

The discovery of apelin signalling began with the cloning of two orphan G protein-coupled receptors (Masri et al., 2005; Audigier, 2006). The amino acid sequence of these two receptors revealed the presence of seven hydrophobic domains which is in agreement with the unique membrane topology of GPCRs made of seven transmembrane segments (TM). These new GPCRs were cloned by a fishing strategy based on the use of degenerate primers directed against consensus sequences located in the transmembrane segments (TM) (Figure 1).
When searching for subtypes of the vasopressin receptors and using degenerate oligos based on the nucleotide sequence encoding the second and the seventh TM regions, one team cloned by serendipity from human genomic DNA a new orphan receptor that was named APJ (O'Dowd et al., 1993). Northern blot analysis with polyadenylated mRNA revealed an expression in different regions of the rat brain.
In order to determine whether GPCR played a role in early embryogenesis, our laboratory looked for DNA fragments amplified from mRNAs extracted from Xenopus gastrulas between primers located in consensus sequences of TM 3 and TM 6 domains. One amplified fragment was used to clone a novel member of the GPCR family in amphibians that we

named X-msr for mesenchyme-associated serpentine receptor (Devic et al., 1996). Interestingly, alignment of the protein sequence and molecular phylogeny analysis clearly demonstrated that the amphibian receptor was homologous to the human APJ receptor and represented its amphibian orthologue. In addition, *in situ* hybridization detected very early transcripts after the midblastula transition, then in the ventro-lateral mesoderm and later in the lateral plate mesoderm.

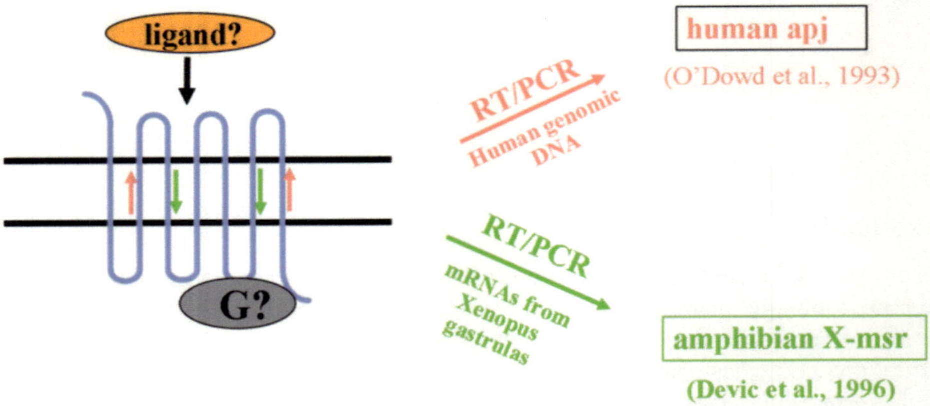

Fig. 1. Cloning of orphan G protein-coupled receptors.
The arrows represent the location of the sequences from which the two primers were designed for PCR amplification. The pink arrows correspond to the primers used for cloning of the human receptor APJ. The green arrows correspond to the primers used for cloning of the amphibian receptor X-msr.

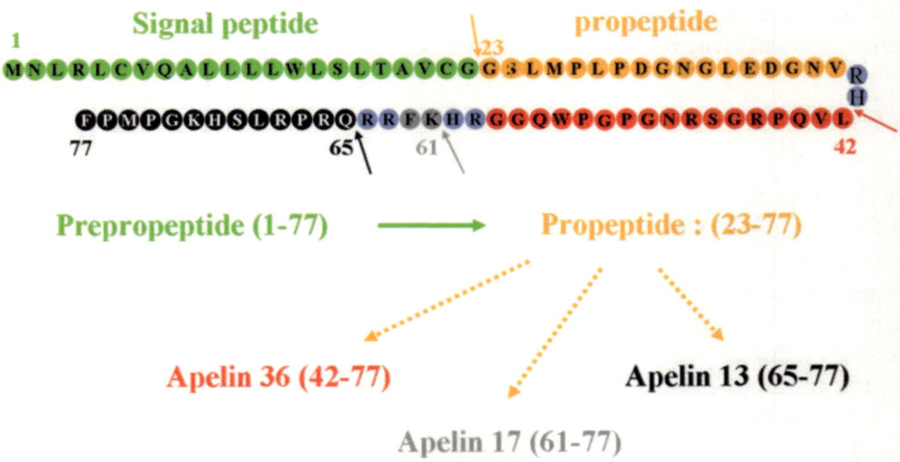

Fig. 2. Isolation of the endogenous ligand.
Apelin gene codes for a peptide of 77 amino acids (AA), which contains a signal sequence of 22 AA (green). Cleavage of this signal peptide generates a propeptide of 55 AA (orange) having three basic doublets (blue). Proteolytic processing at the level of each basic doublet can produce three fragments of different length : apelin36 (red), apelin17 (grey) and apelin13 (black).

These receptors remained orphan until the identification of their endogenous ligand isolated several years later from stomach extracts (Tatemoto et al., 1998). The corresponding gene codes for a prepropeptide of 77 aminoacids (Figure 2) containing a signal peptide which addresses the proapelin to the secretory pathway. Then, the propeptide would be processed by proteolytic cleavage at the level of three basic doublets and thus generate apelin fragments of different size: apelin 36, apelin 17 and apelin 13.

3. Apelin signalling and cell lineages

3.1 Embryogenesis and cell lineages

Although each animal model displays its own advantages and limits, their embryonic development displays strong similarities in the signalling pathways orchestrating and coordinating the migration and the differentiation of the different cell progenitors.

In a schematic manner, embryogenesis begins with a totipotent cell, the fertilized egg, and ends up with the emergence of the different cell types of adult organism and their assembly into specialized organs. The first event is the formation of three embryonic layers, ectoblast, endoblast and mesoblast, which will generate separately and specifically their own cell subpopulations. Gastrulation is the downstream event by which the spatial organization of the cell layers is rearranged with ectoblast outside the embryo, endoblast inside, and the mesoblast in between. Then, each embryonic layer is subdivided into different areas of presumptive territories associated with the commitment of cell progenitors and the formation of cell lineages. Migration of these progenitors and their *in situ* differentiation will initiate the formation of organ *primordia* where several cell subtypes will assemble in a spatial and temporal manner in order to form the outline of the future organ.

Mesoblast provides the best example of this regional subdivision linked to the emergence of pluripotent progenitors before the induction of specific cell lineages (Figure 3). Progressively after gastrulation, the mesoblast splits into several territories with different cell potency : axial, paraxial, intermediate and lateral plate mesoderms.

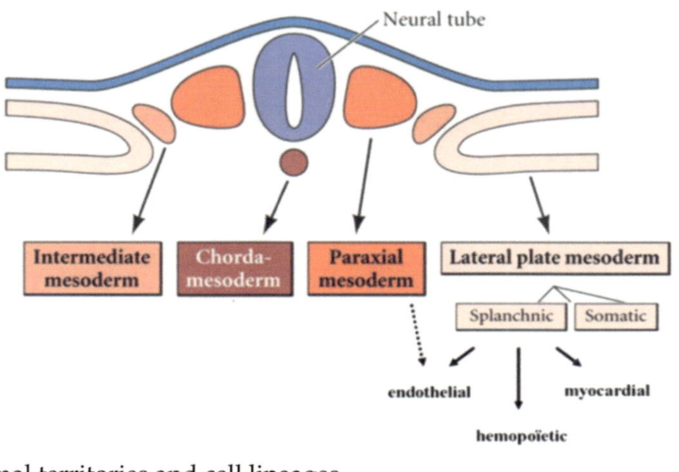

Fig. 3. Mesodermal territories and cell lineages.
After gastrulation, the mesoblast becomes subdivided into different regions that will generate separate progenitors at the origin of specific lineages. A particular emphasis is given for the derivatives of lateral plate mesoderm and the corresponding cell lineages.

The axial mesoderm strictly corresponds to the formation of a transient structure, the notochord. Segmentation of the paraxial mesoderm gives rise to the somites, which then develop into three distinct regions : the sclerotome, which becomes mesenchymal and is the precursor of vertebrae and ribs, the myotome which forms myoblasts (muscle precursors), and the dermatome precursor of subcutaneous tissue and skin. The intermediate mesoblast is linked to the formation of the urogenital system and serves as the origin of the kidney and gonads. The lateral plate mesoderm is composed of two layers : the **somatopleure** close to the ectoblast is involved in the formation of connective tissue and bones; the **splanchnopleure** lying on the endoblast takes part in the formation of the cardiovascular system *via* three cell lineages corresponding to hemopoïetic, myocardial and endothelial progenitors. In most lineages, commitment of mesodermal cells precedes migration of lineage progenitors to the sites of organ formation. At their final destination, these progenitors *in situ* differentiate into the corresponding cell subtype.

3.2 Apelin signalling and endothelial lineage

In Xenopus (Devic et al., 1996) as well as in mouse (Devic et al., 1999) and zebrafish (Scott et al., 2007), mRNA expression of apelin receptors is observed very early and is localized in the ventrolateral mesoderm at gastrulation stage. Accordingly, apelin receptor may represent a **marker** of the different lineages originating from this mesodermal territory, such as hemopoïetic, myocardial and endothelial lineages. In addition, apelin signalling may exert a function in the migration or commitment of these cell progenitors.

Our preliminary experiments on the expression pattern of apelin receptor gene from the gastrulation stage to the larval stage clearly established that its later expression was intimately associated with the formation of blood vessels and heart (Devic et al., 1996). Indeed, the transcripts initially in the ventrolateral mesoderm are later detected in the lateral plate mesoderm at neurula stage and then in procardiac tube and forming blood vessels at larval stage. Interestingly, gene expression is strictly localized in the inner endothelium layer. Accordingly, we proposed that receptor gene expression traces an endothelial lineage originating from uncommitted mesodermal cells and ending in endothelial cells (Figure 4).

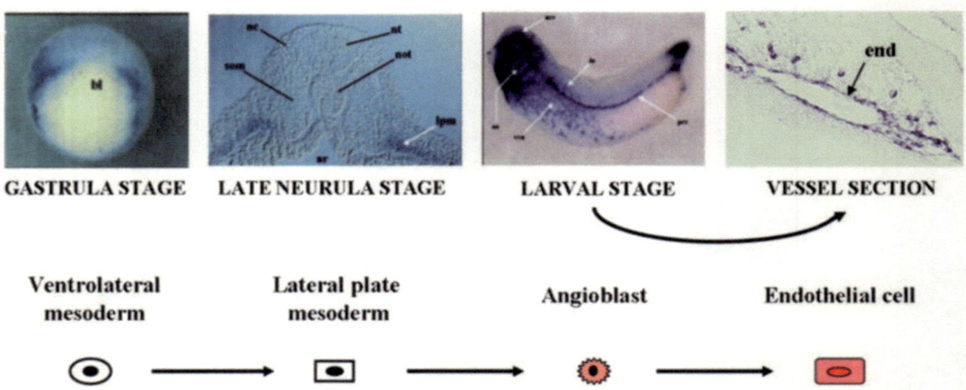

Fig. 4. Expression of apelin receptor and endothelial lineage.
The upper part shows the localization of apelin receptor transcripts determined by *in situ* hybridization during embryogenesis. The arrow from the larval stage shows that the vessel section was performed at this stage. The lower part is a schematic drawing of the cell events occurring along the endothelial lineage.

Indeed, a subpopulation of mesodermal cells are first specified in endothelial progenitors, the angioblasts, which migrate to the sites of vessel formation. Organization of these endothelial progenitors in tubules and their *in situ* differentiation into endothelial cells correspond to the formation of the primary vascular network.
The involvement of apelin signalling in this endothelial lineage is further confirmed by the blockade of gene expression using morpholino antisense probes during Xenopus embryogenesis. This experimental inhibition of the ligand or the receptor mRNA leads to a disruption of embryonic vessels (Cox et al., 2006). An additional proof of the vascular role of apelin signalling is revealed by the phenotype of apelin-deficient mice, which corresponds to a retardation of the development of some retinal vessels (Kasai et al., 2008).

3.3 Apelin signalling and other lineages

As mentioned before, mesodermal cells from the ventrolateral region not only contributes to endothelial lineage but also to hemopoïetic and myocardial lineages. This common origin together with the pluripotency of these cells have fully challenged the idea of lineage specificity. Indeed, the concept of hemangioblast, a bipotential progenitor of hemopoïetic and endothelial lineages has been validated by various approaches (Jaffredo et al., 2000; Mandal et al., 2004).
Interestingly, such a link between the three lineages has been revealed by a study performed on apelin signalling in Xenopus. Gene inactivation of apelin or its receptor results in a severe phenotype, which corresponds to an attenuated expression of endothelial, hemopoïetic and myocardial markers (Inui et al., 2006). Such an unexpected relationship between endothelial and myocardial lineages is further illustrated by the concomitant expression of apelin receptors by myocardial and endothelial progenitors. But apelin receptors are not simple markers and they also play an active role in the migration of myocardial progenitors : functional inactivation of apelin receptors impairs the migration of these progenitors to the sites of heart formation (Scott et al., 2007; Zeng et al., 2007).
A very recent study has identified a common precursor of endothelial and mesenchymal cells, which was named mesenchymoangioblast. Previously, a late mesodermal precursor expressing Flk1 receptor was characterized by its potential to differentiate into endothelial cells, blood cells and mesenchymal cells (Minasi et al., 2002). However, the early precursors of this Flk1+ mesoderm subpopulation remained to be isolated. Surprisingly, it is expression of apelin receptor that identifies this mesodermal population of early bipotential progenitors giving rise to mesenchymal stem cells and angioblasts (Vodyanik et al., 2010).

4. Apelin signalling and the formation of blood vessels

4.1 The embryonic formation of blood vessels

The vasculature of the body is a highly organized system and its anatomy is referred to as the vascular tree. Blood vessels are ranging from the simplest structures with a single endothelial layer, the capillaries, to complex structures, the large vessels made of different cell layers (endothelial, mural and elastic), such as aorta (Figure 5).
The first step of blood vessel formation corresponds to the formation of the primary vascular network and is named vasculogenesis (Figure 6). This process results from the migration of endothelial progenitors, the angioblasts, to the sites of vessel formation and their *in situ* differentiation into endothelial cells. Concomitantly, these angioblasts or endothelial cells assemble together and participate in the formation of tubes or cord-like structures, which will later acquire a lumen.

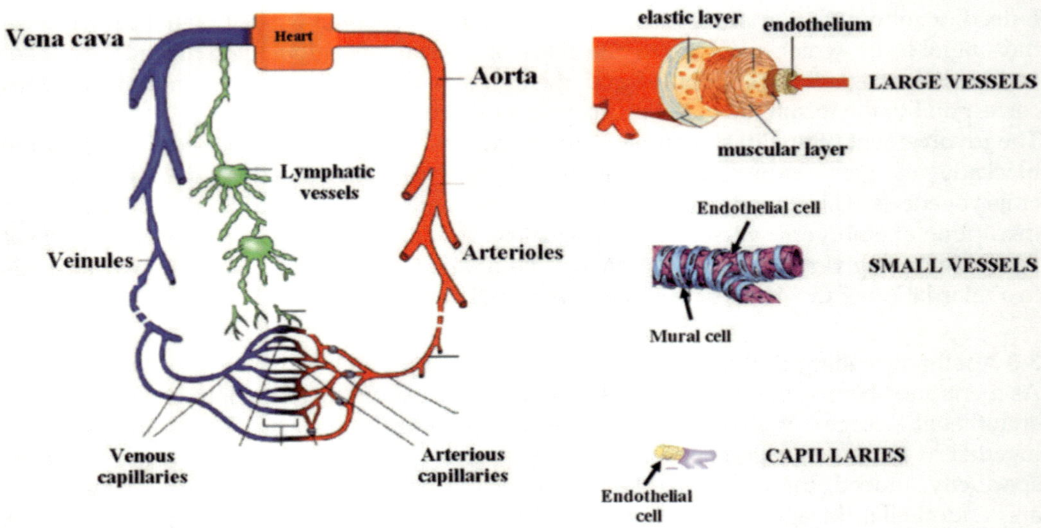

Fig. 5. Vascular tree and vessels.
The left part shows the different arterio-venous elements of the vascular system and includes lymphatic vessels. On the right part are given the vascular structure and layer organization related to the different sizes of vessel .

The second step involves extension and remodelling of the primary network and is named angiogenesis (Figure 6). This process is driven by the increase of embryo size, which requires an adjustment of the oxygen demand and nutrient supply by the vessels to the increased metabolism of the growing tissues and organs. The stability of this mature network is provided by the recruitment of mural cells (pericytes or smooth muscle cells), which will form the second layer of the vessels and induce the quiescence of endothelial cells. Indeed, the proliferation index of the endothelial cells is the lowest among the various cell types of the body.

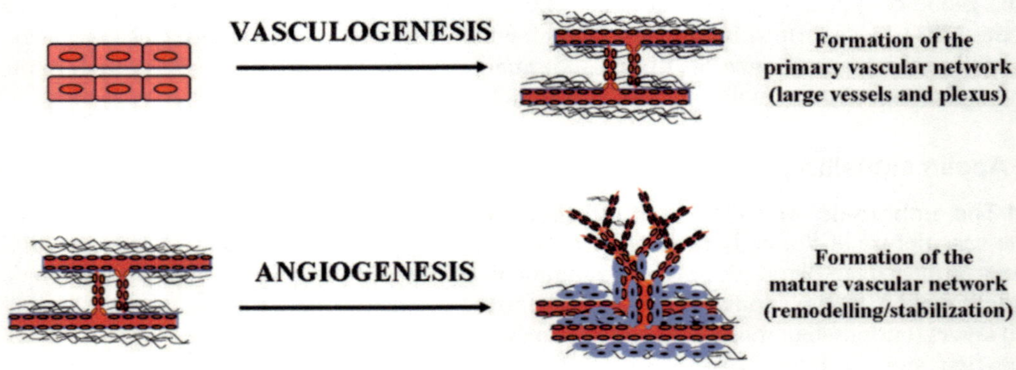

Fig. 6. The two steps of vessel formation.
The upper part describes the first step called vasculogenesis that is involved in the formation of the primary vascular network. The lower part concerns the second step called angiogenesis, which corresponds to remodelling of the primary network and the formation of the mature vascular tree.

All these cell events are orchestrated and finely tuned by various signalling pathways. The VEGF pathway plays a crucial role during vasculogenesis as well as angiogenesis (Ferrara et al., 2003). Through activation of the VEGFR2, Vascular Endothelial Growth Factor (VEGF) induces the differentiation, proliferation and migration of endothelial cells during vessel formation. In the maturation process, the recruitment of mural cells is mediated by the PDGF pathway (Figure 7).

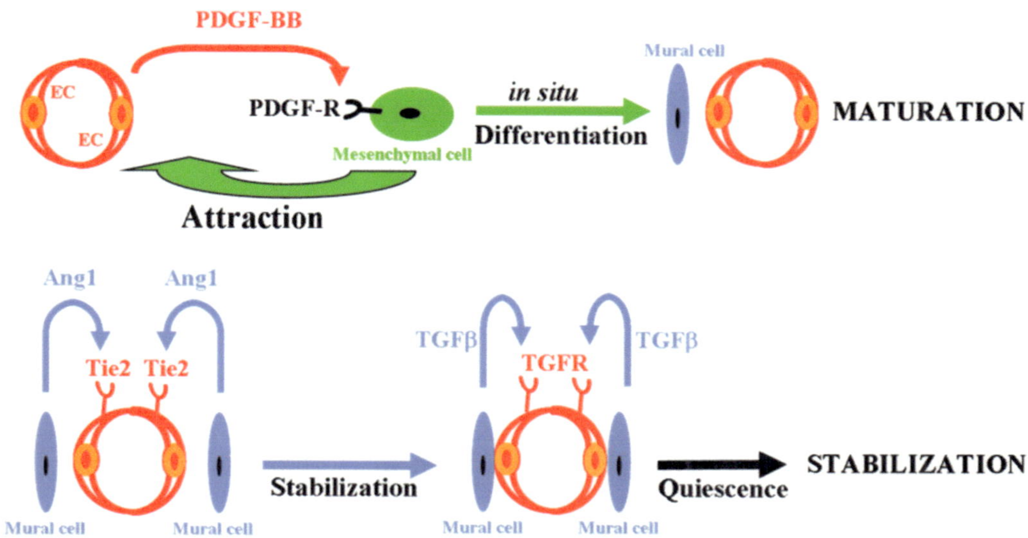

Fig. 7. Maturation and stabilization of vascular structures.
The upper part corresponds to the maturation phase. Endothelial cells (EC) secrete PDGF-BB, which is a chemotactic factor for mesenchymal cells. This migration is followed by an *in situ* differentiation into mural cell. The lower part describes the stabilization phase. The first event is release of angiopoïetin 1 (Ang1) by the mural cell, which then activates its Tie2 receptor expressed at the surface of the endothelial cell. Ang1 pathway strongly reinforces the association between the two cell types. The second event corresponds to the TGFβ-induced quiescence of the endothelial cell whereby TGFβ released by mural cell activates its receptor expressed by EC.

Endothelial cells release Platelet-Derived Growth Factor (PDGF-BB), thereby attracting the mural cells which express its cognate receptors (Lindahl et al., 1997). The stabilization of the vascular structure is accomplished by a strong interaction between the endothelial cell and the mural cell, which relies on angiopoïetin pathway (Figure 7). Cell adhesion between these two cell types results from the angiopoïetin 1 release by mural cell, which then stimulates its Tie2 receptor expressed at the surface of the endothelial cell (Dumont et al., 1994; Sato et al., 1995; Suri et al., 1996). This constitutive dialogue *via* the ligand and its receptor is the molecular basis of the stabilization of vessel structure. The concomitant quiescence of the endothelial cell is induced by another factor, TGFβ which is secreted by the mural cell and activates its receptor expressed at the surface of the endothelial cell (Figure 7).
In parallel, the different caliber of blood vessels must be precisely controlled during the maturation process. Again, the Ang1/Tie2 pathway is a potent regulator of the enlargement of vessel caliber (Suri et al., 1996; Cho et al., 2005; Thurston et al., 2005).

In the adult organism, physiological and pathological situations are associated with regression or extension of the vascular network (see Figure 12). These changes are initiated by disruption of the mural/endothelial interaction, which involves an another angiopoïetin, Ang2, acting as an endogenous antagonist of Tie2 receptor (Maisonpierre et al., 1997). Accordingly, the alternate ligand use in the same pathway either reinforce or disrupt a cell interaction, which is central in the stability of blood vessel and remodelling of the vascular network.

4.2 Apelin signalling and the formation of blood vessels

So far, there is no clear evidence that apelin signalling plays a role during vasculogenesis. As mentioned before, expression of apelin receptors traces the endothelial lineage from unspecified mesodermal cells to differentiated endothelial cells (Devic et al., 1996, 1999). In Xenopus, blockade of gene expression gave controversial results, from full suppression of three cell lineages (Inui 2006) to a restricted angiogenesis defect (Cox et al., 2006). In addition, the phenotypes of gene invalidation in mouse are very mild, ranging from retardation of the formation of retinal network (Kasai et al., 2008) to a mild consequence on blood pressure (Ishida et al., 2004). On the other hand, it has been proposed that the severity of the vascular defects may depend on the genetic background of the invalidated mice. Accordingly, although apelin receptor is a marker of vasculogenesis, it may be a dispensable actor in this early process of vessel formation.

As far as angiogenesis is concerned, the role of apelin signalling is well documented, and a large body of evidence reveals that apelin displays all the properties required for an angiogenic factor. As mentioned before, the endothelial cell is the first cell type which appears during vasculogenesis and represents the organizing center of the vascular structure during angiogenesis. In the adult, proliferation or apoptosis of endothelial cells is also the cell basis of tissue plasticity and vessel remodelling : their proliferation induces extension of the vasculature and their apoptosis promotes regression of the vasculature (see figure 12). Accordingly, it can be assumed that any angiogenic factor must have its cognate receptors expressed by the endothelial cell and that stimulation of these receptors by their ligand promotes a proliferative response. In addition to the characterization of receptor expression by the endothelial cells (Devic et al., 1996, 1999), our laboratory was the first to show that apelin induces the phosphorylation of ERK proteins (Masri et al., 2002, 2006) and behaves as a mitogenic peptide for primary cultured umbilical endothelial cells (Masri et al., 2004) (Figure 8). At the same time, another group published that apelin induces the proliferation of an immortalized endothelial cell line (Kasai et al., 2004).

These results at the cell level have been extended to the whole vessel : a large number of *in vitro* assays such as matrigel plug assay (Kasai et al., 2004) and *in vivo* studies such as ectopic apelin expression (Cox et al., 2006) has strongly confirmed the angiogenic activity of apelin peptide (Figure 8). Altogether, these data clearly demonstrate that apelin signalling fulfil at the protein level all the criteria required for an angiogenic pathway and represents a significant actor of physiological angiogenesis during embryonic development.

A more recent study has revealed that apelin also regulates the caliber size of blood vessels by inducing their enlargement (Kidoya et al., 2008). Indeed, we also observed a similar phenomenon during tumour neoangiogenesis, as overexpression of apelin not only promotes an extension of the vascular network but also increases the number of large vessels (Sorli et al., 2007)(see figure 14). Since the Ang1/Tie2 pathway regulates enlargement of vessel caliber, a link between this pathway and apelin signalling was expected. Indeed, Ang1 was found to upregulate apelin gene expression in endothelial cells (see figure 17) and apelin expression was increased in Ang1 overexpressing transgenic mice (Kidoya et al., 2008).

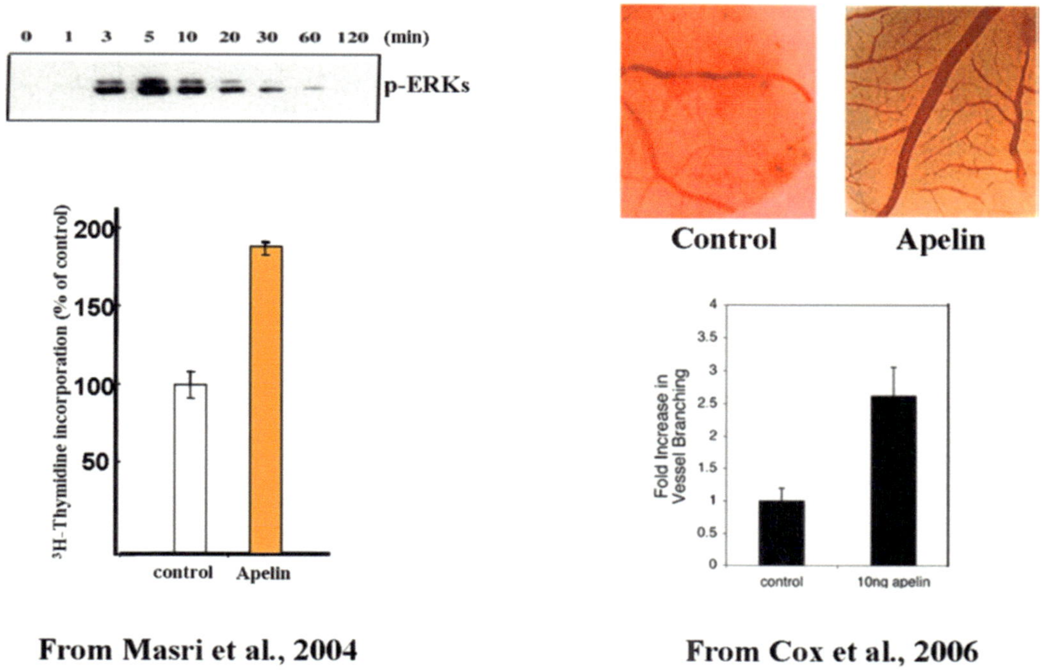

Fig. 8. Mitogenic and angiogenic activities of apelin.
The upper left panel shows the time dependent phosphorylation of ERKs induced by apelin (determined by immunoblotting). The lower left panel corresponds to thymidine incorporation, an index of cell proliferation, measured in umbilical endothelial cells in the absence or presence of apelin. The upper right panel shows the angiogenic effect of apelin in the chorioallantoïc membrane of chicken. The lower right panel gives the quantitative analysis based on the calculation of vessel branching.

4.3 Hypoxia and angiogenesis

In the adult, the vascular system is quiescent and the proliferative index of endothelium is very low. Several physiological or pathological stimuli may promote the proliferation of endothelial cells and reactivate the angiogenic process. But this reactivation should logically recapitulate the same events and use the same mechanisms operating during the embryonic formation of blood vessels.
The formation of retinal vessels has been the cornerstone for two fruitful hypothesis. A first observation was that extension of the retinal vasculature strictly follows the centrifugal extension of the nervous retina (see Figure 10). A proposed explanation was that a vasotropic substance released by neural cells exerted a chemotactic and proliferative effect on the vessel. As it was already discussed, the concept of a vasotropic substance is simply the ancient denomination for an angiogenic factor. More interestingly, the second hypothesis was on the nature of the driving force initiating the angiogenic process. Indeed, extension of nervous tissue increased the oxygen demand and thus the

growth-induced hypoxia might be the stimulus for reactivating angiogenesis. However, the molecular link between hypoxia and the angiogenic factor remained to be characterized.

In 1992, Shweiki et al. described that hypoxia was able to upregulate the expression of the VEGF gene, the major angiogenic factor. Such an upregulation of VEGF gene was also reported in the hypoxic regions inside tumours (Plate et al., 1993). Consequently, it established a direct relationship between hypoxia and angiogenesis and provided an explanation for the adjustment of the vascular network to the increased oxygen consumption resulting from tissue growth (Figure 9).

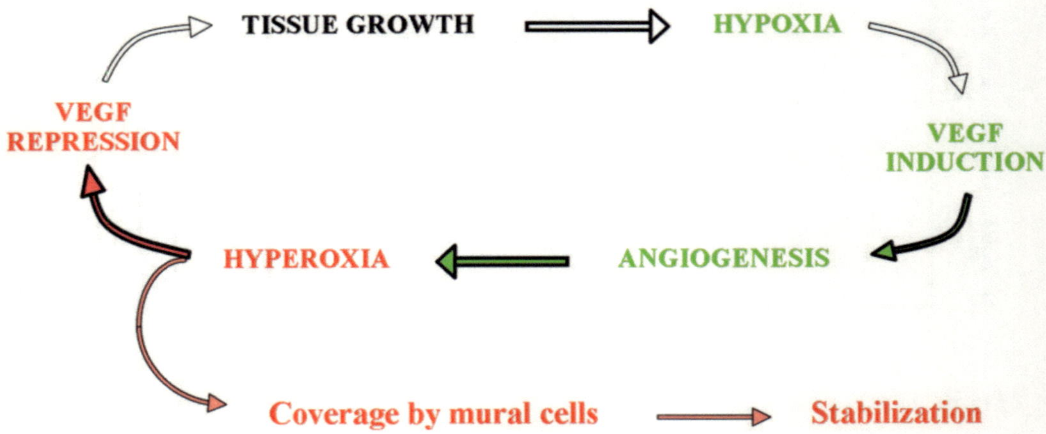

Fig. 9. Hypoxia and vascular homeostasis.
The figure illustrates the relationship between expression levels of VEGF gene and adjustment of vessel number during the angiogenic phase. Tissue growth generates tissue hypoxia which induces expression of VEGF gene. VEGF stimulates the formation of new vessels which become excendentary and thus the subsequent hyperoxia downregulates VEGF expression. Different cycles of VEGF upregulation and downregulation occur until formation of the definitive network, which is then stabilized by coverage of the endothelial layer by mural cells.

More recently, the various intermediates involved in the transduction of the hypoxic stimulus and overexpression of the VEGF gene have been characterized. The central protein in this regulation is a heterodimeric transcription factor named Hypoxia Inducible Factor 1 (HIF-1). The protein complex consists of a hypoxically inducible subunit HIF-1α and a constitutively expressed subunit HIF-1β (Wang et al., 1995). Although the transcription and the synthesis of HIF-1α are constitutive, it has in normoxia a short half-life due to its targeting to and degradation by the proteasome (Wang et al., 1995). Several post-translational modifications are necessary for targeting the α subunit to the proteasome, but the most relevant is hydroxylation by prolyl hydroxylases (Masson et al., 2001). Indeed, this oxygen-dependent modification initiates a complex series of molecular interactions which ultimately end up in subunit ubiquitination and proteasome degradation. As hydroxylation requires sufficient oxygen levels, this reaction is inhibited in hypoxic conditions. Consequently, HIF-1α becomes stabilized and translocates to the nucleus where its

dimerization with HIF-1β generates a transcriptionally active HIF complex (Huang et al., 1996; Kallio et al., 1997).
As many transcription factors, HIF complex selectively recognizes and binds to discrete DNA sequences located in the promoter or enhancer elements of target genes. These consensus sequences have been identified and named Hypoxia Responsive Elements (HRE)(Semenza et al., 1994). As it could be anticipated, the presence of HRE was detected in the genes encoding angiogenic factors, notably that of the VEGF gene (Levy et al., 1995).
All these results provide a very simple and adaptative mechanism, which ensures a direct causal relationship between hypoxia and angiogenesis in order to achieve a fine homeostasis between oxygen demand of growing tissues and oxygen supply by blood vessels.

4.4 Hypoxia and apelin expression

The corollary of the previous findings is that the gene encoding any angiogenic factor has to contain HRE sequences and to be induced by hypoxia.
In view of the angiogenic role of apelin, several studies have been performed in order to characterize an upregulation of apelin gene under hypoxic conditions. The results clearly showed that hypoxia increases apelin mRNA levels via HIF protein in different cell types, but with varying intensity ranging from a 2-fold to 30-fold increase (Cox et al., 2006; Sorli et al., 2007; Ronkainen et al., 2007; Glassford et al., 2007; Sheikh et al., 2008; Eyries et al., 2008).
In addition, gene upregulation at the mRNA level is accompanied by a subsequent increase of peptide synthesis and secretion (Ronkainen et al., 2007; Sheikh et al., 2007).
A bioinformatic analysis has corroborated these experimental data by identifying the presence of putative HRE sequences in apelin gene (Cox et al., 2006). In addition, a functional HRE was mapped within the first intron by reporter constructs and the binding of HIF-1α to this HRE was demonstrated by chromatin immunoprecipitation (Eyries et al., 2008).

4.5 Retinal vessels and endothelial subpopulations

The retinal vasculature of mouse represents an interesting model system used for the study of blood vessel formation. In contrast to the embryo, the vessels are readily accessible as their formation occurs postnatally, and whole mount retinas allow to characterize the spatio-temporal expression of genes by *in situ* hybridization or proteins by immunohistochemistry (Figure 10).
Interestingly, a study on the formation of retinal vessels has revealed the presence of two distinct endothelial populations, which differ in their morphology and their functional specialization (Gerhardt et al., 2003). Endothelial cells at the front of migrating vessels, called tip cells, possess cell protrusions (filipodia) and their function is specialized in the decoding of chemotactic signals and polarized extension of the network (Figure 11). Underneath, the other endothelial cells, called stalk cells, do not have a particular morphology and their function is to proliferate in order to provide the new endothelial cells that are required for extension of retinal vasculature (Figure 11).

4.6 Apelin signalling and endothelial subpopulations

In this retinal model, the spatio-temporal expression of apelin and its receptor displays a very interesting pattern (Saint-Geniez et al., 2002). Ligand and receptor mRNA expression is selectively upregulated during the formation of retinal vessels and downregulated after maturation and stabilization of the retinal network (Figure 10). Again, these observations confirm that apelin signalling is activated during the angiogenic phase and desactivated when the vessels become quiescent.

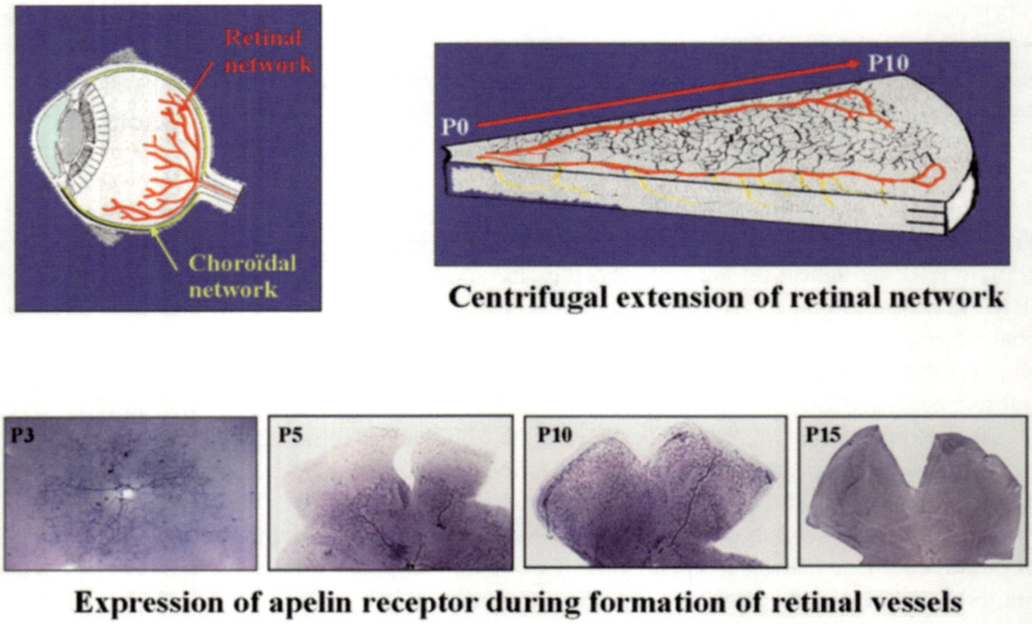

Fig. 10. Retinal model and apelin signalling.
Upper panel illustrates the vascular networks of retina. Nervous retina is irrigated by two vascular networks, the retinal vessels and the choroïdal vessels. In mouse, the postnatal formation of the retinal network proceeds in a centrifugal manner from optic disk at birth to the periphery at postnatal day 10 (P10). Lower panel shows the spatio-temporal expression of apelin receptor gene during formation of retinal vessels. Note the downregulation observed after the onset and stabilization of the retinal network at P15.

In addition, expression pattern of apelin and its receptor was spatially different, even inside the endothelium (Saint-Geniez et al., 2002) (Figure 11). Apelin expressing endothelial cells were localized at the leading edge of the retinal vascular network, whereas receptor expression was mainly observed in the underneath endothelial cells. Using a specific fluorescent lectin for labelling endothelial cells, we detected high apelin expression levels in tip cells easily recognized by their filipodia. On the other hand, we were unable to detect apelin receptor transcripts in this first row of endothelial cells, whereas receptor expression was observed in the other endothelial cells of the vascular network, previously referred to as stalk cells (Sorli et al., 2006).
According to this expression pattern and the proposed role of VEGF as the chemotactic signal for the polarized extension of the vascular network, we proposed a model in which apelin would be the downstream molecule transmitting the proliferative signal from tip cells to downstream stalk cells.

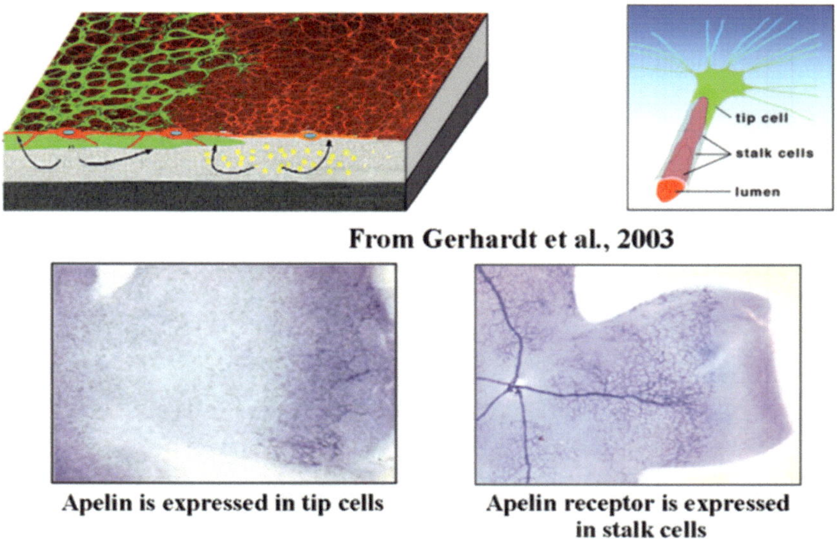

Fig. 11. Apelin signalling and endothelial subpopulations.
The upper left panel is a schematic representation of the formation of retinal vessels (green) driven by extension of the nervous retina (red). The upper right panel is a magnification of the migrating front of endothelial cells, with the tip cells at the leading edge and the underneath stalk cells. The lower part shows the gene expression of apelin in the front at the tip cell level (left) and apelin receptor underneath in the stalk cells (right).

5. Apelin signalling and vascular pathologies

5.1 Vascular pathologies

Besides its involvement in vessel formation, the endothelial cell is the integration center of vascular plasticity. The integration of various environmental stimuli defines its cellular response, proliferation or apoptosis, which will lead to the corresponding modification of the vascular network, extension or regression (Figure 12).
According to the previously described role of Ang2, its expression is increased by these activating environmental stimuli in order to disrupt vessel stability and initiate the vascular plasticity (Maisonpierre et al., 1997). The qualitative change of vascular network depends on the growth factor (GF) "context", which will orientate the vascular system to either extension in high GF levels or regression in low GF levels (Figure 12).
These two different modifications of the vascular network divide the vascular pathologies into ischemic diseases associated with a vessel defect and neovascularisation linked pathologies associated with a vessel excess. The ischemic pathologies primarily concern two organs, heart and leg muscle. The treatment of these pathologies requires therapeutic angiogenesis which is achieved by the use of receptor agonists of angiogenic pathways. The opposite pathologies that are characterized by neovascularisation represent more frequent and severe diseases, such as tumour neovascularisation, diabetic retinopathies and age-related macular degeneration (AMD). For them, the therapeutic strategy is the administration of antiangiogenic molecules, such as antagonists of receptors mediating angiogenic signals.

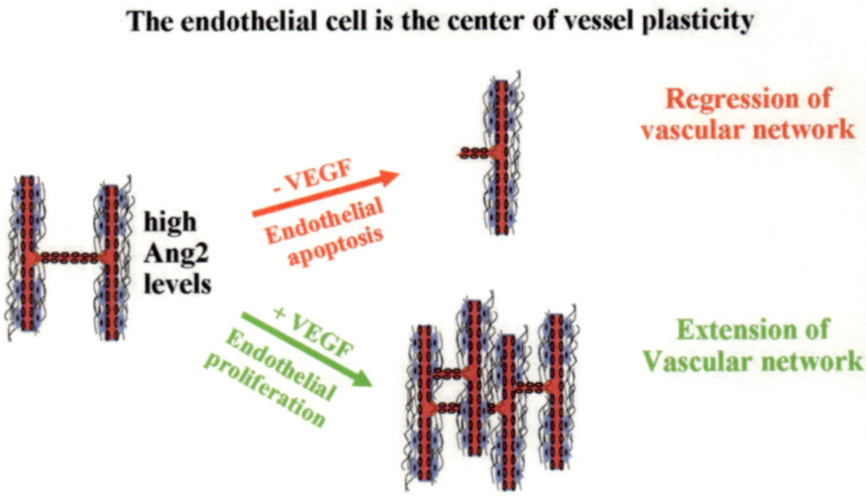

Fig. 12. Vessel plasticity and vascular pathologies.
The figure illustrates how the growth factor "context" drives the fate of vessel plasticity. Destabilization is first initiated by expression of angiopoïetin2 (Ang2) which disrupts the interaction between EC and mural cells. Low levels of VEGF induce endothelial apoptosis and lead to regression of vascular network, a situation that occurs in the ischemic diseases. In high levels of VEGF, endothelial cells proliferate, new vessels are formed, and this abnormal extension of the vascular network recapitulates what happens in the neovascular pathologies.

5.2 Apelin signalling and vascular pathologies

5.2.1 Apelin signalling and ischemic pathologies

Apelin is a potent activator of cardiac contractility (Szokodi et al., 2002), suggesting the possible involvement of apelin signalling in ischemic heart failure. Such a role is corroborated by the upregulation of apelin receptor gene in left ventricule and an increase of apelin plasma levels in left ventricular dysfunction. In addition, apelin released from the endothelium of the coronary arteries would locally act in a paracrine manner on myocardial tissue (Chen et al., 2003).

Similar data have been obtained in ischemic heart failure : total myocardial amounts of apelin and apelin receptor proteins increase in compensation of heart failure (Atluri et al., 2007). The stimuli (including tissue hypoxia) associated with heart failure upregulate transcription of ligand and receptor genes and increase their protein expression (Sheikh et al., 2008). As apelin signalling is activated for protecting the heart against ischemia injury, the effect of infusion of the endogenous agonist apelin13 was tested after ischemia. Interestingly, apelin not only limited infarct size but also improved cardiac postischemic mechanical recovery (Rastaldo et al., 2011)(Figure 13).

In limb ischemia, therapeutic angiogenesis using local delivery of genes encoding angiogenic factors or systemic injection of their recombinant proteins has proved its efficiency in promoting the revascularization of ischemic territories. In a mouse model of limb ischemia, coadministration of apelin and VEGF improves the revascularisation of the ischemic limb and induces an increase of vessel size (Kidoya et al., 2010) (Figure 13).

5.2.2 Apelin signalling and tumour neovascularisation

As formulated by Folkman in 1971, the survival and growth of solid tumours depend on the formation of new vessels, which are necessary to compensate the increased oxygen demand of this highly proliferative tissue. The corollary of this hypothesis is that tumoral cells secrete angiogenic factors in order to attract host vessels and create tumoral vessels. As described for physiological angiogenesis, one activating stimulus is hypoxia occuring in the center of tumour because of its maximal distance from vessel supply.

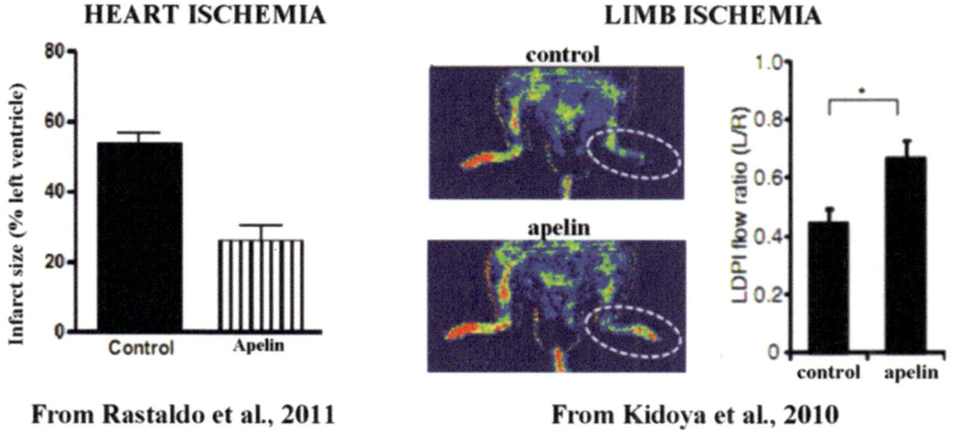

Fig. 13. Effects of apelin in ischemic diseases.
The left part shows that the size of infarct trigged on isolated hearts is reduced by perfusion of apelin. The right part describes the angiogenic effects of apelin in limb ischemia model. Doppler images demonstrates an increase of blood flow following apelin gene transfer, which is confirmed by quantification of laser Doppler-monitored blood flow measurements.

In order to address whether apelin secreted by tumoral cells may possess a neoangiogenic activity, we developed two mouse models of tumour neovascularisation. Stable clones of B16 melanoma cells and TS/A mammary adenocarcinoma cells overexpressing apelin were created and their tumour growth was compared to that of clones transfected with the empty plasmid (named mock) (Sorli et al., 2006, 2007). Apelin overexpression clearly accelerates tumour growth *in vivo* and this effect results from a paracrine action on endothelial cells of host vessels (Sorli et al., 2007) (Figure 14). In addition, the number of small vessels decreases whereas that of large vessels increases (Figure 14).

The pathological relevance of apelin signalling in tumour neovascularisation was suggested by gene upregulation of apelin and its receptor in malignant gliomas, which represent highly vascularised tumours (Kälin et al., 2007). Moreover, a cancer profiling array revealed a clear upregulation of apelin gene in one third of human adenocarcinomas (Sorli et al., 2007). As far as pulmonary tumours are concerned, a recent study has confirmed that apelin mRNA levels were significantly increased in human non-small cell lung cancer (Berta et al., 2010). Interestingly, the extent and the frequency of apelin gene upregulation in a cancer profiling array was dependent on the tissue origin of the tumoral cells, the highest frequency being observed in colon (50%) and pancreas (71%)(Figure 15).

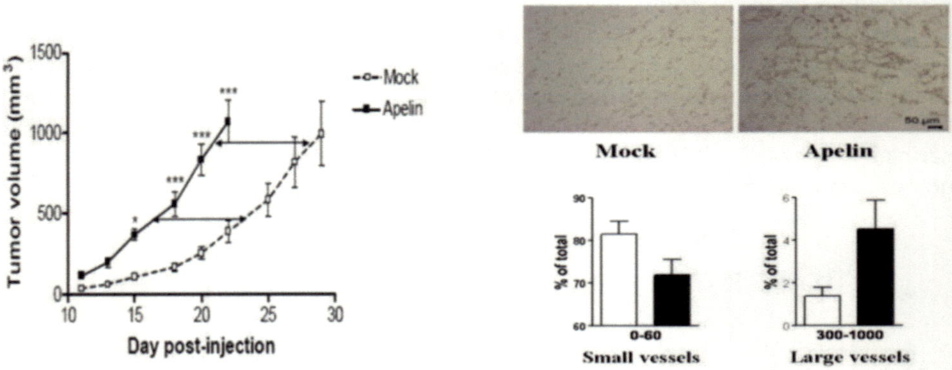

From Sorli et al., 2007

Fig. 14. Apelin overexpression and tumour neovascularisation.
Left part illustrates the acceleration of *in vivo* tumour growth in tumours derived from tumoral cells overexpressing apelin when compared to the animals injected with empty plasmid transfected tumoral cells (Mock). Overexpressed apelin acts on the vascular component of the tumour by increasing the total number of vessels as revealed by immunostaining with the endothelial marker CD31 (upper right panel). As shown in lower right panel, it also modifies caliber of the neovessels by increasing the number of large vessels (300-1000 μ^2).

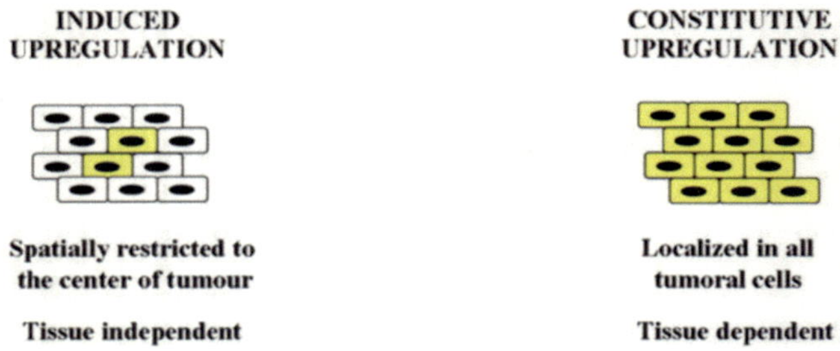

INDUCED UPREGULATION
Spatially restricted to the center of tumour
Tissue independent
CONSTITUTIVE UPREGULATION
Localized in all tumoral cells
Tissue dependent

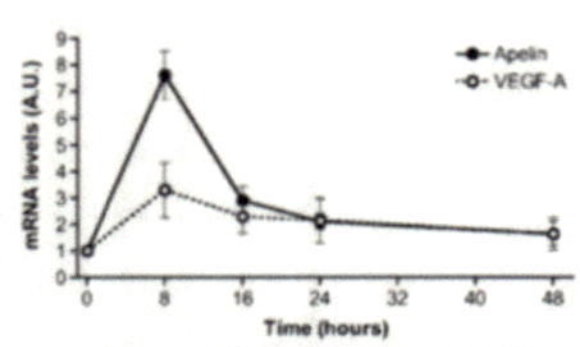

	Stomach	Colon	Pancreas
Frequency	20%	50%	71%
Amplitude	1.77 ± 0.18	1.90 ± 0.20	3.51 ± 0.83

From Sorli et al., 2007 **From Sorli et al., 2007**

Fig. 15. Upregulation of apelin gene and tumour growth.
Two distinct modes of gene upregulation can occur during tumour neovascularisation. The hypoxia-induced upregulation is spatially restricted (yellow cells) and likely independent of the tissue origin of tumoral cells. The lower left panel shows the hypoxia-induced upregulation of apelin gene in TS/A mammary adenocarcinoma cells. On the other hand, gene upregulation may result from the genetic changes leading to the cell transformation and thus becomes constitutive (right panel). In this situation, upregulation is ubiquitous (yellow cells) and tissue dependent. As shown in the lower right panel, upregulation of apelin gene varies in frequency and amplitude from one tumoral tissue to the other.

As the center of all tumours is hypoxic, the tissue dependent variations of gene upregulation may rather be a direct consequence of the genetic alteration(s) occurring in the genomic DNA (Figure 15). Indeed, activation of oncogenes or inactivation of tumour suppressors also leads to the upregulation of genes coding for angiogenic factors (Rak et al., 1995; Brugarolas & Kaelin, 2004). However, such a link between genetic alterations and upregulation of apelin gene remains to be established. Altogether, the variable upregulation of apelin gene observed in human tumours may result from both genetic factors and environmental stimuli, including hypoxia.

5.2.3 Apelin signalling and retinal neovascularisation

Nervous retina is irrigated by two vascular networks, the retinal and the choroïdal vasculatures. The postnatal formation of retinal vessels begins at birth from the optic disk and the growing network extends in a centrifugal manner to the periphery of the retina. During formation of retinal vessels, gene expression of apelin receptor on pup retinas traces the centrifugal extension of this retinal network (see figure 10).

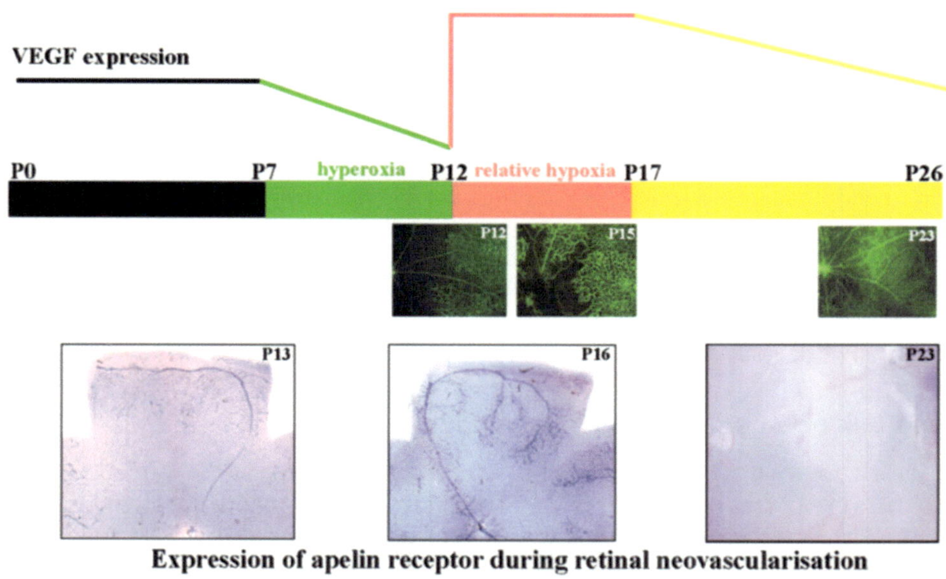

Fig. 16. Apelin signalling and retinal neovascularisation.
The upper part describes the different steps in the mouse model of retinal neovascularisation. Hyperoxia is made between postnatal day 7 (P7) and postnatal day 12 (P12) (green) and leads to vessel regression as shown by a fluorescent marker of endothelial cells. Return to normoxia corresponds to a relative hypoxia, which triggers the formation of neovessels in a centripetal manner (see the network labelled with the fluorescent probe at P15). From P17 to P23, extensive remodelling allows recovery from hyperoxia and the retinal network becomes normal (see the network labelled with the fluorescent probe at P23). In the upper part are reported the concomitant variations of VEGF levels occurring at the different steps of neovascularisation. The lower part shows the variations of apelin receptor expression from return to normoxia until normalization of the vascular network

The main pathological defect affecting this retinal network is observed in diabetic patients where there is an abnormal formation of new retinal vessels leading to cecity. A mouse model reproducing the main features of this retinal pathology has enabled the dissection of the molecular and cellular events during the onset and the development of this pathology (Smith et al., 1994) (Figure 16). Hyperoxia treatment of seven-day-old mice for five days induces endothelial apoptosis and decreases the number of retinal vessels. Return to normoxia corresponds to a form of hypoxia in the mid-retina, which upregulates the expression of VEGF gene and promotes the formation of new vessels. According to the localization of the ischemia in the mid-retina, the normal centrifugal extension of the forming vasculature is reversed to a pathological centripetal extension.

Interestingly, expression of apelin receptor gene is highly upregulated in these new vessels and strictly follows the centripetal extension of the retinal network (Sorli et al., 2006). In addition, quantitative analysis of apelin mRNA levels revealed a very strong increase (31-fold) during the hypoxic phase; furthermore, in apelin-deficient mice, there was no increase in capillary density and abnormal vessels during the hypoxic phase (Kasai et al., 2010). Accordingly, systemic or local injection of antagonists of apelin receptor is a promising therapy for blocking the formation of new retinal vessels in diabetic retinopathies.

5.2.4 Apelin signalling and choroïdal neovascularisation

A frequent pathology of the elderly is the formation of excedentary vessels in the choroïdal network, which is appropriately named age-related macular degeneration (AMD). At the present time, there is no immunohistochemical study on the expression of apelin or its receptor in endothelial cells lining the choroïdal vessels. The only related observation is that apelin induces the proliferation of the immortalized choroïdal endothelial cell line RF/6A, suggesting expression of apelin receptors at the surface of these cells (Kasai et al., 2004). However, it can be assumed that the pathological angiogenesis occuring in AMD should involve the same angiogenic pathways that are activated in the formation of new vessels in the retinal network, including apelin signalling pathway.

6. Cross-talk between angiogenic pathways

Apelin clearly represents one of the various actors that participate in the formation of blood vessels. However, the respective role of each angiogenic pathway, including apelin signalling, as well as their synergic activity, remains to be elucidated.

A specific property of apelin peptide seems to be its ability to regulate the caliber of blood vessels by promoting the formation of enlarged vessels during physiological (Kidoya et al., 2008) and pathological (Sorli et al., 2007) angiogenesis. This vessel enlargement is one mechanism by which hemodynamic changes can respond to an increase of oxygen demand. But this effect may be indirect and due to the consequences of its cross-talk with other angiogenic pathways such as that of VEGF and Ang1 (Figure 17). The initiator of the angiogenic process would be VEGF, which induces the sprouting of endothelial cells from mature vessels and the concomitant expression of apelin receptor. Then, Ang1 *via* activation of its Tie2 receptor triggers the expression of apelin, which becomes secreted outside the endothelial cell. The synergic action of VEGF and apelin would lead to the proliferation of EC and the formation of cell to cell contacts. In this scenario, the precise role of apelin signalling would concern the mobilization of ECs in this assembly process and the construction of enlarged vessels.

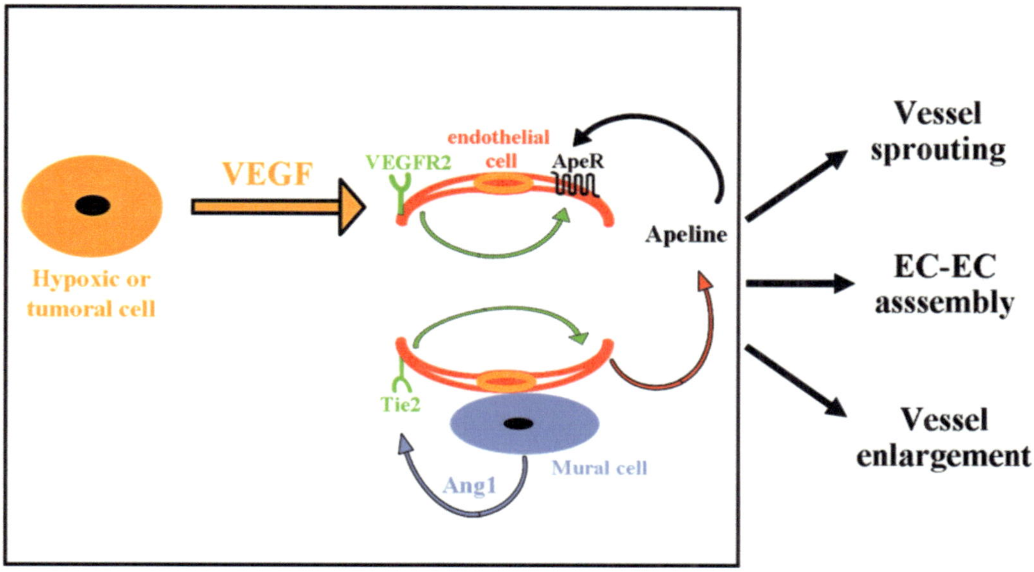

Fig. 17. Cross-talk between angiogenic pathways.
An hypoxic cell or a tumoral cell expresses VEGF gene in an induced or constitutive manner, respectively. Then VEGF activates its receptor expressed by the endothelial cell (EC), leading to increased expression of apelin receptor. In parallel, Ang1 expressed by mural cells stimulates its receptor Tie2 at the surface of EC, leading to an increased release of apelin. Apelin released in the medium can activate the same EC in an autocrine manner or another EC in a paracrine manner. All these interactions between angiogenic pathways result in vascular changes, such as vessel sprouting, EC-EC assembly and vessel enlargement.

As mentioned before, induction of genes encoding angiogenic factors by hypoxia clearly represents a crucial mechanism leading to an increased oxygen supply *via* extension of vascular network. However, the level of hypoxia-induced upregulation in the same cell or in various cell subtypes may vary from one angiogenic factor to the other, and thus their respective contribution may be modulated by the nature of the environmental stimuli. A same statement can be applied to tumoral cells where the genetic alterations may constitutively upregulate some angiogenic genes. In addition, as this transformation-induced modifications are extended to all tumoral cells and not restricted to the center of the tumour, the role of a specific angiogenic factor may be selectively enhanced, thereby representing a more relevant therapeutic target.

7. Therapeutic potential of apelin signalling in vascular diseases

As mentioned before, upregulation of the expression of apelin and its receptor is intimately associated with the angiogenic phase of vessel formation or remodelling, and their downregulation follows maturation and stabilization of the vascular structures.
These two observations have theoretical and practical consequences for vascular pharmacology. First, it reveals that apelin signalling is not a constitutive pathway at the vascular level and rather behaves as an adaptative pathway only activated during vascular

plasticity. Second, the expression upregulation and activation of apelin signalling during angiogenesis imply that receptor antagonists may selectively target the proliferative ECs forming neovessels without affecting the quiescent ECs of stabilized vessels. These spatio-temporal properties of apelin signalling should strongly decrease the secondary effects induced by pharmacological agents targetting this pathway.

At the present time, the pharmacology of this emergent pathway is still in its infancy. The first molecule reported to act on apelin receptors was ALX40-4C, but this peptide had a very low affinity for apelin receptors and a much better affinity for CXCR4 receptors (Zhou et al., 2003). A first receptor antagonist resulting from substitution of apelin C-terminal amino acid was reported to block the hypotensive effects of apelin (Lee et al., 2005). However, in several other assays, this compound behaved as an agonist (Medhurst et al., 2003; Fan et al., 2003). Very recently, bicyclic peptides have been shown to represent competitive antagonists of apelin receptor (Macaluso et al., 2011). All these compounds are promising antiangiogenic agents for the treatment of pathological neovascularisations.

So far, only one agonist molecule has been identified and characterized (Iturrioz et al., 2010). This nonpeptidic compound behaves as an agonist in various assays, but it does not have a very high affinity. Nevertheless, it provides the structural basis for the design of better molecules which will be used for extension of the vascular network and revascularization in ischemic diseases.

8. Conclusion and perspectives

The discovery of new receptors and their ligands open avenues for the design of novel pharmacological agents for treating human diseases. In addition, if the discovered signalling pathway is linked to severe diseases or lethal pathologies, the development of structurally related drugs such as nonpeptidic agonists or antagonists will lead to important clinical applications.

Apelin signalling fulfils these criteria as this emerging pathway represents a promising therapeutic target and requires the design of new pharmacological molecules in order to treat the prime causes of human mortality, such as heart failure and cancer, or severe diseases, such as limb ischemia and AMD.

9. Acknowledgment

I acknowledge the scientific contribution of all the people having worked with me : E. Devic, L. Paquereau, K. Rizzoti, B. Knibiehler, S. Bodin, M. Saint-Geniez, H. Mazarguil, N. Morin, M. Cornu, L. Pedebernade, L. Van den Berghe, C. Sorli, S. Le Gonidec and B. Masri.

I thank I. Scott and D. Stainier (UCSF, California) for our fruitful collaboration and our excellent scientific exchanges.

10. References

Atluri P, Morine KJ, Liao GP, Panlilio CM, Berry MF, Hsu VM, Hiesinger W, Cohen JE & Joseph Woo Y. (2007). Ischemic heart failure enhances endogenous myocardial apelin and APJ receptor expression. *Cell Mol Biol Lett.* 12, 127-38.

Audigier, Y . (2006). Apelin Receptor. *AfCS-Nature Molecule Pages* doi:10.1038/mp.a000304.01

Berta J, Kenessey I, Dobos J, Tovari J, Klepetko W, Jan Ankersmit H, Hegedus B, Renyi-Vamos F, Varga J, Lorincz Z, Paku S, Ostoros G, Rozsas A, Timar J. & Dome B. (2010). Apelin expression in human non-small cell lung cancer: role in angiogenesis and prognosis. *J Thorac Oncol.* 5, 1120-9.

Brugarolas, J. & Kaelin JrWG. (2004). Dysregulation of HIF and VEGF is a unifying feature of the familial hamartoma syndromes. *Cancer Cell* 6, 7–10.

Chen, M. M., Ashley, E. A., Deng, D. X., Tsalenko, A., Deng, A., Tabibiazar, R., Ben-Dor, A., Fenster, B., Yang, E., King, J. Y., *et al.* (2003). Novel role for the potent endogenous inotrope apelin in human cardiac dysfunction. *Circulation* 108, 1432-1439.

Cho CH, Kim KE, Byun J, Jang HS, Kim DK, Baluk P, Baffert F, Lee GM, Mochizuki N, Kim J, Jeon BH, McDonald DM. & Koh GY. (2005). Long-term and sustained COMP-Ang1 induces long-lasting vascular enlargement and enhanced blood flow. *Circ Res.* 97, 86-94.

Devic, E., Paquereau, L., Vernier, P., Knibiehler, B. & Audigier, Y., (1996). Expression of a new G protein-coupled receptor X-msr is associated with an endothelial lineage in Xenopus laevis. *Mech. Dev.* 59, 129–140.

Devic, E., Rizzoti, K., Bodin, S., Knibiehler, B. & Audigier, Y., (1999). Amino acid sequence and embryonic expression of msr/apj, the mouse homolog of Xenopus X-msr and human APJ. *Mech. Dev.* 84, 199–203.

Dumont, D.J., Gradwohl, G., Fong, G.H., Puri, M.C., Gertsenstein, M., Auerbach, A. & Breitman, M.L. (1994). Dominant-negative and targeted null mutations in the endothelial receptor tyrosine kinase, tek, reveal a critical role in vasculogenesis of the embryo. *Genes Dev.* 8, 1897–1909.

Eyries M, Siegfried G, Ciumas M, Montagne K, Agrapart M, Lebrin F. & Soubrier F. (2008). Hypoxia-induced apelin expression regulates endothelial cell proliferation and regenerative angiogenesis. *Circ Res.* 103, 432-40.

Fan X, Zhou N, Zhang X, Mukhtar M, Lu Z, Fang J, DuBois GC. & Pomerantz RJ. (2003). Structural and functional study of the apelin-13 peptide, an endogenous ligand of the HIV-1 coreceptor, APJ. *Biochemistry.* 242, 10163-8.

Ferrara N, Gerber HP. & LeCouter J. (2003). The biology of VEGF and its receptors. *Nat Med.* 6, 669-76.

Folkman J. (1971). Tumor angiogenesis:therapeutic implications. *N Engl J Med* 285, 1182–1186.

Gerhardt H, Golding M, Fruttiger M, Ruhrberg C, Lundkvist A, Abramsson A, Jeltsch M, Mitchell C, Alitalo K, Shima D. & Betsholtz C. (2003) VEGF guides angiogenic sprouting utilizing endothelial tip cell filopodia.. *J Cell Biol* 161, 1163-1177.

Glassford AJ, Yue P, Sheikh AY, Chun HJ, Zarafshar S, Chan DA, Reaven GM, Quertermous T. & Tsao PS. (2007). HIF-1 regulates hypoxia- and insulin-induced expression of apelin in adipocytes.*Am J Physiol Endocrinol Metab.* 293, E1590-6.

Huang LE, Arany Z, Livingston DM. & Bunn HF. (1996). Activation of hypoxia-inducible transcription factor depends primarily upon redox-sensitive stabilization of its alpha subunit. *J Biol Chem.* 271, 32253-9.

Inui, M., Fukui, A., Ito, Y. & Asashima, M. (2006). Xapelin and Xmsr are required for cardiovascular development in Xenopus laevis. *Dev Biol.* 298, 188-200.

Ishida J., Hashimoto T., Hashimoto Y., Nishiwaki S., Iguchi T., Harada S., Sugaya T., Matsuzaki H., Yamamoto R., Shiota N., Okunishi H., Kihara M., Umemura S.,

Sugiyama F., Yagami K. I., Kasuya Y., Mochizuki N. & Fukamizu A. (2004) Regulatory roles for apj, a seven-transmembrane receptor related to angiotensin-type 1 receptor in blood pressure *in vivo*. *J Biol Chem.* 279, 26274-9.

Iturrioz X, Alvear-Perez R, De Mota N, Franchet C, Guillier F, Leroux V, Dabire H, Le Jouan M, Chabane H, Gerbier R, Bonnet D, Berdeaux A, Maigret B, Galzi JL, Hibert M. & Llorens-Cortes C. (2010). Identification and pharmacological properties of E339-3D6, the first nonpeptidic apelin receptor agonist. FASEB J. 5, 1506-17.

Jaffredo, T., Gautier, R., Brajeul, V. & Dieterlen-Lievre, F., (2000). Tracing the progeny of the aortic hemangioblast in the avian embryo. *Dev. Biol.* 224, 204–214.

Kälin RE, Kretz MP, Meyer AM, Kispert A, Heppner FL. & Brändli AW. (2007). Paracrine and autocrine mechanisms of apelin signaling govern embryonic and tumor angiogenesis. *Dev Biol.* 305, 599-614..

Kallio PJ, Okamoto K, O'Brien S, Carrero P, Makino Y, Tanaka H. & Poellinger L. (1998). Signal transduction in hypoxic cells: inducible nuclear translocation and recruitment of the CBP/p300 coactivator by the hypoxia-inducible factor-1alpha. EMBO J. 17, 6573-86.

Kasai, A., Shintani, N., Oda, M., Kakuda, M., Hashimoto, H., Matsuda, T., Hinuma, S. & Baba, A. (2004). Apelin is a novel angiogenic factor in retinal endothelial cells. *Biochem. Biophys. Res. Commun.* 325, 395–400.

Kasai A, Shintani N, Kato H, Matsuda S, Gomi F, Haba R, Hashimoto H, Kakuda M, Tano Y. & Baba A. (2008). Retardation of retinal vascular development in apelin-deficient mice. *Arterioscler Thromb Vasc Biol.* 28, 1717-22.

Kasai A, Ishimaru Y, Kinjo T, Satooka T, Matsumoto N, Yoshioka Y, Yamamuro A, Gomi F, Shintani N, Baba A. & Maeda S. (2010). Apelin is a crucial factor for hypoxia-induced retinal angiogenesis. *Arterioscler Thromb Vasc Biol.* 30, 2182-7.

Kidoya H, Ueno M, Yamada Y, Mochizuki N, Nakata M, Yano T, Fujii R. & Takakura N. (2008). Spatial and temporal role of the apelin/APJ system in the caliber size regulation of blood vessels during angiogenesis. *EMBO J.* 27, 522-34.

Kidoya H, Naito H. & Takakura N. (2010). Apelin induces enlarged and nonleaky blood vessels for functional recovery from ischemia. *Blood.* 115, 3166-74.

Lee DK, Saldivia VR, Nguyen T, Cheng R, George SR. & O'Dowd BF. (2005). Modification of the terminal residue of apelin-13 antagonizes its hypotensive action. *Endocrinology.* 2005 146, 231-6.

Levy AP, Levy NS, Wegner S. & Goldberg MA. (1995). Transcriptional regulation of the rat vascular endothelial growth factor gene by hypoxia. *J Biol Chem.* 270, 13333-40.

Lindahl P, Johansson BR, Levéen P. & Betsholtz C. (1997). Pericyte loss and microaneurysm formation in PDGF-B-deficient mice. *Science* 277, 242-5.

Macaluso NJ, Pitkin SL, Maguire JJ, Davenport AP. & Glen RC. (2011). Discovery of a competitive apelin receptor (APJ) antagonist.ChemMedChem. 6, 1017-23.

Maisonpierre PC, Suri C, Jones PF, Bartunkova S, Wiegand SJ, Radziejewski C, Compton D, McClain J, Aldrich TH, Papadopoulos N, Daly TJ, Davis S, Sato TN. & Yancopoulos GD.(1997). Angiopoietin-2, a natural antagonist for Tie2 that disrupts in vivo angiogenesis. Science 277, 55-60.

Mandal, L., Banerjee, U. & Hartenstein, V. (2004). Evidence for a fruit fly hemangioblast and similarities between lymph-gland hematopoiesis in fruit fly and mammal aorta–gonadal–mesonephros mesoderm. *Nat. Genet.* 36, 1019–1023.

Masri B, Knibiehler B. &Audigier Y (2005). Apelin signalling: a promising pathway from cloning to pharmacology. *Cell Signal* 17, 415-26.

Masri B, Lahlou H, Mazarguil H, Knibiehler B. & Audigier Y (2002). Apelin (65-77) activates extracellular signal-regulated kinases via a PTX-sensitive G protein. *Biochem Biophys Res Commun* 290, 539-45.

Masri B, Morin N, Cornu M, Knibiehler B. &Audigier Y (2004). Apelin (65-77) activates p70 S6 kinase and is mitogenic for umbilical endothelial cells. *Faseb J* 18, 1909-11.

Masri B, Morin N, Pedebernade L, Knibiehler B. & Audigier Y (2006). The apelin receptor is coupled to Gi1 or Gi2 protein and is differentially desensitized by apelin fragments. *J Biol Chem*. 281, 18317-26.

Masson N, Willam C, Maxwell PH, Pugh CW & Ratcliffe PJ. (2001). Independent function of two destruction domains in hypoxia-inducible factor-alpha chains activated by prolyl hydroxylation. *EMBO J*. 20, 5197-206.

Medhurst AD, Jennings CA, Robbins MJ, Davis RP, Ellis C, Winborn KY, Lawrie KW, Hervieu G, Riley G, Bolaky JE, Herrity NC, Murdock P & Darker JG. (2003). Pharmacological and immunohistochemical characterization of the APJ receptor and its endogenous ligand apelin. J Neurochem. 84, 1162-72.

O'Dowd, B.F., Heiber,M., Chan, A., Heng, H.H., Tsui, L.C., Kennedy, J.L., Shi, X., Petronis, A., George, S.R. & Nguyen, T., (1993). A human gene that shows identity with the gene encoding the angiotensin receptor is located on chromosome 11. *Gene* 136, 355–360.

Plate KH, Breier G, Millauer B, Ullrich A. & Risau W (1993). Up-regulation of vascular endothelial growth factor and its cognate receptors in a rat glioma model of tumor angiogenesis. *Cancer Res* 53, 5822-7.

Rak J, Mitsuhashi Y, Bayko L, Filmus J, Shirasawa S, Sasazuki TL. & Kerbel RS. (1995). Mutant ras oncogenes upregulate VEGF/VPF expression : implications for induction and inhibition of tumor angiogenesis. Cancer Res 55, 4575–4580.

Rastaldo R, Cappello S, Folino A. & Losano G. (2011). Effect of apelin-apelin receptor system in postischaemic myocardial protection: a pharmacological postconditioning tool? *Antioxid Redox Signal*. 14, 909-22.

Ronkainen VP, Ronkainen JJ, Hänninen SL, Leskinen H, Ruas JL, Pereira T, Poellinger L, Vuolteenaho O. & Tavi P. (2007). Hypoxia inducible factor regulates the cardiac expression and secretion of apelin. *FASEB J*. 21, 1821-30.

Saint-Geniez M, Masri B, Malecaze F, Knibiehler B. & Audigier Y. (2002). Expression of the murine msr/apj receptor and its ligand apelin is upregulated during formation of the retinal vessels. *Mech Dev* 110, 183–186.

Sato, T.N., Tozawa, Y., Deutsch, U., Wolburg-Buchholz, K., Fujiwara, Y., Gendron-Maguire, M., Gridley, T., Wolburg, H., Risau, W. & Qin, Y. (1995). Distinct roles of the receptor tyrosine kinases Tie-1 and Tie-2 in blood vessel formation. *Nature* 376, 70–74.

Scott IC, Masri B, D'Amico LA, Jin SW, Jungblut B, Wehman AM, Baier H, Audigier Y. & Stainier DY. (2007). The g protein-coupled receptor agtrl1b regulates early development of myocardial progenitors. *Dev Cell*. 12, 403-13.

Semenza GL, Roth PH, Fang HM. & Wang GL. (1994). Transcriptional regulation of genes encoding glycolytic enzymes by hypoxia-inducible factor 1. *J Biol Chem*. 269, 23757-63.

Sheikh AY, Chun HJ, Glassford AJ, Kundu RK, Kutschka I, Ardigo D, Hendry SL, Wagner RA, Chen MM, Ali ZA, Yue P, Huynh DT, Connolly AJ, Pelletier MP, Tsao PS, Robbins RC. & Quertermous T.(2008). In vivo genetic profiling and cellular localization of apelin reveals a hypoxia-sensitive, endothelial-centered pathway activated in ischemic heart failure. *Am J Physiol Heart Circ Physiol.* 294, H88-98.

Shweiki D, Itin A, Soffer D. & Keshet E (1992). Vascular endothelial growth factor induced by hypoxia may mediate hypoxia-initiated angiogenesis. *Nature* 359, 843-5.

Smith LE, Wesolowski E, McLellan A, Kostyk SK, D'Amato R, Sullivan R. & D'Amore PA. (1994). Oxygen-induced retinopathy in the mouse. *Invest Ophthalmol Vis Sci* 35, 101-111.

Sorli SC, van den Berghe L, Masri B, Knibiehler B. & Audigier Y. (2006). Therapeutic potential of interfering with apelin signalling. *Drug Discov Today* 11, 1100–1106.

Sorli SC, Le Gonidec S, Knibiehler B. &Audigier Y. (2007). Apelin is a potent activator of tumour neoangiogenesis. *Oncogene*. 26, 7692-9.

Suri C, Jones PF, Patan S, Bartunkova S, Maisonpierre PC, Davis S, Sato TN. & Yancopoulos GD. (1996). Requisite role of angiopoietin-1, a ligand for the TIE2 receptor, during embryonic angiogenesis. *Cell*. 87, 1171-80.

Szokodi, I., Tavi, P. & Foldes, G., Voutilainen-Myllyla, S., Ilves, M., Tokola, H., Pikkarainen, S., Piuhola, J., Rysa, J., Toth, M. & Ruskoaho, H. (2002). Apelin, the novel endogenous ligand of the orphan receptor APJ, regulates cardiac contractility. *Circ. Res.* 91, 434–440.

Tatemoto, K., Hosoya, M., Habata, Y., Fujii, R., Kakegawa, T., Zou, M.X., Kawamata, Y., Fukusumi, S., Hinuma, S., Kitada, C., Kurokawa, T., Onda, H. & Fujino, M. (1998). Isolation and characterization of a novel endogenous peptide ligand for the human APJ receptor. *Biochem. Biophys. Res. Commun.* 251, 471–476.

Thurston G, Wang Q, Baffert F, Rudge J, Papadopoulos N, Jean-Guillaume D, Wiegand S, Yancopoulos GD. & McDonald DM. (2005). Angiopoietin 1 causes vessel enlargement, without angiogenic sprouting, during a critical developmental period. *Development*. 132, 3317-26.

Vodyanik MA, Yu J, Zhang X, Tian S, Stewart R, Thomson JA. & Slukvin II. (2010). A mesoderm-derived precursor for mesenchymal stem and endothelial cells. *Cell Stem Cell*. 7, 718-29.

Wang GL, Jiang BH, Rue EA. & Semenza GL. (1995). Hypoxia-inducible factor 1 is a basic-helix-loop-helix-PAS heterodimer regulated by cellular O2 tension. *Proc Natl Acad Sci U S A*. 92, 5510-4.

Zeng XX, Wilm TP, Sepich DS. & Solnica-Krezel L. (2007). Apelin and its receptor control heart field formation during zebrafish gastrulation. *Dev Cell*. 12, 391-402.

Zou MX, Liu HY, Haraguchi Y, Soda Y, Tatemoto K. & Hoshino H. (2000). Apelin peptides block the entry of human immunodeficiency virus (HIV). *FEBS Lett*. 473, 15-8.

Part 2

Endothelial Progenitor Cells

5

Regulation of Endothelial Progenitor Cell Function by Plasma Kallikrein-Kinin System

Yi Wu[1] and Jihong Dai[1,2]
[1]*Sol Sherry Thrombosis Research Center,*
Temple University School of Medicine, , Philadelphia, PA,
[2]*Cyrus Tang Hematology Research Center,*
Sooochow University, Suzhou,
[1]*USA*
[2]*China*

1. Introduction

Circulating endothelial progenitor cells (EPCs) are a hierarchy of pluripotent cells in peripheral blood capable of differentiating into mature endothelial cells destined for blood vessel formation[1]. These cells have the ability to be mobilized to the site of vascular injury or tissue ischemia, and they differentiate into mature endothelial cells. They are a major determinant of a postnatal mechanism for neovascularization and vascular remodeling, and play an important role in endothelial cell and vessel maintenance. However, in patients with atherosclerosis and cardiovascular disease, EPCs are reduced in number and impaired in function, which are negatively correlated with the atherosclerotic risk factors, and may contribute to vascular dysfunction[2]. For example, the frequency of circulating EPCs is reduced 50% in patients with coronary artery disease, and their EPCs display an impaired migratory response[3]. Moreover, although EPCs successfully restore endothelial function and enhance angiogenesis after tissue ischemia in animal models, the clinical administration of EPCs to patients has had limited efficacy. It is likely that EPCs are targets of endogenous angiogenic inhibitors elaborated in the setting of atherosclerosis. Therefore, understanding the factors and mechanisms that affect EPC function and number may not only provide new insights into the pathogenesis of vasculogenesis, but also promote development of specific therapies to ultimately correct EPC dysfunction and prevent progression of atherosclerosis.

The plasma kallikrein–kinin system (KKS) consists of the proteins factor XII, prekallikrein, and high molecular weight kininogen (HK)[4-5]. This system widely participates in maintenance of the cardiovascular phenotype, and displays multiple physiologic and pathophysiological activities, such as blood pressure adjustment, modulation of thrombosis, regulation of endothelial cell function and angiogenesis. Plasma HK, which is synthesized and released from the liver, is a major component of the KKS and is responsible for the association of the KKS with cell surface. The plasma membrane of endothelial cells is an important site for the assembly and activation of the KKS. Activation of the KKS is triggered *in vivo* by tissue destruction or by thrombus development, and results in cleavage of HK by kallikrein and generation of two-chain HK (HKa) and a nonapeptide bradykinin[6]. HKa and bradykinin differentially regulate the endothelial cell function, HKa is antiangiogenic, but bradykinin is of proangiogenesis. Unlike HK, HKa exposes its domain 5 to the surface on cleavage, thereby acquiring a function of antiadhesion. This antiadhesive property enables HKa to inhibit endothelial cell proliferation and to induce endothelial apoptosis on extracellular proteins, thus it exhibits potent antiangiogenic activity[7-8]. The inhibitory effect of HKa may result from its inhibition of $\alpha v\beta 3$ integrin function[7, 9], and induction of apoptosis via its interaction with uPAR[10]. Because EPCs express high levels of uPAR, which is a HKa receptor, HKa may exerts inhibitory effect on EPCs[11]. In this chapter, we summarize the recent observations that the KKS regulates EPC function.

Human EPCs can be isolated from adult circulation. If EPCs are to be defined as true progenitor cells with postnatal vasculogenic potential, they should give rise to differentiated progeny with the capacity for vessel formation. In a 3D collage gel, EPCs, but not differentiated endothelial cells such as HAECs and HUVECs, exhibit strong capacity to form vacuoles and tubes in the presence of VEGF[11], suggesting that EPCs are unique in their stronger potential for tubular morphogenesis and are more sensitive to physiological growth factor stimulation.

2. HKa inhibits EPC tube formation via suppression of MMP-2 activation

In the process of neovascularization, invasive endothelial cells secrete MMPs to remodel the extracellular matrix (ECM) and the basal lamina – an important physical barrier between the endothelial and connective tissue[12]. Two members of the MMP family, MMP-2 and MMP-9, display the highest enzymatic activities against the ECM components important in angiogenesis. MMP-2 and MMP-9 participate in the mobilization of EPCs. Recently we have demonstrated that MMP-2 is selectively required for VEGF-stimulated vasculogenic differentiation of EPCs[11]. In the conditioned culture media of EPCs embedded in 3D collagen gel, VEGF selectively stimulated the secretion and activation of MMP-2, but not MMP-9, and VEGF-stimulated proMMP-2 expression and secretion are time-dependent, the secreted proMMP-2 was meanwhile converted into active form. As the specific inhibitor of MMP-2 (444244), but not MMP-9 (444278), concentration-dependently attenuated VEGF-stimulated tube formation by EPCs, suggesting the role of MMP-2 activities in tube formation by EPCs[11]. The requirement of MMP-2 and MMP-9 expression for the tube formation by EPCs is examined by specific siRNA oligonucleotides. VEGF-stimulated tube formation by EPCs was almost completely suppressed by gene silencing of MMP-2, but not of MMP-9. [11] Thus, MMP-2 is selectively required for EPC formation of tubular structures. The inhibitory effect of the MMP-2 gene silencing was more potent than that of the enzymatic inhibitor, suggesting that both the catalytic activity and expression of MMP-2 are necessary for the tubular morphogenesis of EPCs. Indeed, pro-MMP-2 possesses enzymatic activity-independent functions; its interaction with cell-surface proteins may mediate intracellular activation signals. Collectively, as found by using pharmaceutical inhibitors and gene ablation, both the enzymatic activity and expression of MMP-2 are required for EPC differentiation. This observation is consistent with a recent study showing that MMP-2 deficiency reduces the functional activities of EPCs, leading to impaired vasculogenesis[12]. Interestingly, HKa markedly inhibits conversion of pro-MMP-2 to active MMP-2 in EPCs without affecting MMP-2 secretion. In a 3D culture system, HKa significantly decreased VEGF-stimulated tube formation by EPCs at the concentrations of 30 nmol /L, 100 nmol/ L and 300 nmol/ L, representing cleavage of HK of 4.5%, 15% and 45%, respectively, which occurs in experimental inflammatory bowel disease and arthritis[11]. VEGF-stimulated MMP-2 secretion and activation was not detected in the medium of EPCs cultured on collagen-coated surfaces, suggesting that MMP-2 is not involved in EPC activation in a 2D system and HKa did not inhibit endothelial cell function on collagen surfaces[11]. Thus, HKa inhibition of tube formation by EPCs in collagen gel (3D system) reveals a novel mechanism for HKa antiangiogenic activities. In a 3D system MMP-2 activation is very likely a target for HKa. The MMP-2 Inhibitor I (444244) markedly abolished the gelatinolytic activity of both proform and active form of MMP-2. In contrast, HKa treatment only reduced the ratio of active MMP-2 to total MMP-2 (44 ± 7% at 0 nmol/ L vs. 27 ± 6% and 19 ± 3% at 100 and 300 nmol/L, respectively)[11]. Thus, HKa inhibits the conversion of pro-MMP-2 to active MMP-2. In purified systems, HKa at 300 nmol/ L did not have apparent inhibition of catalytic activity of MMP-2 and the conversion of pro-MMP-2 to MMP-2[11]. Collectively, HKa inhibits the conversion of pro-MMP-2 to MMP-2 in EPCs without directly affecting MMP-2 secretion and activity. Because the KKS activation may occur during inflammation and thrombosis, HKa as an activation product of this system may induce EPC dysfunction in the setting of pathological conditions.

3. HKa inhibition of MMP-2 activation in EPCs is dependent on αvβ3 integrin

EPCs expressed a high level of αvβ3 integrin and HKa downregulates αvβ3 integrin ligand binding affinity in endothelial cells, whether HKa inhibition of MMP-2 activation through αvβ3 integrin was examined by an αvβ3CS-1 cell line[11]. In the αvβ3-CS-1 cells, the expression of αvβ3 integrin on the cell surface increased MMP-2 activation and stimulated autoactivation of MMP-2 (conversion of 64-kDa to 62-kDa form)[11]. However, in the presence of HKa, the conversion of proMMP-2 to 64- and 62-kDa forms was inhibited. Correspondingly, HKa blocked the formation of avβ3 integrin-MMP2 complex in EPCs cultured in a 3D gel[11]. HKa disrupts the association between αvβ3 integrin and proMMP-2, which may account for its inhibition of MMP-2 activation[11]. MMP-2-αvβ3 integrin interaction is critical for angiogenesis, HKa inhibition of MMP-2 activation and tube formation by EPCs is, at least in part, mediated through αvβ3 integrin. Therefore, HKa inhibits the vasculogenic differentiation by EPCs via the suppression of MMP-2 activation, which is a novel activity of the KKS system. The inhibitory effect of HKa on MMP-2 is dependent on the presence of αvβ3 integrin and mediated by the dissociation of proMMP-2 from αvβ3 integrin. The αvβ3 integrin is necessary for vascular cell survival, proliferation and invasion during angiogenesis. MMP-2 activation has been suggested to be downstream of αvβ3 integrin activation, and MMP2- αvβ3 binding is required for proper MMP2 function. This is consistent with MMP-2 and αvβ3 integrin being colocalized in a particular membrane fraction caveolae, which enhances cellular protrusive activity. The disruption of MMP-2 binding to αvβ3 integrin blocks angiogenesis *in vitro* and *in vivo;* αvβ3 integrin may serve as an MMP-2 receptor in the process of angiogenesis. In endothelial cells, the primary target for HKa is uPAR and HKa occupancy of uPAR disrupts uPAR-αvβ3 integrin complex formation. HKa seems to indirectly modulate αvβ3 integrin function. In platelets, αIIbβ3 integrin also interacts with the C-terminal hemopexin-like domain of MMP-2, suggesting that MMP-2 is likely to be associated with β3 subunit[13]. In a purified system, αvβ3 integrin did not form a complex with pro-MMP2 or active MMP-2, supporting the observation that MMP-2, which does not have a RGD sequence, indirectly interacts with αvβ3 integrin via a mediatory RGD-bearing molecule. Alternatively, MMP-2 may bind to

$\alpha v\beta 3$ integrin in a RGD-independent manner, as cRGDfK failed to completely prevent the association between proMMP-2 and $\alpha v\beta 3$ integrin. Strikingly, HKa possesses stronger inhibition of both pathways. Taken together, HKa, by interfering with $\alpha v\beta 3$ integrin function, decreases the ligation of proMMP2 or its associated molecule to $\alpha v\beta 3$ integrin in EPCs, thereby suppressing MMP-2 activation. The inhibitory effect of HKa on MMP-2, at least in part, accounts for its inhibition of EPC vasculogenic differentiation.

HKa inhibition of the tube forming capacity of EPCs reveals a novel activity of the components of the KKS in vascular dysfunction and expands our understanding of the pathophysiological activities of this system. Local EPCs recruited after early arterial injury incorporate into foci of postnatal vasculogenesis and exhibit strong potential for vascular repair. A study using kininogen-deficient mice indicates that the KKS activation, in the process of vascular injury, induces arterial thrombosis[6]. Thus, developing thrombus in atherosclerotic lesions may form a surface that promotes the assembly of the components of the KKS, leading to a secondary activation of this system and further production of HKa. HKa inhibition of vasculogenesis of EPCs proposes a novel concept that activation of the KKS may contribute to EPC dysfunction. Although it remains to be determined whether and how HKa inhibition of EPCs is involved in the disordered vascular remodeling *in vivo*, recognition of components of plasma KKS modulation of EPC function allows for the beginning of understanding its pathophysiologic activities in atherosclerosis.

4. HKa suppresses clonogenic capacity of EPCs

Clonogenic capacity of EPCs can be analyzed using a single-cell assay. [14]. To test whether HKa affects the clonal expansion potential of EPCs, a single-cell suspension of EGFP-EPCs was seeded into 96-well culture plate precoated with collagen, in order to test whether HKa affects the clonal expansion potential of EPCs. The culture medium EGM-2 was replaced every 2 days. After culture for 14 days, EGFP-EPCs formed large colonies, and ≈85% of colonies contained more than 200 cells (large colonies). However, in the presence of 50 nmol/L HKa, the percentage of large colonies was markedly reduced to <6% ($P<0.001$), indicating that HKa strongly inhibits clonogenic capacity of EPCs[14].

5. HKa inhibits EPC proliferation without induction of apoptosis

HKa inhibition of EPC colony formation suggested that HKa suppresses proliferation of EPCs. The effect of HKa on proliferative capacity of EPCs was examined using a 5-bromo-2'-deoxyuridine (BrdU) incorporation assay. Treatment of EPCs with HKa for 72 hours significantly inhibited vascular endothelial growth factor–stimulated BrdU incorporation into EPCs, and the inhibition was concentration-dependent, whereas the significant inhibitory effect of HKa was detectable only at 100 nmol/L after treatment for 48 hours. In contrast to its significant effects on proliferation, HKa at the same concentrations did not inhibit EPC adhesion to collagen[14], suggesting that HKa inhibition of EPC proliferation does not result from an antiadhesion activity. Because HKa induces apoptosis of differentiated endothelial cells on vitronectin-coated surfaces, the effect of HKa on EPC apoptosis was examined. HKa did not induce EPC apoptosis on collagen surfaces, although its effect on induction of EPCs apoptosis on vitronectin-coated plates was significant. Therefore, HKa inhibition of EPC colony formation and proliferation is not subject to antiadhesive activity and induction of apoptosis.

6. HKa accelerates the onset of EPC senescence and suppresses telomerase activity

Reduction of EPCs in number and activity is associated with EPC senescence. The common features of senescent endothelial cells include the enhanced presence of acidic β-galactosidase activity, an increase in lysosomal mass, and formation of autophagic vacuoles. To determine whether HKa induces EPC senescence, the activity of acidic β-galactosidase was measured, the former referred as senescence-associated-β-galactosidase (SA-β-gal). Although a small portion of EPCs were positive for SA-β-gal staining after culture for 14 days, in the presence of 50 nmol/L HKa the majority of EPCs became positive for SA-β-gal staining[14]. Moreover, EPCs treated with 50 nmol/L HKa displayed a unique flattened and enlarged morphology and formed intracellular vacuoles[14], HKa treatment significantly resulted in an increase in SA-β-gal-positive cells, 17.2±2.6% vs 52.3±3.7% on day 7 and 22.3±2.7% vs 85.5±7.9% on day 14[14]. Acceleration of the onset of EPC senescence is known to be critically influenced by the level of telomerase activity, which elongates telomeres, thereby counteracting telomere length reduction induced by each cell division. Therefore, whether HKa treatment was capable of regulating telomerase activity in EPCs was tested. Treatment of EPCs with 50 nmol/L HKa for 14 days markedly diminished telomerase activity by >60% ($P<0.005$)[14], serving as additional evidence for HKa acceleration of EPC senescence.

7. HKa increases intracellular ROS production, contributing to EPC senescence

Cell senescence is tightly associated with intracellular ROS production. Whether HKa exposure increases intracellular ROS in EPCs was tested using the 2'-7'-dichlorodihydrofluorescein diacetate (H_2DCF-DA) labeling assay. In a concentration-dependent manner, HKa significantly increased H_2DCF-DA oxidation level in exposed EPCs[14]. Further whether HKa accelerates EPC senescence via ROS production was tested in an inhibition assay using the ROS scavengers Mn(III)tetrakis(4-benzoic acid)porphyrin chloride (MnTBAP) and *N*-acetylcysteine (NAC). MnTBAP is a cell-permeable superoxide dismutase mimetic and peroxynitrite scavenger. NAC is an efficient free radical scavenger and contributes to production of other antioxidant species. Treatment with either 100 μmol/L NAC or 10 μmol/L MnTBAP significantly attenuated the increase in ROS production in EPCs treated with 100 nmol/L HKa for 12 hours[14]. Moreover, 100 μmol/L NAC or 10 μmol/L MnTBAP significantly reduced both the percentage of senescent cells and ROS production in EPCs treated with 50 nmol/L HKa for 14 days[14]. These observations suggest that HKa generation of ROS is involved in the acceleration of EPC senescence.

8. HKa upregulates p38 kinase phosphorylation and $p16^{INK4a}$ expression

To investigate the mechanism for HKa acceleration of EPC senescence, we measured the levels of p38 kinase activation and prosenescence molecule $p16^{INK4a}$ expression, which are downstream of ROS generation in the process of cellular senescence. Immunoblotting analysis indicated that treatment with HKa at 30 and 100 nmol/L for 7 days increased p38 kinase phosphorylation[14]. Concomitantly, HKa upregulated $p16^{INK4a}$ expression at the protein and mRNA levels. Since 10 μmol/L SB203580, a specific p38 kinase inhibitor, markedly suppressed HKa-induced p16^{INK4a} expression as well as EPC senescence, HKa upregulates p16^{INK4a} expression via its activation of p38 kinase[14].

The above observation demonstrates novel activities of HKa in regulating several key elements of EPC biology. Aging is associated with an increased risk for atherosclerosis, and insufficient repair of damaged vascular walls by a diminished number or dysfunction in EPC is one of many possible causes. A reduction in EPC number and activity has been associated with EPC senescence. Because senescence limits the ability of EPCs to sustain ischemic tissue repair, a full characterization of the pathophysiological factors leading to EPC senescence, as well as the related underlying mechanisms, is clearly important. Our current study demonstrating HKa acceleration of EPC senescence not only expands our understanding of the KKS activation in the regulation of vascular biology but also reveals a potential novel endogenous inducer of EPC senescence.

The in vivo activation of the KKS and cleavage of HKa has been widely detected in numerous pathophysiological conditions, such as thrombosis, arthritis, inflammatory bowel disease, vasculitis, sepsis, systemic amyloidosis, and preeclampsia[4]. However, how the KKS activation products initiate and regulate downstream effects remains elusive. The plasma concentration of HK is 660 nmol/L. In patients with sepsis and autoimmune diseases, more than 30% of plasma HK was cleaved[15]. Because the minimal concentration of HKa that significantly induced EPC senescence was 30 nmol/L, the circulating levels of HKa in the pathological settings could affect EPC function. This HKa-mediated effect was associated with profoundly impaired EPC clonal expansion potential and resulted in a low overall proliferative capacity of the EPC progeny. Because HK is localized at sites of vascular injury, such as atherosclerotic lesions, it might become cleaved over the abundant negative-charged surfaces to release HKa. The observation that HKa potently inhibited the clonogenic capacity of EPCs suggests that HKa is possibly involved in the vascular dysfunction by blocking EPC aggregation and expansion. Because HKa inhibition of EPC function is not dependent on its antiadhesion activity, HKa in plasma may attack circulating EPCs. Whether the blockade of HK cleavage prevents EPC senescence remains to be determined using an in vivo model.

EPC senescence can be triggered by a variety of factors, such as proinflammatory cytokines, DNA damage, hyperoxia, and hyperglycemia. All these factors increase oxidative stress, by which they induce EPC senescence and suppress telomerase activity. The mechanism by which HKa accelerates the onset of senescence of EPCs seems to be tightly associated with ROS production. NAC and MnTBAP, which quench ROS, significantly attenuated HKa-induced EPC senescence. A previous study has shown that HKa inhibits Akt phosphorylation and endothelial nitric oxide synthase phosphorylation, which may inhibit the production of nitric oxide (NO). Although NO prevents endothelial cell senescence, the NO donor *S*-nitrosopenicillamine did not prevent HKa-accelerated onset of EPCs senescence. Thus, HKa regulation of EPC senescence appears independent of the NO pathway. Accumulation of ROS in most cell types is associated with high expression of p16^{INK4a}, which leads to the arrest of the cell cycle at the G_1 phase and accelerates senescence of cells.The expression of p16^{INK4a} increases with age and contributes to age-dependent stem and progenitor cell senescence. It can be deduced that accumulative ROS exposure, caused by various atherosclerotic risk factors, may also increase the expression of p16^{INK4a} in EPCs, contributing to EPC senescence. We found that HKa increased expression of p16^{INK4a} at the mRNA and protein level, demonstrating that HKa accelerates EPC senescence by the regulation of p16^{INK4a} expression. We previously have found that p38 kinase is responsible for mediating the effect of HKa in other cells. Our observations in this study indicate that HKa enhances phosphorylation of p38 kinase, and the inhibition of p38 kinase prevented both HKa-induced $p16^{INK4a}$ expression and EPC senescence. Therefore, HKa-induced ROS seems to act through p38 kinase to upregulate prosenescence molecule $p16^{INK4a}$ expression, which may further regulate telomerase activity and result in EPC senescence.

9. Bradykinin upregulates CXCR4 mRNA expression and stimulates transendothelial migration (TEM) of EPCs

TEM is an essential step for the EPC homing to sites of inflammatory and ischemic tissues. In a TEM assay using 96-transwell filters, EPCs were cultured on collagen-coated transwell filters until becoming confluent, CFDA-SE-labeled EPCs in endothelial basal medium (EBM-2) containing 2% FBS were placed on top of the lung microvessel endothelial cells (LMEC) monolayer. EBM-2 containing 2% FBS and bradykinin was added to the lower compartment. After incubation at 37°C for 18 hrs, the filters were fixed with 2% PFA. EPCs migrating into the lower side of the filters were visualized with a fluorescent microscope and counted in 6 random microscopic fields. Bradykinin (a B2R agonist) dose-dependently increased the transmigration of EPCs. In contrast, des-Arg9-BK (a B1R agonist) did not have such effect (data not shown). B2R predominantly mediates transmigration of normal EPCs. Treatment with bradykinin dose-dependently increased CXCR-4 mRNA expression in EPCs, but not the expression of other homing receptors such as E-selectin and α4-integrin.

In conclusion, HKa inhibits vasculogenic differentiation of EPCs and accelerates the onset of their senescence, and bradykinin upregulates transendothelial migration capacity. These activities of HKa and bradykinin reveal a novel link between KKS activation and EPC function, and it expands our understanding of the additional pathophysiological activities of this system. Although it remains to be determined whether and how HKa and bradykinin regulate the function of EPCs in the disordered vascular remodeling that occurs in vivo, our novel recognition that components of plasma KKS modulate EPC function allows for focused determination of the pathophysiologic activities of plasma KKS in atherosclerosis in future studies, provides an improved understanding of the contribution of the KKS cascade to EPC dysfunction in vitro and suggest candidate pathways for investigation of EPC dysfunction in subjects with vascular pathology.

10. References

[1] Yoder, M.C., et al., *Redefining endothelial progenitor cells via clonal analysis and hematopoietic stem/progenitor cell principals.* Blood, 2007. 109(5): p. 1801-1809.

[2] Hill, J.M., et al., *Circulating Endothelial Progenitor Cells, Vascular Function, and Cardiovascular Risk.* New England Journal of Medicine, 2003. 348(7): p. 593-600.

[3] Schmidt-Lucke, C., et al., *Reduced Number of Circulating Endothelial Progenitor Cells Predicts Future Cardiovascular Events.* Circulation, 2005. 111(22): p. 2981-2987.

[4] Colman, R.W. and A.H. Schmaier, *Contact System: A Vascular Biology Modulator With Anticoagulant, Profibrinolytic, Antiadhesive, and Proinflammatory Attributes.* Blood, 1997. 90(10): p. 3819-3843.

[5] Schmaier, A.H. and K.R. McCrae, *The plasma kallikrein-kinin system: its evolution from contact activation.* Journal of Thrombosis and Haemostasis, 2007. 5(12): p. 2323-2329.

[6] Merkulov, S., et al., *Deletion of murine kininogen gene 1 (mKng1) causes loss of plasma kininogen and delays thrombosis.* Blood, 2008. 111(3): p. 1274-1281.

[7] Colman, R.W., Y. Wu, and Y. Liu, *Mechanisms by which cleaved kininogen inhibits endothelial cell differentiation and signalling.* Thromb Haemost, 2010. 104(5): p. 875-85.

[8] Liu, Y., et al., *The inhibition of tube formation in a collagen-fibrinogen, three-dimensional gel by cleaved kininogen (HKa) and HK domain 5 (D5) is dependent on Src family kinases.* Exp Cell Res, 2008. 314(4): p. 774-88.

[9] Wu, Y., et al., *Kininostatin associates with membrane rafts and inhibits alpha(v)beta3 integrin activation in human umbilical vein endothelial cells.* Arterioscler Thromb Vasc Biol, 2007. 27(9): p. 1968-75.

[10] Cao, D.J., Y.-L. Guo, and R.W. Colman, *Urokinase-Type Plasminogen Activator Receptor Is Involved in Mediating the Apoptotic Effect of Cleaved High Molecular Weight Kininogen in Human Endothelial Cells.* Circulation Research, 2004. 94(9): p. 1227-1234.

[11] Wu, Y., et al., *Cleaved high molecular weight kininogen inhibits tube formation of endothelial progenitor cells via suppression of matrix metalloproteinase 2.* J Thromb Haemost, 2010. 8(1): p. 185-93.

[12] Yoon, C.-H., et al., *Synergistic Neovascularization by Mixed Transplantation of Early Endothelial Progenitor Cells and Late Outgrowth Endothelial Cells.* Circulation, 2005. 112(11): p. 1618-1627.

[13] Choi, W.S., et al., *MMP-2 regulates human platelet activation by interacting with integrin* $\alpha IIb\beta 3$. Journal of Thrombosis and Haemostasis, 2008. 6(3): p. 517-523.

[14] Dai, J., et al., *Cleaved high-molecular-weight kininogen accelerates the onset of endothelial progenitor cell senescence by induction of reactive oxygen species.* Arterioscler Thromb Vasc Biol, 2011. 31(4): p. 883-9.

[15] Asmis, L.M., et al., *Contact system activation in human sepsis - 47kD HK, a marker of sepsis severity?* Swiss Med Wkly, 2008. 138(9-10): p. 142-9.

6

Vasculogenesis in Diabetes-Associated Diseases: Unraveling the Diabetic Paradox

Carla Costa
Faculty of Medicine of the University of Porto, Departament of Biochemistry (U38-FCT)
Department of Experimental Biology
Portugal

1. Introduction

During several decades it was thought that in the adult, vascular growth and remodelling was exclusively dependent on the activation of angiogenesis, being the process of vasculogenesis restricted to embryonic life (Risau & Flamme, 1995; Risau, 1997). This long-lasting belief has come to an end in the late nineties, with the isolation from adult peripheral blood (PB) of angioblast-like circulating Endothelial Progenitor Cells (EPCs) (Asahara et al., 1997). The discovery of bone marrow (BM)-derived EPCs with angioblastic morphological and functional properties was a landmark in vascular biology that forever has changed the concept of neovascularization. Numerous studies have demonstrated that EPCs residing in the BM could be mobilized to the peripheral circulation, migrate to neoangiogenic sites and partake *in vivo* in the pathophysiological development of vascular networks, by differentiating into functional, mature endothelial cells (ECs) (Asahara et al., 1999a, 1999b; Goon et al., 2007; Grant et al., 2002; Lyden et al., 2001; Takahashi et al., 1999). However, much controversy has accompanied this field over time, particularly regarding the phenotypic characterization of EPCs. In fact, this cell population does not have specific cell surface markers, sharing a diversity of membrane receptors with other BM-derived cells (Hristov et al., 2003; Peichev et al., 2000). Additionally, several subsets of EPCs have been identified and together with other lineages of precursor cells were found to be differentially recruited to neovascular foci contributing synergistically to vasculogenic neoformation (Gulati et al., 2003; Hur et al., 2004; Lyden et al., 2001; Yoder et al., 2007; Yoon et al., 2005a). Since their identification, an increasing body of evidence has definitely revealed the important properties and roles played by EPCs in several vascular-related diseases, such as peripheral vascular disease (Asahara et al., 1999a, 1999b; Takahashi et al., 1999), tumor neovascularisation (Asahara et al., 1999a, 1999b; Lyden et al., 2001) and vascular complications associated to diabetes (Goon et al., 2007; Grant et al., 2002; Egan et al., 2008; Fadini et al., 2005). The metabolic alterations present in diabetic individuals are known to profoundly affect vascular biology, being responsible for the impairment of macro- and microvascular beds (Fadini et al., 2006a; Werner et al., 2005). Diabetes associated vascular complications involve distinct modifications in neovascular formation, which is reduced in ischemic heart and limbs and increased in the retina, defining the diabetic paradox (Ciulla et al., 2003). The vasculogenic process seems to play a central dual role in this paradoxal puzzle: systemically, diabetes-associated hyperglycemia, insulin resistance, hypertension and oxidative stress, can simultaneoulsy injure the endothelium and deliteriously affect EPCs biological functions, impairing efficient systemic vascular repair and promoting peripheral vasculopathy (Povsic & Goldschmidt-Clermont, 2008); locally in the retina, the specific microenvironment may contribute to the local recruitment of EPCs, promoting increased vessel growth (Goon et al., 2007; Grant et al., 2002). Although still under investigation, these divergent features seem related to a differential regulation of neovascular mechanisms, which responde differently to ischemia-induced depletion of angiogenic factors in systemic conditions, or to the local induction of vascular growth factors in the diabetic retina (Duh & Aiello, 1999). Due to the growing importance of vasculogenesis in diabetic vascular complications, interventions differentially modulating EPCs levels/functions may be regarded as therapeutic strategies. Systemically, vasculoprotective agents provided with beneficial cardiovascular effects, have showed to improve endothelium-dependent vascular function, by restoring EPCs properties and actions (Liang et al., 2009). Local delivery of anti-angiogenic drugs to the retina may have positive effects by hampering EPCs recruitment in proliferative diabetic retinopathy (PDR) (Chung et al., 2011). However, one might not neglect that diabetic patients frequently display both neovascular peripheral decrease and retinal increase of vessel growth. So, important questions are raised regarding the therapeutic use of EPCs in the promotion of periptheral vascularization and the impairment of EPCs-induced retinal neovascular formation and increased ischemia. Several issues need to be addressed in order to optimize the therapeutic use of EPCs and to get further information on the putative harmful side effects. Future research is mandatory in order to elucidate the complex molecular mechanisms governing the diabetic-vasculogenic paradigm, bringing novel insights into the safety on the therapeutic modulation of EPCs in diabetes vascular disorders.

2. Endothelial progenitor cells (EPCs) and postnatal vasculogenesis

Vasculogenesis and angiogenesis are the fundamental processes by which new blood vessels are formed. Vasculogenesis is defined as the differentiation of EPCs or angioblasts into ECs and the *de novo* formation of a primitive vascular network, whereas angiogenesis is the growth of new capillaries from pre-existing blood vessels (Risau & Flamme, 1995; Risau, 1997). In the embryo, blood vessels form through both vasculogenesis and angiogenesis. Vasculogenesis occurs during early embryonic development and mediates the *de novo* vessel formation from angioblasts of mesodermal origin, which differentiate into mature ECs assembling into a primary capillary plexus (Risau & Flamme, 1995). Subsequently, this primitive vascular network expands by angiogenesis, where new blood vessels arise from the proliferation and migration of the pre-existing ECs (Folkman, 1984; Risau, 1997). During several decades it was thought that in the adult, vascular growth and remodelling was exclusively dependent on the activation of angiogenesis, and that the process of vasculogenesis was restricted to embryonic life. This prevailing dogma has come to an end over a decade ago, with the identification of circulating BM-derived EPCs in 1997 by Asahara and collaborators, which have isolated a population of angioblast-like CD34+ circulating EPCs from adult PB. In *in vitro* cultures, these cells presented an increased proliferation rate and exhibited endothelial morphological and functional properties (Asahara et al., 1997). However, this pioneering work was criticized and the true identity of the putative EPCs was questioned. In fact, besides the functional characteristics of these progenitor cells, namely their high proliferative capacity, this report did not provide any additional information regarding other specific functional characteristics. Additionaly, in

Asahara's work the CD34 antigen was used to select EPCs, however the authors did not present a defined set of other phenotypic markers that could unambiguously identify this cell population allowing their sole isolation. In fact, CD34 is also expressed in sub-groups of hematopoietic stem/progenitor cells and mature ECs and does not specifically discriminate EPCs. Nevertheless, the work of Asahara *et al.* set a landmark in the field of vascular biology, for being the first to suggest that vasculogenesis could occur during adult life. Besides the controversy, after this initial report, a boom of novel studies corroborated Asahara's hypothesis, presenting novel evidence for the existence of postnatal EPCs and their functional role in pathophysiological neovascular processes. Several reports demonstrated that a population of EPCs residing in the BM could be mobilized to the peripheral circulation, migrate to neoangiogenic foci and partake *in vivo* in the development of vascular networks, by differentiating into functional matured ECs and incorportating the vasculature (Asahara et al., 1999a, 1999b; Lyden et al., 2001; Shi et al., 1998). EPCs mobilization from the BM and homing to neovascular foci occurred in response of progenitor cells to specific angiogenic stimuli. The initial steps in mobilization involved the activation of matrix metalloproteinase (MMP)-9, which catalyses the conversion of membrane-bound Kit ligand to soluble Kit ligand. The subsequent cKit-positive progenitor cells are disengaged and can then move from the osteoblastic to the vascular zone of the BM. This process is enhanced by elevated levels of the chemokines Stromal Derived Factor (SDF)-1 and Vascular Endothelial Growth Factor (VEGF) (Heissig et al., 2002) and appears to be endothelial Nitric Oxide (eNO) dependent (Aicher et al., 2003). Increased eNO levels stimulate the passage of EPCs through BM sinusoidal endothelium and their entrance in the blood stream, where they are further recruited to neoangiogenic foci (Aicher at el., 2003, 2005).

3. EPCs phenotypic and functional properties

Since their identification, the phenotypic characterization of EPCs has emerged a major setback in the field. Their isolation, identification and characterization were mostly hampered by the lack of EPCs-specific surface markers. Over time some consensus has apparently been reached and EPCs were considered to be the cell population characterized by the concomitant expression of: the early hematopoietic stem cell markers CD34 and CD133 (former AC133) and VEGF receptor-2 (VEGFR-2) (Hristov et al., 2003; Peichev et al., 2000). However, it has been suggested that human CD34+CD133+VEGFR2+ cells comprise a population of cells that are not only EPCs, but distinct primitive hematopoietic progenitors, which also express markers such as CD45 and are devoid of vessel formation capabilities (Case et al., 2007; Timmermans et al., 2007). Other findings have demonstrated the existence of novel subsets of progenitor cells with an involvement in vascular repair. It was reported the presence in PB of a stem cell population which lack the CD34 antigen and is able to differentiate into CD34+CD133+ EPCs, and acquire a more mature endothelial phenotype (Friedrich et al., 2006). Additionally, other populations with endothelial repair capabilities which express additional cell surface markers, including the receptor for SDF-1, the chemokine (C-X-C motif) receptor (CXCR)-4 have also been identified (Egan et al., 2008). The characterization of these different subpopulations of EPCs is due to the different methodology used for cell isolation. To date, there are three main techniques that have been used to select, identify and characterize EPCs (Hirschi et al., 2008; Yoder, 2009). The cell types isolated using the different protocols are not phenotypically similar and as such, their potential to influence neovascularization and/or vascular repair may vary. Consequently, this may offer an explanation as to the differences observed amongst similar studies which presented divergent results.

3.1 Methods for EPCs isolation and characterization

3.1.1 Culture of isolated mononuclear cells

This method involves the isolation of mononuclear cells from PB or BM using density gradient centrifugation and the platting of these cells on fibronectin-coated substracts and cultured in medium supplemented with endothelial growth factors. Approximately 3 days later, non-adherent cells are removed from the culture and fresh media is added to the remaining cells which continue to be cultured and futher analysed. These spindle shaped-adherent cells express EC markers and functional qualities, such as endocytosis and acetylated low-density lipoprotein (LDL) uptake. However, unlike progenitor cells they display low proliferative capacity, cannot form EC tube-like structures in an *in vitro* angiogenesis assay model, but do display panleukocyte and monocytic/macrophage markers, such as CD14 and CD45 (Rehman et al., 2003; Zhang et al., 2006, 2007). In support of this finding, previous data showed that monocytes have high affinity for fibronectin, and that 90% of cells from PB samples which adhere to coated dishes are of monocytic origin (Freundlich & Avdalovic, 1983). Moreover, a recent study by Prokopi *et al.* suggested how these putative EPCs may acquire EC markers. According to their data, the method used for mononuclear cell isolation from PB leads to the contamination of cells with platelets, which also express endothelial markers such as CD31 and von Willebrand factor (vWF) (Prokopi et al., 2009). During a 7 day mononuclear cell culture, the platelets are degraded into microparticles, vesicles which retain specific antigens from the cell of origin. So, adherent day 1 mononuclear cells presented as CD31 negative, but by day 7 expressed the CD31 antigen, along with platelet-specific markers, following the uptake of degraded platelet microparticles and a transfer of cell antigens. Additionally, depletion of platelet microparticles from the EPCs culture media also removed the angiogenic properties often attributed to EPC culture medium, indicating that this *in vitro* property may be dependent on initial platelet presence following mononuclear cell isolation (Kirton & Xu, 2010; Rehman et al., 2003; Urbich et al., 2005).

3.1.2 Fluorescence activated cell sorting (FACS) and *in vitro* culture

One of the most currently used methods for EPCs separation, involves cell labelling with antigen specific antibodies and FACS analysis. This was the technique used by Asahara *et al.* in their pioneering work to isolate CD34+ mononuclear cells (Asahara et al., 1997). Since as aforementioned, CD34 does not selectively discriminate EPCs, following studies also included the use of CD133 combined with CD34 and VEGFR-2 (Peichev et al., 2000), to ensure that only progenitor cells were isolated as apposed to circulating ECs that have detached from the vessel wall (Blann & Pretorius, 2006; Ingram et al., 2005). These cells were cultured for 2 days and non-adherent cells re-plated for further 14 days, giving similar clustered colonies. Upon differentiating into mature ECs, EPCs lose the expression of CD133 and start exhibiting classical EC morphology and features, such as the expression of the endothelial markers vWF and vascular endothelial cadherin (VE-cadherin) and the capacity to uptake acetylated LDL (Peichev et al., 2000; Shi et al., 1998). Several subsequent studies successfully isolated this cell type from adult PB, umbilical cord blood and fetal liver, using a combination of these three markers (Timmermans et al., 2009). However, further controversy has arised since, it was reported that CD34+CD133+VEGFR2+ cells comprise a mixed population of EPCs and primitive hematopoietic progenitors, which express also CD45 and also lack the ability to form vessel-like structures (Case et al., 2007; Timmermans et al., 2007).

3.1.3 *In vitro* colony forming cell assays

Using this technique independent groups have shown that in adult PB mononuclear cells there are two distinct EPCs populations, which form *in vitro* Early Outgrowth Colonies (EOCs) and Late Outgrowth Colonies (LOCs) (Gulati et al., 2003; Hur et al., 2004). Additional studies have used different designations for these cell types: EOCs were also named early EPCs (eEPCs) and LOCs are also known as Outgrowth Endothelial Cells (OECs) (Medina et al., 2010, Yoon et al., 2005a) Although the biology of these endothelial progenitor-like cells is still under investigation, they seem to present different phenotypes, surface antigens and display diverse vasculogenic features *in vitro*. EOCs and LOCs are primarily characterized based on their morphology and chronology of appearance following *in vitro* culture. EOCs appear in culture within 7 days, emanating from a central cluster of cells, exhibiting spindle-shaped morphology and having a peak growth at 2-3 weeks after which they cannot be further expanded (Gulati et al., 2003; Hur et al., 2004). LOCs generally appear after 3 weeks and exhibit a "classic endothelial" phenotype, having an increased expansion potential. LOCs seem more capable of *in vitro* morphogenesis into capillary tubes, the best approximate true definition of an EPC, a competent progenitor cell whose terminally differentiated progeny are mature ECs (Gulati et al., 2003; Hur et al., 2004; Yoder et al., 2007). This capillary-forming capacity is minimal or nonexistent within EOCs, which are thought to have a paracrine role by supporting LOCs differentiation and capillary formation, through the release of pro-angiogenic molecules and by inducing the activation of MMPs (Gulati et al., 2003; Hur et al., 2004; Yoon et al., 2005a). Phenotypically, EOCs additionally express the monocyte/macrophage marker CD14, which is absent among mature LOCs, and both populations may concomitantly express CD34 and VEGFR-2 (Yoon et al., 2005a). However, besides the reported alterations in phenotypic markers and the dissimilar biological properties, there was a lack of information regarding molecular differences between EOCs and LOCs. Recently, a study has provided a detailed molecular fingerprint of these two EPC subtypes, designated in this report by eEPCs and OECs. Medina and collaborators have shown that eEPCs and OECs have strikingly different gene/protein expression signatures (Medina et al., 2010). As evaluated by microarrays, many highly expressed transcripts in eEPCs were hematopoietic specific, including the Runt-related transcription factor (RUNX1) and the protein tyrosine kinase LYN; and with links to immunity and inflammation (Toll-Like Receptors, TLRs; CD14; Human Leukocyte Antigens, HLAs). On the other hand, OECs presented several highly expressed transcripts involved in vascular development and angiogenesis-related signaling pathways, such as the receptor tyrosine kinase Tie2, eNOS and Ephrins. Similarly, proteomic analysis revealed that 90% of spots identified by 2D gel electrophoresis analysis were common between OECs and endothelial cells while eEPCs shared 77% with monocytes. This study provided evidence that eEPCs are hematopoietic cells with a molecular phenotype linked to monocytes; whereas OECs exhibit commitment to the endothelial lineage, corroborating at the molecular level all the previous studies that have phenotypically characterized these cell populations. These findings indicate that OECs are the subtype with vasculogenic capability and that functionally integrates neovascular foci, and it should be an attractive cell candidate for inducing therapeutic angiogenesis.

Overall, these reports indicate that EPCs represent a heterogeneous population of cells, some of monocytic nature and others with a pro-angiogenic potential. Depending on the study model, cell isolation method and cell subtype used, the pro-angiogenic effects are a consequence of the direct vascular integration, the paracrine release of growth factors and cytokines, or the complex interactions with other cellular components like monocytes or platelets. Nonetheless, most of the reports involving *in vitro* and *in vivo* EPCs studies do not usually make a distinction between EOCs (eEPCs) and LOCs (OECs), analyzing both populations as a whole. As aforementioned, this may explain divergences observed amongst similar studies.

4. Vasculogenesis and *in vivo* neovascular formation in pathophysiological processes

Studies carried on experimental models have shown that postnatal vasculogenesis could take place under certain physiological and pathological settings. Further, it was also suggested that other BM-derived hematopoietic stem/myeloid progenitor cells, named as accessory cells, could be co-recruited to neoangiogenesis foci, and support vascular growth in a paracrine fashion through the release of pro-angiogenic factors or by contributing to extracellular matrix remodeling (De Palma et al., 2005; Fang & Salven, 2011; Grunewald et al., 2006; Kaplan et al., 2005; Lyden et al., 2001; Takakura, 2006). Due to the relevant role of neovascularization for tumor growth and metastization, several pre-clinical studies evaluated EPCs functions and their contribution for malignant development (Asahara et al., 1999a, 1999b; Lyden et al., 2001). Additionally and corroborating experimental data, it was also reported that a percentage of BM-derived EPCs can integrate human tumour-associated neovasculature (Peters et al., 2005). Nonethess, despite all these evidence Purhonen et al. have suggested that BM-derived circulating EPCs do not contribute to vascular endothelium and are not needed for tumor development, raising novel controversy in the field (Purhonen et al., 2008). Besides tumor neovascular formation, further studies confirmed that EPCs play also a role in: vascular homeostasis and repair (Asahara et al., 1999a; Kirton & Xu, 2010; Shantsila et al., 2007), wound healing (Asahara et al., 1999b), bone regeneration (Matsumoto et al. 2008), myocardial infaction (Porto et al., 2011; Shintani et al., 2001), limb ischemia (Asahara et al., 1999a, 1999b; Takahashi et al., 1999), burn individuals and escharectomy (Foresta et al., 2011; Gill et al., 2001) and vascular complications associated to diabetes (Goon et al., 2007; Grant et al., 2002; Egan et al., 2008; Fadini et al., 2005).

5. Vasculogenesis and the diabetic paradox

Diabetes mellitus (DM) is a common costly chronic disease and its incidence is rapidly increasing worldwide. Once considered primarily as a risk factor for heart disease, diabetes has now become a high profile public health concern in its own right, due to the escalating epidemic of diabetes in older people, and the emergence of type 2 DM (T2DM) in children. In fact, individuals with T2DM account for most of this augmentation in the general population. An important part of this rise is attributed to changing living conditions, including overweight and obesity, sedentary behaviour, and unhealthy lifestyle (Perkins,

2004; Zimmet et al., 2001). Vascular complications in T2DM are a significant cause of human morbidity and mortality, by affecting multiple organs, in particular the cardiovascular system, through the promotion of atherosclerosis (Haffner et al., 1998; Nakagami et al., 2005; Werner et al., 2005). Diabetic vascular alterations in different organs occur by distinct modifications in neovascular formation, which is decreased in systemic cardiovascular disease (CVD) and increased in DR. This diabetic paradox has been attributed to the differential regulation of neovascular mechanisms, which responde differently to ischemia in diabetic conditions (Duh & Aiello, 1999). The vasculogenic process seems to play a central dual role in this paradoxal puzzle: by one hand diabetes-associated hyperglycemia, insulin resistance, hypertension and oxidative stress, can simultaneoulsy injure the endothelium and deliteriously affect EPCs functions, thus preventing efficient systemic vascular repair, favoring the development of peripheral vasculopathy (Povsic & Goldschmidt-Clermont, 2008); on the other hand the specific retinal *millieu* may promote the local recruitment of EPCs, contributing to increased vessel growth in PDR (Goon et al., 2007; Grant et al., 2002). Althought the complex mechanisms governing this diabetic-vasculogenic paradox are still under investigation, novel evidence links alterations in EPCs biological functions to diabetic vascular complications, and will be further discussed.

6. Diabetic vasculopathy and altered vasculogenesis

Diabetes is characterized by a systemic pro-inflammatory state and generalized endothelial dysfunction (EDys). EDys ultimately represents the unbalance between endothelium injury and the endogenous capacity for endothelial repair (Costa et al., 2007). Compelling evidence suggested that hyperglycemia, insulin resistance, hypertension and oxidative stress, simultaneously promote endothelial damage and deliteriously affect EPCs functions, thus preventing efficient vascular repair and favoring the development of atherosclerotic lesions (Madonna & De Caterina, 2011; Povsic & Goldschmidt-Clermont, 2008). Amongst all these risk factors, increased glycemic levels and excessive oxidative stress seem to be the major causal factors underlying both endothelial injury and vasculogenic impairment (Callaghan et al., 2005). Nonetheless, the complex interplay between all the aforementioned conditions is thought to sinergistically decrease endothelial regeneration by altering EPCs biological activities, such as: reducing EPCs migration (Kränkel et al., 2005; Vasa et al., 2001); impairing their mobilization (Fadini et al., 2006b; Gallagher et al., 2007; Kang et al., 2009; Yao et al., 2006); promoting premature senescence (Higashi et al., 2002); inhibiting integrative and morphogenic capacities (defective adhesion, colony-forming ability and tubulization) (Fadini et al., 2006a; Tepper et al., 2002) and inducing EPCs apoptosis (Chen et al., 2010; Shen et al., 2010). These alterations on EPCs features have been associated with deficient endogenous re-endothelialization/neovascularization, being a potential indicator of diabetic CVD severity (Egan et al., 2008; Fadini et al., 2005; 2006b). In conjunction with deficient EPCs functions, the production of chemotactic/angiogenic factors is inhibited in diabetic peripheral ischemic tissues; contributing both to poor collateral formation and insufficient perfusion. It has been shown that the expression of angiogenic factors such as, VEGF and Hypoxia-Inducible Factor (HIF)-1α are reduced in the heart of diabetic patients during acute coronary syndromes (Marfella et al., 2004). Recently, it was also demonstrated that following the onset of acute myocardial infarction in T2DM patients, the numbers of CD133+ progenitor cells are reduced and their chemotactic responsiveness attenuated (Vöö et al., 2009). Both the defective expression of angiogenic factors and the dysfunction in EPCs account for the delayed post-ischemic vascular healing and myocardial recovery in patients with DM. Diabetic cardiomyopathy is also characterized by an early and progressive decline in myocardial VEGF expression and reduced circulating EPCs, which contributes to diminished capillary density, decreased myocardial perfusion and impaired contractility (Yoon et al., 2005b). A significant decline in circulating EPCs was also reported in diabetic patients with peripheral arterial disease (PAD), particularly in individuals with ischemic foot lesions. EPCs levels correlated with the ankle-brachial index, the most objective diagnostic and prognostic test for lower extremity arterial disease. It was also demonstrated that decreased EPCs closely correlated with the severity of both carotid and lower limb atherosclerosis. Higher degrees of carotid stenosis, as well as, worse stages of leg claudication and ischemic lesions, were associated with lower levels of EPCs. This suggested that EPCs counts could be considered a valuable marker for atherosclerotic involvement (Fadini et al., 2005). Additionally, EPCs isolated from diabetic patients with PAD exhibited poor endothelial differentiation capacity, impaired proliferation and deficient adhesion to mature endothelium (Fadini et al., 2006a; 2006c). Recently, a study evaluated circulating levels of CD34-CD133+VEGFR-2+ EPCs in diabetic patients with CVD, revealing a decrease in this subpopulation caused by diabetes-induced apoptosis (Jung et al., 2010). Similarly, it was also proposed that a subset of CXCR-4+ progenitor cells with vascular repair capability, were decreased in the PB of T2DM patients (Egan et al., 2008). In ischemic conditions, reduced levels of CXCR-4+ precursors may responde poorly to SDF-1, preventing their efficient mobilization and recruitment from the BM niche to ischemic sites. In addition, it seems relevant to mention novel data disclosing the effects of hyperglycemia in EPCs in intrauterine life. Interestingly, the exposure to high glucose levels in a diabetic intrauterine environment was shown to diminish the clonogenic potential of neonatal EPCs, providing a new insight into the long-term cardiovascular complications observed in newborns of diabetic pregnancies (Ingram et al., 2008). Since it was reported that hyperglycemia, insulin resistance, hypertension and oxidative stress, are key factors on promoting endothelial damage and by altering EPCs functions, it will be further discussed how these conditions deleteriously affect vasculogenic events associated to peripheral vasculopathy (Madonna & De Caterina, 2011; Povsic & Goldschmidt-Clermont, 2008)

6.1 Hyperglycemia

Hyperglycemia is one of the major causal factors implicated in the development of vascular alterations (Aronson, 2008). High glucose levels are involved in the generation of advanced glycation end products (AGEs), which accumulate in the vessel wall, and by interacting with its receptors (RAGE) induce oxidative stress, increase inflammation and promote EDys (Jandeleit-Dahm & Cooper, 2008). Hyperglycemia is thought to maintain EDys conditions by directly impairing most EPCs-driven functional capabilities. Hyperglycemia was demonstrated to: decrease EPCs migration and integrative capacities (Kränkel et al., 2005); shift their differentiation into a pro-inflammatory phenotype (Loomans et al., 2009); reduce EPCs mobilization (Gallagher et al., 2007); accelerate the onset of progenitor cell senescence (Chen et al., 2007); induce apoptotsis (Chen et al., 2010); inhibit EPCs colony-forming ability; decrease the number and proliferation of both early and late EPCs (EOCs and LOCs) and to impair the migration and vasculogenesis activities of LOCs, the subtype with vasculogenic-associated morphogenesis capability (Chen et al., 2007). Decreased vascular progenitor cells migration and inhibition of functional incorporation into tubular structures, were suggested to occur through hyperglycemia-induced decrease in NO production and MMP-9 activity (Kränkel et al., 2005). Reduced mobilization of EPCs was showed to occur due to modifications in eNOS phosphorylation and activation status within the BM microenvironment, unabling efficient EPCs release from the marrow niche to the peripheral circulation (Gallagher et al., 2007; Ingram et al., 2008). Hyperglycemia-induced EPCs senescence was demonstrated to take place through multiple mechanisms such as, by promoting telomere shortening, and alterations in the p38 MAPK and NO-mediated pathways (Chen et al., 2007; Ingram et al., 2008; Kuki et al., 2006). Additionally, a novel molecular link between high glucose levels and EPCs-increased senescence has been unveilled, as it was demonstrated that the Sirtuin 1 (SIRT1) gene, which regulates cell cycle, premature senescence and apoptosis, is downregulated in EPCs. SIRT1 low expression levels impair the important cascade of intracellular events, culminating with EPCs early senescence (Balestrieri et al., 2008a). Highlighting the crucial effects of high glicemic levels, it was also reported that the number of EPCs in T2DM was significantly decreased as compared with healthy controls. Additionally, an inverse correlation between EPCs numbers, plasma glucose and glycated hemoglobin (HbA1C) was found. Further, the number and function of EPCs in patients with good glycemic control were recovered compared with those with poor glycemic control. When glucose was supplemented to *in vitro* cultures, there was a negative effect on the proliferation and viability of EPCs, in a dose-dependent manner, whereas the enhancement of apoptosis was observed (Churdchomjan et al., 2010). All these deleterious effects were reported to occur due to a direct effect of elevated glucose levels on EPCs (Chen et al., 2007), however it was also suggested that hyperglycemia may promote EPCs dysfunction indirectly through the induction of Reactive Oxygen Species (ROS) overproduction and increased oxidative stress (Callaghan et al,. 2005). Moreover, anti-diabetic treatments were reported to improve the re-endothelialization capacity of EPCs from diabetic individuals (Gensch et al., 2007).

6.2 Insulin resistance (IR)

Approximately 80% of all T2DM coexist with IR (Zimmet et al.; 2001). Several studies have proposed that IR may affect unfavourably the balance between endothelial injury and endogenous repair, promoting EDys and contributing to premature atherosclerosis (Dandona et al., 2003; 2004). Apparently, IR aids EDys perpectuation (Kim et al., 2006) by modulating vasculogenesis-associated EPCs capability of effectively promoting endothelium regeneration. Althought the direct mechanisms by which IR alters EPCs functions are still unclear, it was recently suggested that the chronic inflammatory environment present in T2DM leads to insulin signaling defects in EPCs, thereby reducing their survival (Desouza et al., 2011). Additionally, it was also reported that after arterial injury in hemizygous knockout mice for the insulin receptor (IRKO), EPCs activities were altered and endothelial regeneration delayed. This defective endothelial repair could be normalized by transfusion of progenitor cells from insulin-sensitive animals, but not from insulin-resistant animals (Kahn et al., 2011). However, it is thought that EPCs biological modifications are mostly affected by IR in an indirect fashion, through the increase in ROS and also by the activation of pro-inflammatory cytokines (Cubbon et al., 2007; 2009; Houstis et al., 2006). In fact, IR states are closely linked to the increased production of ROS, which is a characteristic feature of IR and thought to play a causal role in its development (Houstis et al., 2006). The deleterious effects of oxidative stress in EPCs biological characteristics have been established and will be contemplated in section 6.4. Although further direct cause-effect between IR and EPCs alterations is currently under investigation, it has been shown that treatments with insulin sensitizing drugs may improve EPCs functional parameters, independently of glycemic levels and/or redox status (Schoonjans & Auwerx, 2001). Nonetheless, further studies are necessary to clarify the molecular links between IR and vasculogenic impairment.

6.3 Hypertension

High blood pressure levels are associated with significant mechanical endothelial injury and dysfunction (Spieker et al., 2000). Disruption of endothelial homeostasis in hypertensive patients is thought to worsen their cardiovascular prognosis (Perticone et al., 2001) and contribute to increased blood pressure levels (Schiffrin, 2001). Alterations in vasculogenesis-related mechanisms have been associated to hypertension-induced EDys (You et al., 2008mi; Watson et al., 2008). A clinical study in patients with coronary artery disease (CAD) concluded that hypertension was a major independent risk factor predictor of impaired EPCs-induced migration (Vasa et al., 2001). It was reported that the functional activity of EPCs is reduced in experimental model settings and in hypertensive patients, due to increased EPC-induced senescence (Imanishi et al., 2005). Recently, it was shown that *in vivo* endothelial repair capacity of early EPCs was reduced in patients with pre-hypertension and hypertension, due to EPC senescence and impaired endothelial function, which potentially represents an early event in the development of hypertension (Giannotti et al., 2010). Although it is still unclear, hypertension does not seem to have a direct action on EPCs reduction of half-life, which may be caused by telomerase inactivation associated with the increase in oxidative stress associated with hypertension (Higashi et al., 2002; Imanishi et al., 2005; Touyz et al., 2004). Further, studies showed that in patients with arterial hypertension, no association was observed between the number of circulating vascular progenitor cells and hypertension, suggesting that cell mobilization may not be affected (Delva et al., 2007; Werner et al., 2005). Inconsistently, it was also reported that reduced levels of circulating CD34+VEGFR-2+ EPCs were detected in hypertensive patients as compared to normotensive individuals (Pirro et al., 2007). Lower levels of peripheral EPCs correlated with a downregulation in the homeobox A9 (HOXA9) gene expression, which is critical for endothelial commitment during progenitor cell maturation (Pirro et al., 2007). Further studies are required to clarify the role of hypertension in EPCs functions. Nonetheless, it was also reported that anti-hypertensive drugs, besides its blood pressure lowering effect, may also improve vascular function through EPC activation (Cacciatore et al., 2011; de Ciuceis et al., 2011; Yao et al., 2007).

6.4 Oxidative stress

Increased oxidative stress has been proposed as an important molecular mechanism for vascular complications associated with DM, IR, and hypertension (Aronson, 2008; Houstis et al., 2006; Yanai et al., 2008), by exerting a direct cytotoxic effect on the vascular monolayer (Griendling & FitzGerald, 2003). ROS may directly harm the vascular endothelium while superoxide reacts with NO to form peroxynitrite anion (ONOO−), a powerful oxidant (Griendling & FitzGerald, 2003; Kuzkaya et al., 2003). Diminished release of eNO caused either by excessive oxidative degradation or impaired local production has been implicated in endothelial lining damage and insufficient repair capability due to deficient EPCs mobilization/functional status (Craeger et al., 2003; Yao et al., 2006). In fact, oxidative stress-induced reduction of NO bioavailability represents the major mechanism leading to impaired EPCs *in vivo* re-endothelialization capacity and *in vitro* function (Fleissner & Thum, 2010; Sorrentino et al., 2007). NO deficient release by the vasculature is thought to impair EPCs migratory function and colony-forming ability, indicating a central role for eNO activity in EPC biology in increased oxidative stress conditions (Hill et al., 2003). Additonally, it was recently shown in patients with metabolic syndrome (MetS) and CAD, that oxidative stress may directly induce DNA damage on EPCs, by promoting telomere shortening with a consequent increase in their senescence rate, which contributed to the progression of atherosclerosis (Fleissner & Thum, 2010; Satoh et al., 2008). Accordingly, anti-oxidant therapies, which exert cellular protective effects by directly scavenging ROS reducing their damaging action, can also improve EPCs functions and regenerative abilities (Marrotte et al., 2010).

7. EPCs and diabetic retinopathy (DR)

DR, the leading cause of visual impairment in the western world, will occur in the majority of T1DM patients and about 20–30% will advance to the blinding stage of the disease. It is expected that over 60% of patients with T2DM will develop retinopathy and with the global epidemic of obesity and subsequently of T2DM this predicament is likely to worsen (Fong et al., 2002). Retinal neovascularization in diabetes is stringently affected by alterations in the local microenviroenment. Hyperglycemia damages retinal microvasculature, which results in increased permeability, blood and serum leakage to the extravascular space, and progressive decline in retinal blood flow; as well as closure of the retinal microvasculature leading to DR. Retinal ischemia and release of angiogenic factors stimulate the proliferation of microvessels, leading to proliferative DR (PDR). Dysfunctional new vessel growth destroys the normal retinal architecture and capillary leakage causes diabetic macular edema (DME), the principal cause of vision loss in diabetes (Li Calzi et al., 2010). Up until recently, angiogenesis was thought to be the only process governing aberrant diabetic retinal neovascularization. However, retinal ischemia-induced release of specific factors may stimulate both local growth of vessels and the mobilization of BM-derived EPCs, which contribute to the development of PDR. Initial studies in PDR experimental models have shown that EPCs could be recruited to retinal sites of ischemic injury, playing a role in the revascularization of the retina (Goon et al., 2007; Grant et al., 2002). Although the mechanisms underlying EPCs roles are still under evaluation, it was reported that they may be mobilized and recruited to the diabetic retina in response to local secretion of VEGF and SDF-1. Moreover, studies in PDR experimental models and in diabetic patients presenting this complication have shown that SDF-1 seems to be the most important chemokine involved in the mobilization of EPCs to the retina (Butler et al., 2005; Csaky et al., 2004). In addition, the concentration of SDF-1 increases with the severity of DR, as evaluated in vitreous samples of T2DM individuals (Butler et al., 2005). Recently, it was also proposed that retinal neuronal tissue could play a role in promoting EPCs-mediated neovascularization (Liu et al., 2010). This study has demonstrated that higher levels of the neurotrophins Nerve Growth Factor (NGF) and Brain-Derived Neurotrophic Factor (BDNF) are present in the PB of DR patients, but not in non-diabetic controls or DM-PAD patients. Additionally, a strong correlation between these neurotrophins and EPC levels in DR patients was found, suggesting that retinal ischemia serves as a signal to stimulate BM-EPCs through selected strong neurotrophic factors that are released into the systemic circulation. Recently, two reports conveyed more important information on the role of different progenitor cells in various stages of DR in T1DM and T2DM patients (Brunner et al., 2009, 2011). In T1DM, it was demonstrated that in non-PDR patients there was a reduction in circulating EPCs, and that in PDR there was a dramatic increase of mature EPCs (Brunner et al., 2009). In addition, circulating EPCs of T1DM patients with PDR were reported to have increased clonogenic potential (Asnaghi et al., 2006). In T2DM patients with DR, circulating angiopoietic cells as EPCs, and mature EPCs had different regulations in PDR depending on each individual's macrovascular comorbidities (Brunner et al., 2011). Recent findings in diabetic patients have corroborated gathered experimental data, demonstrating that BM-derived CD133+ EPCs, as well as, CD14+ monocytes could be mobilized to diabetic epiretinal membranes, contributing to vasculogenesis in PDR (Abu El-Asrar et al., 2011). Taken together, these data strengthen the importance of EPCs in the development of human PDR, highlighting the crucial role played by both the local retinal and the systemic environment.

8. Modulating EPCs functions as therapeutic strategy

It seems paradoxal that diabetic vascular complications, as PDR and PAD, may both affect the same patient, and alterations in EPCs exhibit opposing roles. This contradictory puzzle will most certainly have an influence when considering the modulating of EPCs levels/functions as therapeutic intervention. It has been shown that several vasculoprotective agents provided with beneficial cardiovascular effects, such as statins, thiazolidinediones (peroxisome proliferators-activated receptor-gamma; PPAR-γ), and anti-oxidants have been shown to improve endothelium-dependent vascular function and prevent atherosclerotic disease progression, by restoring EPCs properties and actions (Chen et al., 2011; Kusuyama et al., 2006; Schoonjans & Auwerx, 2000). Additionally, and althougth there are no conclusive answers on the safety on EPCs therapies and of their potential undesidered side effects, pre-clinical and clinical studies have highlighted that autologous transplantation of several stem and progenitor cell populations ameliorated diabetic peripheral vascular complications (Procházka et al., 2009; Zhou et al., 2007). Nonetheless, the dysfunction of endogenous EPCs may limit the feasibility and efficiency of this approach, since their biological features are altered, which reduces their capacity to significantly improve therapeutic neovascularization. In addition, one might not neglect that there are several EPCs subtypes, which raises the question on what might be the best reparative BM-derived EPCs population (Figure 1). Further, would EPCs-based therapies provide any beneficial effects in retinal neovascularization? As aforementioned, retinal new vessel growth associated to diabetes is dysfunctional, destroying the normal retinal architecture. So we may assume that improving diabetic EPCs functions/transplanting non-diabetic EPCs to the retina may promote the re-endothelialization of acellular capillaries and the elimination of retinal ischemia. In fact, if intra-retinal neovascularization could be harnessed at the appropriate stage, ischemia could be contained or reversed (Figure 2). However, since the intravitreal delivery of anti-angiogenic drugs may provide multiple benefits on DME and PDR (Arevalo et al., 2011; Chung et al., 2011), would the therapeutic use of EPCs be a better strategy for the treatment of DR? Many questions are still answered and in order to promote efficient EPCs-based therapies and to prevent harmful side effects, it is needed to go deeper into the molecular events accompanying alterations in diabetic vascular complications governing the diabetic-vasculogenic paradox.

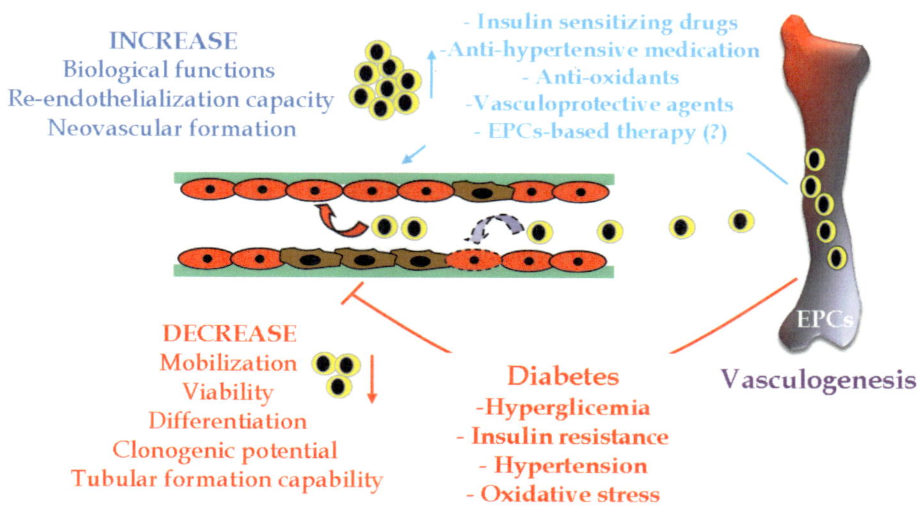

Fig. 1. Diabetes and peripheral vasculopathy. Diabetes related metabolic disorders decrease EPCs number and function being associated with impaired re-endothelialization and neovascular formation. Several agents may increase EPCs functions improving their re-vascularization capabilities. Adapted from Costa & Vendeira, 2007.

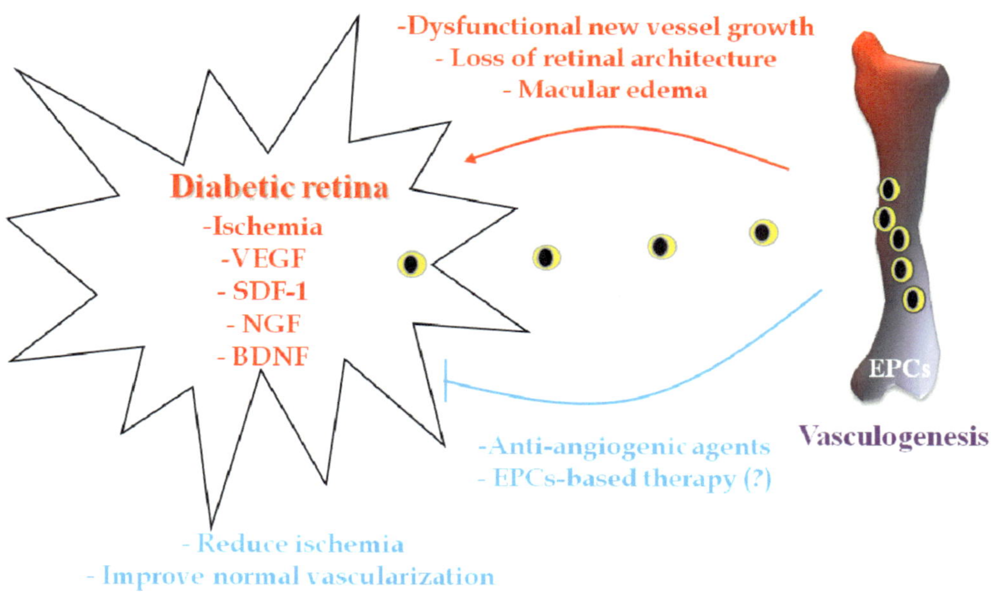

Fig. 2. Diabetic retinopathy. The ischemic retinal microenvironment and the production of vascular and neurothrophic factors promote increased EPCs recruitment and dysfunctional neovascular formation. Anti-angiogenic agents may improve retinal vascular architecture.

9. Concluding remarks

Even though EPCs constitute a relatively small percentage of circulating cells, they can specifically and effectively home to sites of injury and partake in the regeneration and repair of endothelial beds. Besides the initially identified population of CD34+AC133+VEGFR-2+ EPCs, other subsets of EPCs and progenitor cells with vascular repair capability have been described. We have discussed the most recent data demonstrating that dysfunctions of several EPCs subpopulations may have a prominent role in the pathogenesis of diabetes systemic and retinal vascular complications. Both the decrease and increase of neovascular formation in diabetes seem differentially regulated by dysfunctional EPCs, which respond selectively to the local depletion/accumulation of growth factors, explaining the reasons why peripheral ischemia cannot stimulate EPCs recruitment, in opposition to what occurs in the retina. Further studies are required to identify the beneficial effects/safety of EPCs-based therapies. Additionally, it is mandatory to investigate the efficient use of EPCs in promoting neovascularization in peripheral vascular disease and the abrogation of retinal ischemia and altered vascular architecture. This carefull evaluation is crucial to further unveil the diabetic-vasculogenic paradox.

10. References

Abu El-Asrar AM, Struyf S, Verbeke H, Van Damme J, Geboes K (2011). Circulating bone-marrow-derived endothelial precursor cells contribute to neovascularization in diabetic epiretinal membranes. *Acta Ophthalmol.*, 89(3), pp. (222-228), 1755-375X

Aicher A, Heeschen C, Mildner-Rihm C, Urbich C, Ihling C, Technau-Ihling K, Zeiher AM, Dimmeler S (2003). Essential role of endothelial nitric oxide synthase for mobilization of stem and progenitor cells. *Nat Med.*, 9(11), pp. (1370-1376), 1078-8956

Aicher A, Zeiher AM, Dimmeler S (2005). Mobilizing endothelial progenitor cells. *Hypertension*, 45(3), pp. (321-325), 0194911X

Arevalo JF, Sanchez JG, Lasave AF, Wu L, Maia M, Bonafonte S, Brito M, Alezzandrini AA, Restrepo N, Berrocal MH, Saravia M, Farah ME, Fromow-Guerra J, Morales-Canton V (2011). Intravitreal Bevacizumab (Avastin) for Diabetic Retinopathy: The 2010 GLADAOF Lecture. *J Ophthalmol.*, 2011, pp. (584238), 2090-0058

Aronson D (2008). Hyperglycemia and the pathobiology of diabetic complications. *Adv Cardiol.*, 45, pp. (1-16), 0065-2326

Asahara T, Murohara T, Sullivan A, Silver M, van der Zee R, Li T, Witzenbichler B, Schatteman G, Isner JM (1997). Isolation of putative progenitor endothelial cells for angiogenesis. *Science*, 275(5302), pp. (964-967), 0036-8075

Asahara T, Takahashi T, Masuda H, Kalka C, Chen D, Iwaguro H, Inai Y, Silver M, Isner JM (1999a). VEGF contributes to postnatal neovascularization by mobilizing bone marrow-derived endothelial progenitor cells. *EMBO J.*, 18(14), pp. (3964-3972), 0261-4189

Asahara T, Masuda H, Takahashi T, Kalka C, Pastore C, Silver M, Kearne M, Magner M, Isner JM (1999b). Bone marrow origin of endothelial progenitor cells responsible for postnatal vasculogenesis in physiological and pathological neovascularization. *Circ Res.*, 85(3), pp. (221-228), 0009-7300

Asnaghi V, Lattanzio R, Mazzolari G, Pastore MR, Ramoni A, Maestroni A, Ruggieri D, Luzi L, Brancato R, Zerbini G (2006). Increased clonogenic potential of circulating endothelial progenitor cells in patients with type 1 diabetes and proliferative retinopathy. *Diabetologia*, 49(5), pp. (1109-1111), 0012-186X

Balestrieri ML, Rienzo M, Felice F, Rossiello R, Grimaldi V, Milone L, Casamassimi A, Servillo L, Farzati B, Giovane A, Napoli C (2008a). High glucose downregulates endothelial progenitor cell number via SIRT1. *Biochim Biophys Acta.*, 1784(6), pp. (936-945), 0006-3002

Blann AD, Pretorius A (2006). Circulating endothelial cells and endothelial progenitor cells: two sides of the same coin, or two different coins? *Atherosclerosis*, 188(1), pp. (12-18), 0021-9150

Brunner S, Schernthaner GH, Satler M, Elhenicky M, Hoellerl F, Schmid-Kubista KE, Zeiler F, Binder S, Schernthaner G (2009). Correlation of different circulating endothelial progenitor cells to stages of diabetic retinopathy: first in vivo data. *Invest Ophthalmol Vis Sci.*, 50(1), pp. (392-398), 0146-0404

Brunner S, Hoellerl F, Schmid-Kubista KE, Zeiler F, Schernthaner G, Binder S, Schernthaner GH. Circulating angiopoietic cells and diabetic retinopathy in T2DM patients with and without macrovascular disease. *Invest Ophthalmol Vis Sci.* 2011 Mar 11. [Epub ahead of print], 0146-0404

Butler JM, Guthrie SM, Koc M, Afzal A, Caballero S, Brooks HL, Mames RN, Segal MS, Grant MB, Scott EW (2005). SDF-1 is both necessary and sufficient to promote proliferative retinopathy. *J Clin Invest.*, 115(1), pp. (86-93), 0021-9738

Cacciatore F, Bruzzese G, Vitale DF, Liguori A, de Nigris F, Fiorito C, Infante T, Donatelli F, Minucci PB, Ignarro LJ, Napoli C. Effects of ACE inhibition on circulating endothelial progenitor cells, vascular damage, and oxidative stress in hypertensive patients. Eur J Clin Pharmacol. 2011, [Epub ahead of print], 0031-6970

Callaghan MJ, Ceradini DJ, Gurtner GC (2005). Hyperglycemia-induced reactive oxygen species and impaired endothelial progenitor cell function. *Antioxid Redox Signal.*, 7(11-12), pp. (1476-1482), 1523-0864

Case J, Mead LE, Bessler WK, Prater D, White HA, Saadatzadeh MR, Bhavsar JR, Yoder MC, Haneline LS, Ingram DA (2007). Human CD34+AC133+VEGFR-2+ cells are not endothelial progenitor cells but distinct, primitive hematopoietic progenitors. *Exp Hematol.*, 35(7), pp. (1109-1118), 0301-472X

Chen YH, Lin SJ, Lin FY, Wu TC, Tsao CR, Huang PH, Liu PL, Chen YL, Chen JW (2007). High glucose impairs early and late endothelial progenitor cells by modifying nitric oxide-related but not oxidative stress-mediated mechanisms. *Diabetes*, 56(6), pp. (1559-1568), 0012-1797

Chen J, Song M, Yu S, Gao P, Yu Y, Wang H, Huang L (2010). Advanced glycation endproducts alter functions and promote apoptosis in endothelial progenitor cells through receptor for advanced glycation endproducts mediate overpression of cell oxidant stress. *Mol Cell Biochem.*, 335(1-2), pp. (137-146), 0300-8177

Chen LL, Yu F, Zeng TS, Liao YF, Li YM, Ding HC (2011). Effects of gliclazide on endothelial function in patients with newly diagnosed type 2 diabetes. *Eur J Pharmacol.*, 659(2-3), pp. (296-301), 0014-2999

Chung EJ, Kang SJ, Koo JS, Choi YJ, Grossniklaus HE, Koh HJ (2011). Effect of intravitreal bevacizumab on vascular endothelial growth factor expression in patients with proliferative diabetic retinopathy. *Yonsei Med J.*, 52(1), pp. (151-157), 0513-5796

Churdchomjan W, Kheolamai P, Manochantr S, Tapanadechopone P, Tantrawatpan C, U-Pratya Y, Issaragrisil S (2010). Comparison of endothelial progenitor cell function in type 2 diabetes with good and poor glycemic control.*BMC Endocr Disord.*, 10:5, (1472-6823), 1472-6823

Ciulla TA, Amador AG, Zinman B (2003). Diabetic retinopathy and diabetic macular edema: pathophysiology, screening, and novel therapies. *Diabetes Care*, 26(9), pp. (2653-2664), 0149-5992

Costa C, Incio J, Soares, R (2007). Angiogenesis and chronic inflammation: cause or consequence? *Angiogenesis*, 10(3), pp. (149-166), 0969-6970

Costa C, Vendeira P. (2007). Penis and endothelium - Extra genital aspects of erectile dysfunction. *Rev Int Androl.*, 5(1), pp. (50-58), 1698-031X

Creager MA, Luscher TF, Cosentino F, Beckman JA (2003). Diabetes and vascular disease: pathophysiology, clinical consequences, and medical therapy, part I. *Circulation*, 108(12), pp. (1527-1532), 0009-7322

Csaky KG, Baffi JZ, Byrnes GA, Wolfe JD, Hilmer SC, Flippin J, Cousins SW (2004). Recruitment of marrow-derived endothelial cells to experimental choroidal neovascularization by local expression of vascular endothelial growth factor. *Exp. Eye Res.*, 78(6), pp. (1107-1116), 0014-4835

Cubbon RM, Rajwani A, Wheatcroft SB (2007). The impact of insulin resistance on endothelial function, progenitor cells and repair. *Diab Vasc Dis Res.*, 4(2), pp. (103-111), 1479-1641

Cubbon RM, Kahn MB, Wheatcroft SB (2009). Effects of insulin resistance on endothelial progenitor cells and vascular repair. *Clin Sci (Lond).*, 117(5), pp. (173-190), 0143-5221

Dandona P, Aljada A, Chaudhuri A, Bandyopadhyay A (2003). The potential influence of inflammation and insulin resistance on the pathogenesis and treatment of atherosclerosis-related complications in type 2 diabetes. *J Clin Endocrinol Metab.*, 88(6), pp. (2422-2429), 0021-972X

Dandona P, Aljada A, Bandyopadhyay A (2004). Inflammation: the link between insulin resistance, obesity and diabetes. *Trends Immunol.*, 25(1), pp. (4-7), 1471-4906

de Ciuceis C, Pilu A, Rizzoni D, Porteri E, Muiesan ML, Salvetti M, Paini A, Belotti E, Zani F, Boari GE, Rosei CA, Rosei EA (2011). Effect of antihypertensive treatment on circulating endothelial progenitor cells in patients with mild essential hypertension. *Blood Press.*, 20(2), pp. (77-83), 0803-7051

De Palma M, Venneri MA, Galli R, Sergi Sergi L, Politi LS, Sampaolesi M, Naldini L (2005). Tie2 identifies a hematopoietic lineage of proangiogenic monocytes required for tumor vessel formation and a mesenchymal population of pericyte progenitors. *Cancer Cell*, 2005; 8(3), pp. (211-226), 1535-6108

Delva P, Degan M, Vallerio P, Arosio E, Minuz P, Amen G, Di Chio M, Lechi A (2007). Endothelial progenitor cells in patients with essential hypertension. *J Hypertens.*, 25(1) , pp. (127-132), 0263-6352

Desouza CV, Hamel FG, Bidasee K, O'Connell K (2011). Role of inflammation and insulin resistance in endothelial progenitor cell dysfunction. *Diabetes.*, 60(4), pp. (1286-1294), 0012-1797

Duh E, Aiello LP (1999). Vascular endothelial growth factor and diabetes: the agonist versus antagonist paradox. *Diabetes*, 48(10), pp. (1899-1906), 0012-1797

Egan CG, Lavery R, Caporali F, Fondelli C, Laghi-Pasini F, Dotta F, Sorrentino V (2008). Generalised reduction of putative endothelial progenitors and CXCR4-positive peripheral blood cells in type 2 diabetes. *Diabetologia*, 51(7), pp. (1296-1305), 0012-186X

Fadini GP, Miorin M, Facco M, Bonamico S, Baesso I, Grego F, Menegolo M, de Kreutzenberg SV, Tiengo A, Agostini C, Avogaro A (2005). Circulating endothelial progenitor cells are reduced in peripheral vascular complications of type 2 diabetes mellitus. *J Am Coll Cardiol.*, 45(9), pp. (1449-1457), 0735-1097

Fadini GP, Sartore S, Albiero M, Baesso I, Murphy E, Menegolo M, Grego F, Vigili de Kreutzenberg S, Tiengo A, Agostini C, Avogaro A (2006a). Number and function of endothelial progenitor cells as a marker of severity for diabetic vasculopathy. *Arterioscler Thromb Vasc Biol.*, 26(9), pp. (2140-2146), 1079-5642

Fadini GP, Sartore S, Schiavon M, Albiero M, Baesso I, Cabrelle A, Agostini C, Avogaro A (2006b). Diabetes impairs progenitor cell mobilisation after hindlimb ischaemia-reperfusion injury in rats. *Diabetologia*, 49(12), pp. (3075-3084), 0012-186X

Fadini GP, Sartore S, Baesso I, Lenzi M, Agostini C, Tiengo A, Avogaro A (2006c). Endothelial progenitor cells and the diabetic paradox. *Diabetes Care*, 29(3), pp. (714-716), 0149-5992

Fang S, Salven P (2011). Stem cells in tumor angiogenesis. *J Mol Cell Cardiol.*, 50(2), pp. (290-295), 0022-2828

Fleissner F, Thum T. Critical Role of the Nitric Oxide/Reactive Oxygen Species Balance in Endothelial Progenitor Dysfunction. Antioxid Redox Signal. 2010 Dec 13. [Epub ahead of print], 1523-0864

Folkman J (1984). What is the role of endothelial cells in angiogenesis? *Lab Invest.*, 51(6), pp. 601-604, 0023-6837

Fong DS, Sharza M, Chen W, Paschal JF, Ariyasu RG, Lee PP (2002). Vision loss among diabetics in a group model Health Maintenance Organization (HMO). *Am J Ophthalmol.*, 133(2), pp. (236-241), 0002-9394

Foresta C, Schipilliti M, De Toni L, Magagna S, Lancerotto L, Azzena B, Vindigni V, Mazzoleni F (2011). Blood levels, apoptosis, and homing of the endothelial progenitor cells after skin burns and escharectomy. *J Trauma*, 70(2), pp. (459-465), 0022-5282

Freundlich B, Avdalovic N (1983). Use of gelatin/plasma coated flasks for isolating human peripheral blood monocytes. *J Immunol Methods*, 62(1), pp. (31–37), 0022-1759

Friedrich EB, Walenta K, Scharlau J, Nickenig G, Werner N (2006). CD34-/CD133+/VEGFR-2+ endothelial progenitor cell subpopulation with potent vasoregenerative capacities. *Circ Res.*, 98(3), pp. (e20-25), 0009-7330

Gallagher KA, Liu ZJ, Xiao M, Chen H, Goldstein LJ, Buerk DG, Nedeau A, Thom SR, Velazquez OC (2007). Diabetic impairments in NO-mediated endothelial progenitor cell mobilization and homing are reversed by hyperoxia and SDF-1 alpha. *J Clin Invest.*, 117(5), pp. (1249-1259), 0021-9738

Gensch C, Clever YP, Werner C, Hanhoun M, Böhm M, Laufs U (2007). The PPAR-gamma agonist pioglitazone increases neoangiogenesis and prevents apoptosis of endothelial progenitor cells. *Atherosclerosis.*, 192(1), pp. (67-74), 0021-9150

Giannotti G, Doerries C, Mocharla PS, Mueller MF, Bahlmann FH, Horvàth T, Jiang H, Sorrentino SA, Steenken N, Manes C, Marzilli M, Rudolph KL, Lüscher TF, Drexler H, Landmesser U (2010). Impaired endothelial repair capacity of early endothelial progenitor cells in prehypertension: relation to endothelial dysfunction. *Hypertension*, 55(6), pp. (1389-1397), 0194911X

Gill M, Dias S, Hattori K, Rivera ML, Hicklin D, Witte L, Girardi L, Yurt R, Himel H, Rafii S (2001). Vascular trauma induces rapid but transient mobilization of VEGFR2(+)AC133(+) endothelial precursor cells. *Circ Res.*, 88(2), pp. (167-174), 0009-7330

Goon PK, Lip GY (2007). Involvement of circulating endothelial progenitor cells and vasculogenic factors in the pathogenesis of diabetic retinopathy. *Eye*, 21(6), pp. (838-839), 0950-222X

Grant MB, May WS, Caballero S, Brown GA, Guthrie SM, Mames RN, Byrne BJ, Vaught T, Spoerri PE, Peck AB, Scott EW (2002). Adult hematopoietic stem cells provide functional hemangioblast activity during retinal neovascularization. *Nat. Med.*, 8(6), pp. (607-612), 1078-8956

Griendling KK, FitzGerald GA (2003). Oxidative stress and cardiovascular injury. Part II. Animal and human studies. *Circulation*, 108(17), pp. (2034-2040), 0009-7322

Grunewald M, Avraham I, Dor Y, Bachar-Lustig E, Itin A, Jung S, Chimenti S, Landsman L, Abramovitch R, Keshet E (2006). VEGF-induced adult neovascularization: recruitment, retention, and role of accessory cells. *Cell*, 124(1), pp. (175-189), 0092-8674

Gulati R, Jevremovic D, Peterson TE, Chatterjee S, Shah V, Vile RG, Simari RD (2003). Diverse origin and function of cells with endothelial phenotype obtained from adult human blood. *Circ Res.*, 93(11), pp. (1023-1025), 0009-7300

Haffner SM, Lehto S, Rönnemaa T, Pyörälä K, Laakso M (1998). Mortality from coronary heart disease in subjects with type 2 diabetes and in nondiabetic subjects with and without prior myocardial infarction. *N Engl J Med.*, 339(4), pp. (229-234), 0028-4793

Heissig B, Hattori K, Dias S, Friedrich M, Ferris B, Hackett NR, Crystal RG, Besmer P, Lyden D, Moore MA, Werb Z, Rafii S (2002). Recruitment of stem and progenitor cells from the bone marrow niche requires MMP-9 mediated release of kit-ligand. *Cell*, 109(5), pp. (625-37), 0092-8674

Higashi Y, Sasaki S, Nakagawa K, Matsuura H, Oshima T, Chayama K (2002). Endothelial function and oxidative stress in renovascular hypertension. *N Engl J Med.*, 346(25), pp. (1954-1962), 0028-4793

Hill JM, Zalos G, Halcox JP, Schenke WH, Waclawiw MA, Quyyumi AA, Finkel T (2003). Circulating endothelial progenitor cells, vascular function, and cardiovascular risk. *N Engl J Med.*, 348(7), pp. (593-600), 0028-4793

Hirschi KK, Ingram DA, Yoder MC (2008). Assessing identity, phenotype, and fate of endothelial progenitor cells. *Arterioscler Thromb Vasc Biol.*, 28(9), pp. (1584–1595), 1079-5642

Houstis N, Rosen ED, Lander ES (2006). Reactive oxygen species have a causal role in multiple forms of insulin resistance. *Nature.*, 440(7086), pp. (944-948), 0028-0836

Hristov M, Erl W, Weber PC (2003). Endothelial progenitor cells: isolation and characterization. *Trends Cardiovasc Med.*, 13(5), pp. (201-206), 1050-1738

Hur J, Yoon CH, Kim HS, Choi JH, Kang HJ, Hwang KK, Oh BH, Lee MM, Park YB (2004). Characterization of two types of endothelial progenitor cells and their different contributions to neovasculogenesis. *Arterioscler Thromb Vasc Biol.*, 24(2), pp. (288-293), 1079-5642

Imanishi T, Moriwaki C, Hano T, Nishio I (2005). Endothelial progenitor cell senescence is accelerated in both experimental hypertensive rats and patients with essential hypertension. *J Hypertens.*, 23(10), pp. (1831-1837), 0263-6352

Ingram DA, Mead LE, Moore DB, Woodard W, Fenoglio A, Yoder MC (2005). Vessel wall-derived endothelial cells rapidly proliferate because they contain a complete hierarchy of endothelial progenitor cells. *Blood*, 105(7), pp. (2783-2786), 0006-4971

Ingram DA, Lien IZ, Mead LE, Estes M, Prater DN, Derr-Yellin E, DiMeglio LA, Haneline LS (2008). In vitro hyperglycemia or a diabetic intrauterine environment reduces neonatal endothelial colony-forming cell numbers and function. *Diabetes*, 57(3), pp. (724-731), 0012-1797

Jandeleit-Dahm K, Cooper ME (2008). The role of AGEs in cardiovascular disease. *Curr Pharm Des.*, 14(10), pp. (979-986), 1381-6128

Jung C, Rafnsson A, Shemyakin A, Böhm F, Pernow J (2010). Different subpopulations of endothelial progenitor cells and circulating apoptotic progenitor cells in patients with vascular disease and diabetes. *Int J Cardiol.*, 143(3), pp. (368-372), 0167-5273

Kahn MB, Yuldasheva NY, Cubbon RM, Smith J, Rashid ST, Viswambharan H, Imrie H, Abbas A, Rajwani A, Aziz A, Baliga V, Sukumar P, Gage M, Kearney MT, Wheatcroft SB (2011). Insulin resistance impairs circulating angiogenic progenitor cell function and delays endothelial regeneration. *Diabetes*, 60(4), pp. (1295-1303), 0012-1797

Kang L, Chen Q, Wang L, Gao L, Meng K, Chen J, Ferro A, Xu B. (2009). Decreased Mobilization of Endothelial Progenitor Cells Contributes to Impaired neovascularization in Diabetes. *Clin Exp Pharmacol Physiol.*, 36(10), pp. (e47-56), 0143-9294

Kaplan RN, Riba RD, Zacharoulis S, Bramley AH, Vincent L, Costa C, MacDonald DD, Jin DK, Shido K, Kerns SA, Zhu Z, Hicklin D, Wu Y, Port JL, Altorki N, Port ER, Ruggero D, Shmelkov SV, Jensen KK, Rafii S, Lyden D (2005). VEGFR1-positive haematopoietic bone marrow progenitors initiate the pre-metastatic niche. *Nature*, 438(7069), pp. (820-827), 0028-0836

Kim JA, Montagnani M, Koh KK, Quon MJ (2006). Reciprocal relationships between insulin resistance and endothelial dysfunction: molecular and pathophysiological mechanisms. *Circulation*, 113(15), pp. (1888-1904), 0009-7322

Kirton JP, Xu Q (2010). Endothelial precursors in vascular repair. *Microvasc Res.*, 79(3), pp. (193-199), 0026-2862

Kränkel N, Adams V, Linke A, Gielen S, Erbs S, Lenk K, Schuler G, Hambrecht R (2005). Hyperglycemia reduces survival and impairs function of circulating blood-derived progenitor cells. *Arterioscler Thromb Vasc Biol.*, 25(4), pp. (698-703), 1079-5642

Kuki S, Imanishi T, Kobayashi K, Matsuo Y, Obana M, Akasaka T (2006). Hyperglycemia accelerated endothelial progenitor cell senescence via the activation of p38 mitogen-activated protein kinase. *Circ J.*, 70(8), pp. (1076-1081), 1346-9843

Kusuyama T, Omura T, Nishiya D, Enomoto S, Matsumoto R, Murata T, Takeuchi K, YoshikawaJ, Yoshiyama M (2006). The effects of HMG-CoA reductase inhibitor on vascular progenitor cells. *J. Pharmacol. Sci.*, 101(4), pp. (344-349), 1347-8613

Kuzkaya N, Weissmann N, Harrison DG, Dikalov S (2003). Interactions of peroxynitrite, tetrahydrobiopterin, ascorbic acid, and thiols: implications for uncoupling endothelial nitric-oxide synthase. *J Biol Chem.*, 278(25), pp. (22546-2254), 0021-9258

Li Calzi S, Neu MB, Shaw LC, Grant MB (2010). Endothelial progenitor dysfunction in the pathogenesis of diabetic retinopathy: treatment concept to correct diabetes-associated deficits. *EPMA J.*, 1(1), pp. (88-100), 1878-5077

Liang C, Ren Y, Tan H, He Z, Jiang Q, Wu J, Zhen Y, Fan M, Wu Z (2009). Rosiglitazone via upregulation of Akt/eNOS pathways attenuates dysfunction of endothelial progenitor cells, induced by advanced glycation end products. *Br J Pharmacol.*, 158(8), pp. (1865-1873), 0007-1188

Liu X, Li Y, Liu Y, Luo Y, Wang D, Annex BH, Goldschmidt-Clermont PJ (2010). Endothelial progenitor cells (EPCs) mobilized and activated by neurotrophic factors may contribute to pathologic neovascularization in diabetic retinopathy. *Am J Pathol.*, 176(1), pp. (504-515), 0002-9440

Loomans CJ, van Haperen R, Duijs JM, Verseyden C, de Crom R, Leenen PJ, Drexhage HA, de Boer HC, de Koning EJ, Rabelink TJ, Staal FJ, van Zonneveld AJ (2009). Differentiation of bone marrow-derived endothelial progenitor cells is shifted into a proinflammatory phenotype by hyperglycemia. *Mol Med.*, 15(5-6), pp. (152-159), 1528-3658

Lyden D, Hattori K, Dias S, Costa C, Blaikie P, Butros L, Chadburn A, Heissig B, Marks W, Witte L, Wu Y, Hicklin D, Zhu Z, Hackett NR, Crystal RG, Moore MA, Hajjar KA, Manova K, Benezra R, Rafii S (2001). Impaired recruitment of bone-marrow-derived endothelial and hematopoietic precursor cells blocks tumor angiogenesis and growth. *Nat. Med.*, 7(11), pp. (1194-1201), 1078-8956

Madonna R, De Caterina R. Cellular and molecular mechanisms of vascular injury in diabetes - Part II: Cellular mechanisms and therapeutic targets. *Vascul Pharmacol.* 2011 Mar 29. [Epub ahead of print], 1537-1891

Marfella R, Esposito K, Nappo F, Siniscalchi M, Sasso FC, Portoghese M, Di Marino MP, Baldi A, Cuzzocrea S, Di Filippo C, Barboso G, Baldi F, Rossi F, D'Amico M, Giugliano D (2004). Expression of angiogenic factors during acute coronary syndromes in human type 2 diabetes. *Diabetes*, 53(9), pp. (2383-2391), 0012-1797

Marrotte EJ, Chen DD, Hakim JS, Chen AF (2010). Manganese superoxide dismutase expression in endothelial progenitor cells accelerates wound healing in diabetic mice. *J Clin Invest.*, 120(12), pp. (4207-4219), 0021-9738

Matsumoto T, Mifune Y, Kawamoto A, Kuroda R, Shoji T, Iwasaki H, Suzuki T, Oyamada A, Horii M, Yokoyama A, Nishimura H, Lee SY, Miwa M, Doita M, Kurosaka M, Asahara T (2008). Fracture induced mobilization and incorporation of bone marrow-derived endothelial progenitor cells for bone healing. *J Cell Physiol.*, 215(1), pp. (234-242), 0021-9541

Medina RJ, O'Neill CL, Sweeney M, Guduric-Fuchs J, Gardiner TA, Simpson DA, Stitt AW (2010). Molecular analysis of endothelial progenitor cell (EPC) subtypes reveals two distinct cell populations with different identities. *BMC Med Genomics*, 3, pp. (18), 1755-8794

Nakagami H, Kaneda Y, Ogihara T, Morishita R (2005). Endothelial dysfunction in hyperglycemia as a trigger of atherosclerosis. *Curr Diabetes Rev.*, 1(1), pp. (59-63), 1573-3998

Peichev M, Naiyer AJ, Pereira D, Zhu Z, Lane WJ, Williams M, Oz MC, Hicklin DJ, Witte L, Moore MA, Rafii S (2000). Expression of VEGFR-2 and AC133 by circulating human CD34(+) cells identifies a population of functional endothelial precursors. *Blood*, 95(3), pp. (952-958), 0006-4971

Perkins I (2004). Diabetes mellitus epidemiology-classification, determinants, and public health impacts. *J Miss State Med Assoc.*, 45(12), pp. (355-362), 0026-6396

Perticone F, Ceravolo R, Pujia A, Ventura G, Iacopino S, Scozzafava A, Ferraro A, Chello M, Mastroroberto P, Verdecchia P, Schillaci G (2001). Prognostic significance of endothelial dysfunction in hypertensive patients. *Circulation*, 104(2), pp. (191-196), 0009-7322

Peters BA, Diaz LA, Polyak K, Meszler L, Romans K, Guinan EC, Antin JH, Myerson D, Hamilton SR, Vogelstein B, Kinzler KW, Lengauer C (2005). Contribution of bone marrow-derived endothelial cells to human tumor vasculature. *Nat Med.*, 11(3), pp. (261-262), 1078-8956

Pirro M, Schillaci G, Menecali C, Bagaglia F, Paltriccia R, Vaudo G, Mannarino MR, Mannarino E (2007). Reduced number of circulating endothelial progenitors and HOXA9 expression in CD34+ cells of hypertensive patients. *J Hypertens.*, 25(10), pp. (2093-2099), 0263-6352

Porto I, Leone AM, De Maria GL, Craig CH, Tritarelli A, Camaioni C, Natale L, Niccoli G, Biasucci LM, Crea F. Are endothelial progenitor cells mobilized by myocardial ischemia or myocardial necrosis? A cardiac magnetic resonance study. *Atherosclerosis*. 2011 Feb 17. [Epub ahead of print], 0021-9150

Povsic TJ, Goldschmidt-Clermont PJ (2008). Endothelial progenitor cells: markers of vascular reparative capacity. *Ther Adv Cardiovasc Dis.*, 2(3), pp. (199-113), 1753-9447

Procházka V, Gumulec J, Chmelová J, Klement P, Klement GL, Jonszta T, Czerný D, Krajca J (2009). Autologous bone marrow stem cell transplantation in patients with end-stage chronical critical limb ischemia and diabetic foot. *Vnitr. Lek.*, 55(3), pp. (173-178), 0042-773X

Prokopi M, Pula G, Mayr U, Devue C, Gallagher J, Xiao Q, Boulanger CM, Westwood N, Urbich C, Willeit J, Steiner M, Breuss J, Xu Q, Kiechl S, Mayr M (2009). Proteomic analysis reveals presence of platelet microparticles in endothelial progenitor cell cultures. *Blood*, 114(3), pp. (723-732), 0006-4971

Purhonen S, Palm J, Rossi D, Kaskenpää N, Rajantie I, Ylä-Herttuala S, Alitalo K, Weissman IL, Salven P (2008). Bone marrow-derived circulating endothelial precursors do not contribute to vascular endothelium and are not needed for tumor growth. *Proc Natl Acad Sci U S A.*, 105(18), pp. (6620-6625), 0027-8424

Rehman J, Li J, Orschell CM, March KL (2003). Peripheral blood "endothelial progenitor cells" are derived from monocyte/macrophages and secrete angiogenic growth factors. *Circulation*, 107(8), pp. (1164–1169), 0009-7322

Risau W, Flamme I (1995). Vasculogenesis. *Annu Rev Cell Dev Biol.*, 11, pp. (73-91), 1081-0706

Risau, W. Mechanisms of angiogenesis (1997). *Nature*, 386(6626), pp. (671-674), 0028-0836

Satoh M, Ishikawa Y, Takahashi Y, Itoh T, Minami Y, Nakamura M (2008). Association between oxidative DNA damage and telomere shortening in circulating endothelial progenitor cells obtained from metabolic syndrome patients with coronary artery disease. *Atherosclerosis*, 198(2), pp. (347-353), 0021-9150

Schiffrin EL (2001). A critical review of the role of endothelial factors in the pathogenesis of hypertension. *J Cardiovasc Pharmacol.*, 38(Suppl 2), pp. (S3-S6), 0160-2446

Schoonjans K, Auwerx J (2000). Thiazolidinediones: an update. *Lancet*, 355(9208), pp. (1008-1110), 0140-6736

Shantsila E, Watson T, Lip GY (2007). Endothelial progenitor cells in cardiovascular disorders. *J Am Coll Cardiol.*, 49(7), pp. (741-752), 0735-1097

Shen C, Li Q, Zhang YC, Ma G, Feng Y, Zhu Q, Dai Q, Chen Z, Yao Y, Chen L, Jiang Y, Liu N (2010). Advanced glycation endproducts increase EPC apoptosis and decrease nitric oxide release via MAPK pathways. *Biomed Pharmacother.*, 64(1), pp. (35-43), 0753-3322

Shi Q, Rafii S, Wu MH, Wijelath ES, Yu C, Ishida A, Fujita Y, Kothari S, Mohle R, Sauvage LR, Moore MA, Storb RF, Hammond WP (1998). Evidence for circulating bone marrow-derived endothelial cells. *Blood*, 92(2), pp. (362-367), 0006-4971

Shintani S, Murohara T, Ikeda H, Ueno T, Honma T, Katoh A, Sasaki K, Shimada T, Oike Y, Imaizumi T (2001). Mobilization of endothelial progenitor cells in patients with acute myocardial infarction. *Circulation*, 103(23), pp. (2776-2779), 0009-7322

Sorrentino SA, Bahlmann FH, Besler C, Müller M, Schulz S, Kirchhoff N, Doerries C, Horváth T, Limbourg A, Limbourg F, Fliser D, Haller H, Drexler H, Landmesser U (2007). Oxidant stress impairs in vivo reendothelialization capacity of endothelial progenitor cells from patients with type 2 diabetes mellitus: restoration by the peroxisome proliferator-activated receptor-gamma agonist rosiglitazone. *Circulation*, 116(2), pp. (163-173), 0009-7322

Spieker LE, Noll G, Ruschitzka FT, Maier W, Luscher TF (2000). Working under pressure: the vascular endothelium in arterial hypertension. *J Hum Hypertens.*, 14(10-11), pp. (617-630), 0950-9240

Takahashi T, Kalka C, Masuda H, Chen D, Silver M, Kearney M, Magner M, Isner JM, Asahara T (1999). Ischemia- and cytokine-induced mobilization of bone marrow-derived endothelial progenitor cells for neovascularization. *Nat. Med.*, 5(4), pp. (434-438), 1078-8956

Takakura N (2006). Role of hematopoietic lineage cells as accessory components in blood vessel formation. *Cancer Sci.*, 97(7), pp. (568-574), 1347-9032

Tepper OM, Galiano RD, Capla JM, Kalka C, Gagne PJ, Jacobowitz GR, Levine JP, Gurtner GC (2002). Human endothelial progenitor cells from type II diabetics exhibit impaired proliferation, adhesion, and incorporation into vascular structures. *Circulation*, 106(22), pp. (2781-2786), 0009-7322

Timmermans F, Van Hauwermeiren F, De Smedt M, Raedt R, Plasschaert F, De Buyzere ML, Gillebert TC, Plum J, Vandekerckhove B (2007). Endothelial outgrowth cells are not derived from CD133+ cells or CD45+ hematopoietic precursors. *Arterioscler Thromb Vasc Biol.*, 27(7), pp. (1572-1579), 1079-5642

Timmermans F, Plum J, Yöder MC, Ingram DA, Vandekerckhove B, Case J (2009). Endothelial progenitor cells: identity defined? *J Cell Mol Med.*, 13(1), pp. (87–102), 1582-1838

Touyz RM, Schiffrin EL (2004). Reactive oxygen species in vascular biology: implications in hypertension. *Histochem Cell Biol.*, 122(4), pp. (339-352), 0948-6143

Urbich C, Aicher A, Heeschen C, Dernbach E, Hofmann WK, Zeiher AM, Dimmeler S. (2005). Soluble factors released by endothelial progenitor cells promote migration of endothelial cells and cardiac resident progenitor cells. *J Mol Cell Cardiol.*, 39(5), pp. (733-742), 0022-2828

Vasa M, Fichtlscherer S, Aicher A, Adler K, Urbich C, Martin H, Zeiher AM, Dimmeler S (2001). Number and migratory activity of circulating endothelial progenitor cells inversely correlate with risk factors for coronary artery disease. *Circ Res.*, 89(1), pp. (E1-7), 0009-7300

Vöö S, Dunaeva M, Eggermann J, Stadler N, Waltenberger J (2009). Diabetes mellitus impairs CD133+ progenitor cell function after myocardial infarction. *J Intern Med.*, 265(2), pp. (238-249), 0954-6820

Watson T, Goon PK, Lip GY (2008). Endothelial progenitor cells, endothelial dysfunction, inflammation, and oxidative stress in hypertension. *Antioxid Redox Signal.*, 10(6), pp. (1079-1088), 1523-0864

Werner N, Kosiol S, Schiegl T, Ahlers P, Walenta K, Link A, Böhm M, Nickenig G (2005). Circulating endothelial progenitor cells and cardiovascular outcomes. *N Engl J Med.*, 353(10), pp. (999-1007), 0028-4793

Yanai H, Tomono Y, Ito K, Furutani N, Yoshida H, Tada N (2008). The underlying mechanisms for development of hypertension in the metabolic syndrome. *Nutr J.*, 7, pp. (10-15), 1475-2891

Yao EH, Yu Y, Fukuda N (2006). Oxidative stress on progenitor and stem cells in cardiovascular diseases. *Curr Pharm Biotechnol.*, 7(2), pp. (101-108), 1389-2010

Yao EH, Fukuda N, Matsumoto T, Kobayashi N, Katakawa M, Yamamoto C, Tsunemi A, Suzuki R, Ueno T, Matsumoto K (2007). Losartan improves the impaired function of endothelial progenitor cells in hypertension via an antioxidant effect. *Hypertens Res.*, 30(11), pp. (1119-1128), 0916-9636

Yoder MC, Mead LE, Prater D, Krier TR, Mroueh KN, Li F, Krasich R, Temm CJ, Prchal JT, Ingram DA (2007). Redefining endothelial progenitor cells via clonal analysis and hematopoietic stem/progenitor cell principals. Blood, 109(5), pp. 1801-1819, 0006-4971

Yoder MC (2009). Defining human endothelial progenitor cells. *J Thromb Haemost.*, 7(Suppl 1), pp. (49-52), 1538-7933

Yoon CH, Hur J, Park KW, Kim JH, Lee CS, Oh IY, Kim TY, Cho HJ, Kang HJ, Chae IH, Yang HK, Oh BH, Park YB, Kim HS (2005a). Synergistic neovascularization by mixed transplantation of early endothelial progenitor cells and late outgrowth endothelial cells: the role of angiogenic cytokines and matrix metalloproteinases. *Circulation*, 112(11), pp. (1618-1627), 0009-7322

Yoon YS, Uchida S, Masuo O, Cejna M, Park JS, Gwon HC, Kirchmair R, Bahlman F, Walter D, Curry C, Hanley A, Isner JM, Losordo DW (2005b). Progressive attenuation of myocardial vascular endothelial growth factor expression is a seminal event in diabetic cardiomyopathy: restoration of microvascular homeostasis and recovery of cardiac function in diabetic cardiomyopathy after replenishment of local vascular endothelial growth factor. *Circulation*, 111(16), pp. (2073-2085), 0009-7322

You D, Cochain C, Loinard C, Vilar J, Mees B, Duriez M, Lévy BI, Silvestre JS (2008). Hypertension impairs postnatal vasculogenesis: role of antihypertensive agents. *Hypertension*, 51(6), pp. (1537-1544), 0194-911X

Zhang SJ, Zhang H, Wei YJ, Su WJ, Liao ZK, Hou M, Zhou JY, Hu SS (2006). Adult endothelial progenitor cells from human peripheral blood maintain monocyte/macrophage function throughout in vitro culture. *Cell Res.*, 16(6), pp. (577-584), 1001-0602

Zhang SJ, Zhang H, Hou M, Zheng Z, Zhou J, Su W, Wei Y, Hu S (2007). Is it possible to obtain "true endothelial progenitor cells" by in vitro culture of bone marrow mononuclear cells? *Stem Cells Dev.*, 16(4), pp. (683-690), 1547-3287

Zhou B, Cao XC, Fang ZH, Zheng CL, Han ZB, Ren H, Poon MC, Han ZC (2007). Prevention of diabetic microangiopathy by prophylactic transplant of mobilized peripheral blood mononuclear cells. *Acta. Pharmacol. Sin.*, (1), pp. (89-97), 1671-4083

Zimmet P, Alberti KG, Shaw J (2001). Global and societal implications of the diabetes epidemic. *Nature*, 414(6865), pp. (782-787), 0028-0836

Part 3

Cancer Research

7

Modeling Tumor Angiogenesis with Zebrafish

Alvin C.H. Ma, Yuhan Guo, Alex B.L. He and Anskar Y.H. Leung
The University of Hong Kong,
Hong Kong

1. Introduction

Angiogenesis is process by which new blood vessels arise from endothelial cells in the existing vessels. In normal circumstances, the initiation, formation, maturation, remodeling and regression of endothelial cells in this process are strictly regulated. During tumor formation, the regulation of angiogenesis is disrupted and endothelial remodeling and regression are usually absent. Therefore, study on angiogenesis is of important relevance to cancer biology and therapeutic intervention (Carmeliet & Jain, 2000), especially in cancers where tumor growth depends on extensive vascularization (Folkman, 2002).

A number of in vitro and in vivo models have been used for the study of angiogenesis. These include an endothelial cell line derived from **h**uman **u**mbilical cord **v**ein **e**ndothelial **c**ells (HUVEC) (Jaffe et al., 1973) as well as a number of organ specific endothelial cell lines. With these cell lines, endothelial cell proliferation, differentiation and migration have been characterized. However, information about how endothelial cells interact with their neighboring cells is often lacking. In this regards, explant cultures (Brown et al., 1996; Jung et al., 2001) might be more representative of the complex interaction between endothelial and the supporting cells. Nevertheless, the issues of incomplete microenvironment, animal to animal variability and technical difficulties from relatively time-consuming and labor-intensive tissue isolation and culture might limit the application of these models.

In vivo models of angiogenesis have also been developed using chick embryo, rabbit and mouse (reviewed by Staton et al., 2009). They provide a more accurate physiological model of angiogenesis and when implanted with primary tumors or cancer cell lines, they can also provide important mechanistic insights to tumor angiogenesis. However, large-scale chemical screening with these models is difficult due to the cost and space needed for husbandry facilities.

Zebrafish has emerged as a model organism for the study of genetics and human diseases. Compare with other vertebrate models, this small tropical fish offers distinctive advantages. Firstly, zebrafish embryos are externally fertilized and optically transparent, allowing direct visualization during embryonic development. Secondly, these embryos are amenable to reverse genetic manipulation including gene knock-down, over-expression or transgenesis by microinjection. Thirdly, the high fecundity of zebrafish enables adequate experimental duplicates and facilitates high through-put forward genetic screening. Mating a single pair of adult zebrafish can produce hundreds of eggs in one day. Fourthly, stable tissue-specific transgenic fish-lines are available, allowing direct visualization of various developmental processes. Lastly, husbandry and maintenance of zebrafish colonies are space and cost effective.

Early zebrafish embryonic vascular development begins at around 12 hour-post-fertilization (hpf) when hemangioblasts first exist along the lateral plate mesoderm. Later at around 24 hpf, the development of dorsal aorta (DA) and dorsal vein (DV), forming the first circulation loop. Subsequently, angiogenesis including the development of inter-segmental vessels (ISV) and sub-intestinal veins (SIV) occurs. Important growth factors and associated receptor tyrosine kinases as well as Notch signaling pathway regulating mammalian vascular development are conserved in zebrafish (Liang et al., 1998; Habeck et al., 2002; Goishi and Klagsbrun, 2004; Siekmann and Lawson ND, 2007). Here, we explore the potential of using zebrafish in vivo to model and more importantly to screen potential therapeutic agents targeting tumor angiogenesis.

2. Zebrafish embryonic angiogenesis

During zebrafish embryonic development, angiogenesis is characterized by the sprouting of inter-segmental vessels in the trunk between each somite initiated around 24 hpf as well as the development of sub-intestinal veins initiated around 48 hpf (Isogai et al., 2001; Lawson and Weinstein, 2002a). Although some argued the sprouting of ISV would represent type II vasculogenesis (Childs et al., 2002), these two processes are well accepted to represent early embryonic angiogenesis.

Traditional assay to examine zebrafish angiogenesis includes alkaline-phosphatase (AP) staining of endothelial cells and whole-mount in situ hybridization of genes associated with vascular development such as *fli1*, *flk1*, *flt4*, *efnb2a* etc. Although in situ hybridization could provide more specific information such as artery or vein specification (Lawson and Weinstein, 2002a), these methods preclude direct and real-time visualization of the vasculature. Also, it takes days to complete staining protocols. These shortcomings have limited the application of zebrafish model until the recent advancement in zebrafish transgenesis and the availability of tissue-specific stable fluorescent reporter transgenic lines. With the use of fluorescent report transgenic zebrafish line such as Tg(*fli1:egfp*) (Lawson and Weinstein, 2002b) or Tg(*flk1:egfp*) (Jin et al., 2005), embryonic angiogenesis could be easily monitored real-time under fluorescent microscope. Figure 1 demonstrates the development of ISV and SIV at 48 and 72 hpf with Tg(*flk1:egfp*) and Tg(*fli1:egfp*).

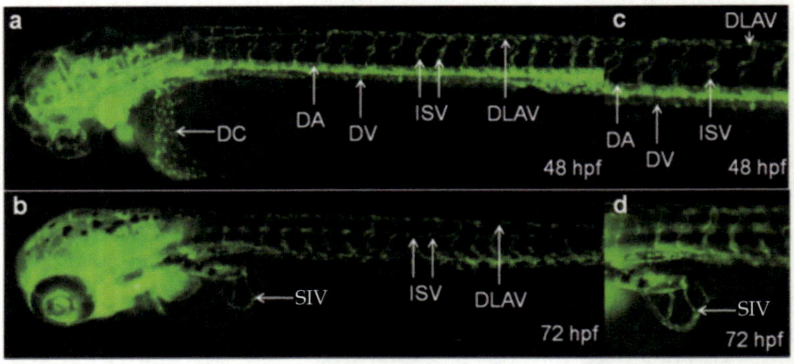

Fig. 1. Endothelial fluorescent transgenic zebrafish embryos showing vascular development at (a, c) 48 and (b, d) 72 hpf. (a, c): Tg(*flk1:egfp*); (b, d): Tg(*fli1:egfp*). DC: Duct of Curvier; DA: Dorsal aorta; DLAV: dorsal longitudinal anastomotic vessels; DV: Dorsal vein; ISV: Inter-segmental vessel; SIV: sub-intestinal vessels.

3. Modeling tumor angiogenesis in zebrafish

3.1 Gene regulation of zebrafish angiogenesis

While angiogenesis is important for tumor growth and metastasis (Folkman, 2002), the precise mechanism and regulation of tumor angiogenesis remains unclear. Therefore, understanding angiogenesis during normal embryonic development might provide insight into how this process would be perturbed during tumor growth. Previous studies have demonstrated that genes that are involved in tumor angiogenesis such as *galectin-1* (Thijssen et al., 2006), *CXCR7* (Miao et al., 2007), *angiomodulin* (Hooper et al., 2009) and *PDGFR-β/B-Raf* (Murphy et al., 2010) may also play a role in embryonic angiogenesis. The zebrafish is unique in this respect because the circulatory system is dispensable during the first few days of embryonic development, enabling study of genes by specific knock-down that is otherwise lethal in the mammalian system.

3.2 Survivin and zebrafish angiogenesis

We have previously identified zebrafish survivin-1 (Ma et al., 2007a) as an important regulator of embryonic angiogenesis. Survivin exerts its effect through anti-apoptosis and interaction with VEGF receptor kinase pathway. Survivin is the smallest member of the inhibitor of apoptosis (IAP) gene family with a single Baculovirus IAP Repeat (BIR) domain and an extended -COOH terminal α-helical coiled coil (Altieri, 2004). While it is not expressed in most normal adult tissues, survivin is highly expressed in solid and hematological malignancies, where it has been linked to tumor angiogenesis and represented a potential target for anti-cancer therapy (Graaf et al., 1998; Altieri, 2003). During human and murine embryonic development, survivin is ubiquitously expressed (Adida et al., 1998). However, homozygous knock-out of *survivin* in mouse ES cells results in disrupted microtubule formation and polyploidy as well as early embryonic fatality, precluding characterization of its functions during murine development (Uren et al., 2000) and therefore zebrafish embryo was considered an alternative embryonic model.

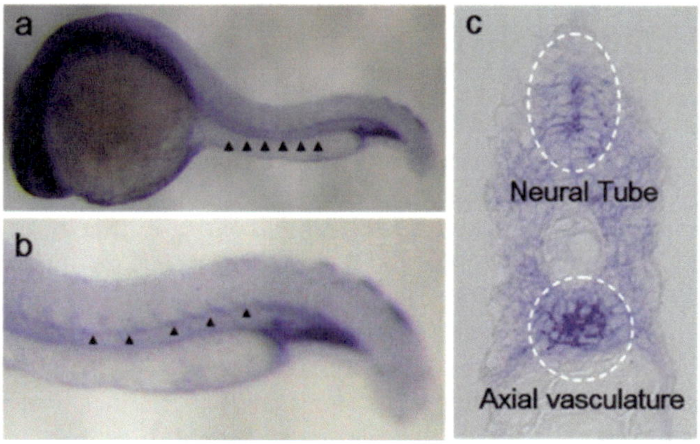

Fig. 2. Expression of *survivin-1* in zebrafish embryo as shown by ISH at 26 hpf. (a,b) Lateral view of whole-mount ISH and black arrowheads denote expression along axial vasculatures. (c) Transverse section of whole-mount ISH showing expression at neural tube and axial vasculatures. Adopted and modified from figure originally published in Ma et al 2007a (with permission).

In zebrafish embryos, *survivin* gene is duplicated into *survivin-1* and *survivin-2*. During embryonic development, *survivin-1* and *survivin-2* are differentially expressed with distinctive functions in the vasculature and hematopoietic tissues (Ma et al., 2007a; Ma et al., 2009). Both survivin-1 and survivin-2 share a highly homologous functional BIR-domain and similar functions at cellular level. Therefore, the distinctive roles of survivin-1 and survivin-2 during embryonic development may be related to a large extent to their difference in spatial expression (Ma et al., 2009). In particular, *survivin-1* predominantly expressed along the neural tube and axial vasculature at 26 hpf (Figure 2). Knock-down of *survivin-1* with anti-sense morpholino gives rise to defective angiogenesis as shown by defective spouting of ISV as well as SIV (Figure 3). Vasculogenesis, demonstrated by the formation of axial vasculatures, was not affected.

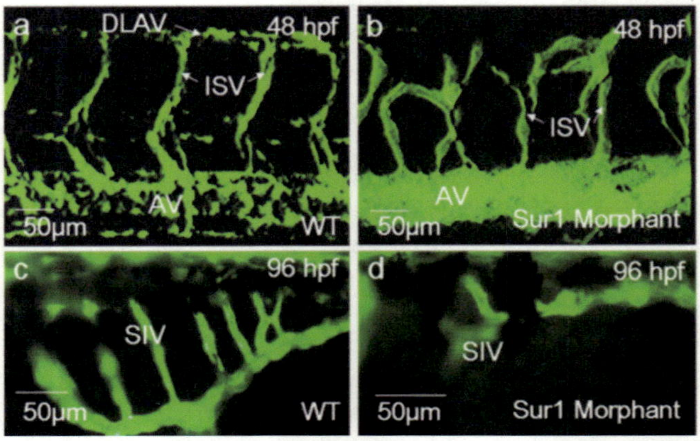

Fig. 3. Effect of *survivin-1* knock-down on zebrafish embryonic angiogenesis. (a, b): Confocal microscopy of *Tg(fli1:egpf)* embryos at 48 hpf either (a) uninjected or (b) injected with *survivin-1* morpholino (MO). Noted the defective sprouting of ISV and the failure to form dorsal longitudinal anastomotic vessels (DLAV) in *survivin-1* (Sur1) morphant. AV: Axial vasculatures. (c, d): *Tg(fli1:egfp)* embryos at 96 hpf showing failure to develop the SIV in Sur1 morphant. Adopted and modified from figure originally published in Ma et al 2007a (with permission).

In vitro and tumorigenesis studies have shown that survivin mediates the angiogenic effects of VEGF (Tran et al., 1999; Mesri et al., 2001; Beierle et al., 2005). In zebrafish embryos, VEGF signaling is also important for angiogenesis. The *schwentine* mutant with defective VEGFR tyrosine kinase, flk1 (Habeck et al., 2002) has perturbed angiogenesis. In addition, phospholipase C-γ (*plc-γ*) mutant (*y10*) (Lawson et al., 2003) as well as knock-down morphant (Ma et al., 2007b) also exhibit specific defects in angiogenesis. VEGF induces ectopic angiogenesis and up-regulates *survivin-1* mRNA expression (Figure 4a-c), suggesting that survivin-1 may mediate the angiogenic effect of VEGF. For instance, we only detect modest apoptotic TUNEL staining in the axial vasculature of *survivin-1* morphant (Figure 4d, e) but not a direct causal link between increased apoptosis and the angiogenesis defect. VEGF might prevent apoptosis (Gupta et al., 1999) and VEGF inhibitors exert pro-apoptotic effect on endothelial cells (reviewed by Epstein, 2007). While apoptotic signal was readily detected along the neural tube of *survivin-1* morphant (Figure 4d, e), survivin-1 might exert its anti-apoptotic effect in a non-cell autonomous fashion downstream of VEGF, regulating the signaling cues for angioblasts to migrate from aorta to the dorsal aspect of the neural tube and to the inter-phase between notochord and the somites before ISV sprouting (Childs et al., 2002).

3.3 Zebrafish xenograft model of tumor angiogenesis

Recently, zebrafish xenograft models have been developed through xenotransplantation of human primary tumor cells or cancer cell lines into yolk sac of 48 hpf zebrafish embryos (Lee LM et al., 2005; Haldi et al., 2006; Topczewska et al., 2006; Nicoli et al., 2007; Marques et al., 2009). Without a functional immune system at this early embryonic stage, immuno-suppression is not needed. The experimental procedures of transplanting fluorescent labeled human cancer cells into perivitelline space of 48 hpf zebrafish embryos was subsequently published (Nocoli and Presta, 2007). In these models, cancer cells were shown to be engrafted into the yolk sac with proliferation and migration. More importantly, angiogenesis were induced in SIV with infiltration of blood vessels into the cancer mass. Combining with fluorescent reporter transgenic lines, these models serve as a promising platform to study the biology of tumor angiogenesis and its microenvironment including hypoxia (Lee SL et al., 2009) and LIM domain kinase 1 and 2 (Vlecken and Bagowski, 2009).

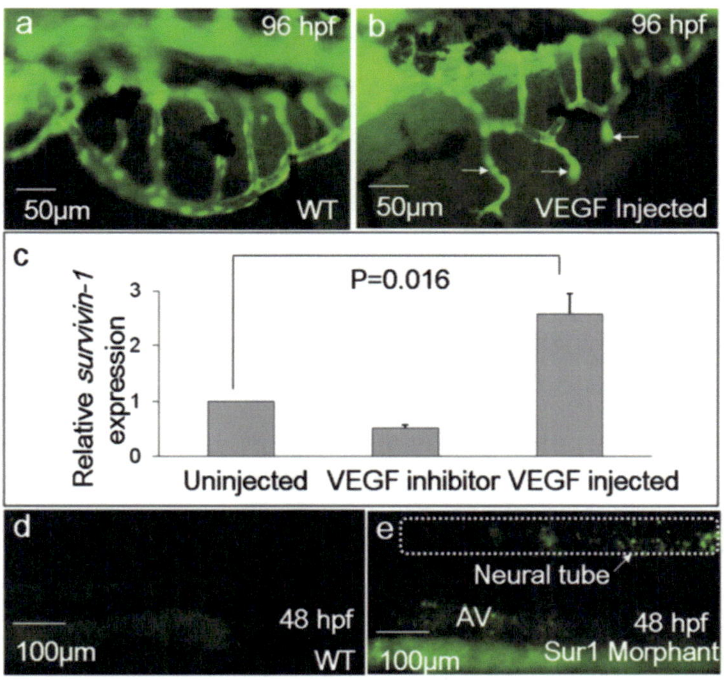

Fig. 4. Survivin-1 interact with VEGF signaling and exert anti-apoptotic activity during zebrafish embryonic angiogenesis. (a, b): Microscopy of *Tg(fli1:egpf)* embryos at 96 hpf either (a) uninjected or (b) injected with human VEGF (2 ng) protein, which induces ectopic angiogenesis (white arrows). (c): relative expression of *survivin-1* mRNA measured by quantitative RT-PCR. (d, e): Whole-mount TUNEL assay in embryos injected with either (e) random sequence or (b) Sur1 MO, which shows positive staining in the area of developing neural tube and at the vicinity of the axial vasculatures (AV) in Sur1 morphant. Adopted and modified from figure originally published in Ma et al 2007a (with permission).

4. Screening potential therapeutic agents with zebrafish embryos

4.1 Large-scale chemical screening platform

Since angiogenesis is crucial for tumor growth and progression, anti-angiogenic agents have been investigated as potential anti-cancer therapies (Demetri et al., 2002; Cunnigham et al., 2004; Shepherd et al., 2005; Van et., al 2007; Hudes et al., 2007). Chemical screening based on in vivo tumor xenograft models are often limited by the relatively low throughput and long read-out time. In this respect, the zebrafish embryo is uniquely suitable for large-scale chemical screening because of the advantages aforementioned. In particular, using the Tg(*flk1:egfp*) or Tg(*fli1:egfp*) embryos, one could conduct large-scale in vivo screening against chemical libraries in a cost-effective way. To examine their effects on the initiation and regression of angiogenesis, embryos will be exposed to chemicals at different concentrations and developmental stages, either before angiogenesis (12 hpf), or after sprouting of ISV and development of SIV (48 hpf). Chemicals that specifically inhibit ISV and SIV formation after 12 hpf likely inhibit the initiation of angiogenesis and those that affect ISV and SIV after their formation at 48 hpf likely induce vascular regression (Figure 5).

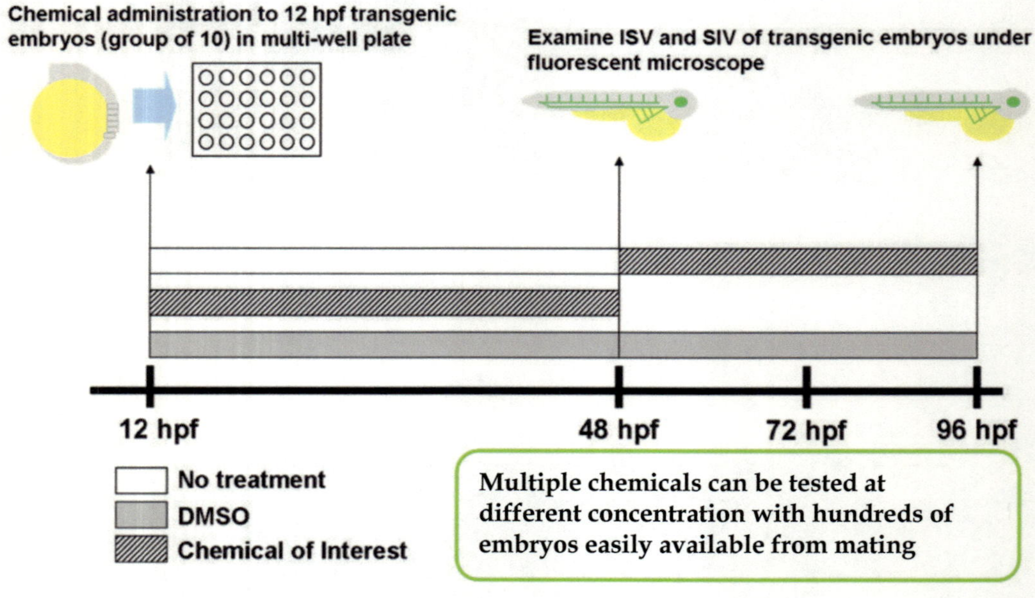

Fig. 5. Cost-effective anti-angiogenic chemicals screening platform with zebrafish embryos.

Both anti-angiogenic mechanisms are considered important component in cancer therapy. This protocol may enable identification of potential anti-angiogenic compounds at high throughput and provide us with novel information about the link between embryonic and tumor angiogenesis. Figure 6 shows the use of Tg(*flk1:egfp*) embryos as a platform to demonstrate anti-angiogenic activity of VEGFR tyrosine kinase inhibitor and anti-cancer drugs (multi-kinase inhibitors) sorafenib and sunitinib.

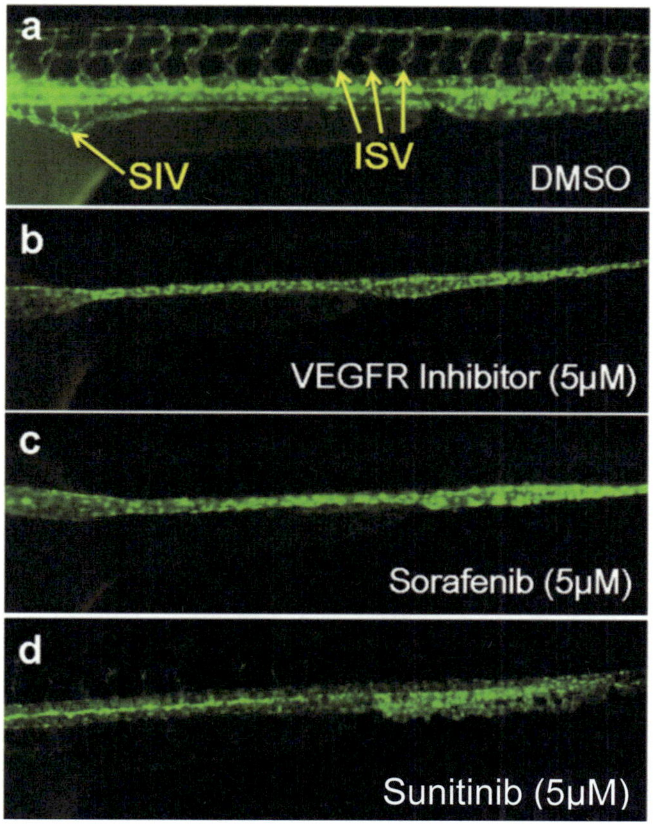

Fig. 6. Demonstration of anti-angiogenic effect of kinase inhibitors with transgenic zebrafish embryos. Microscopy of Tg(*flk1:egfp*) embryos at 48 hpf treated with (a) DMSO, (b) VEGFR tyrosine kinase inhibitor, (c) sorafenib and (d) sunitinib. Treatment with these inhibitors significantly perturbed zebrafish embryonic angiogenesis as shown by development of ISV and SIV.

5. Conclusion

Since angiogenesis is crucial for tumor growth and progression, it may present a potential target for cancer therapy. A number of anti-angiogenic agents targeting at the VEGF signaling pathway are being evaluated and large-scale chemical screening is needed to provide more candidates that can be tested in clinical trials. In this respect, the zebrafish embryos have emerged as a promising model that can shed important lights to the biology of physiological and tumor angiogenesis at whole organism level and allow cost-effective high throughput chemical screening. A number of new genetic modification technologies are now available that can specifically interrogate gene function related to angiogenesis. For instance, artificial endonucleases constructed by fusing non-specific nuclease domain with specific DNA binding domains (Ekker, 2008; Foley et al., 2009a; Foley et al., 2009b; Miller et al., 2011; Cermak et al., 2011; Sander et al., 2011) can now be used to target specific genes from zebrafish genome. An in vivo protein trap mutagenesis system (Clark et al., 2011) is also available that can simultaneously reveal spatio-temporal protein expression dynamics and assess gene function in zebrafish embryos. These new technologies greatly improve the efficiency of zebrafish genetic modifications and forward genetic screening, making zebrafish a more powerful model organism for angiogenesis.

6. References

Adida C, Crotty PL, Berrebi MD, Diebold J and Altieri DC. (1998). Developmentally regulated expression of the novel cancer anti-apoptosis gene survivin in human and mouse differentiation. *American Journal of Pathology,* Vol.152, No.1, pp.43-49, ISSN 0002-9440

Altieri DC. (2003). Validating survivin as a cancer therapeutic target. *Nature Reviews Cancer,* Vol.3, No.1, pp.46-54, ISSN 1474-175X

Altieri DC. (2004). Molecular circuits of apoptosis regulation and cell division control: The survivin paradigm. *Journal of Cellular Biochemistry,* Vol.92, No.4, pp.656-663, ISSN 0730-2312

Beierle EA, Nagaram A, Dai W, Iyenger M and Chen MK. (2005). VEGF-mediated survivin expression in neuroblastoma cells. *Journal of Surgical Research,* Vol.127, N0.1, pp.21-28, ISSN 0022-4804

Brown KJ, Maynes SF, Bezos A, Maguire DJ, Ford MD and Parish CR. (1996) A novel in vitro assay for human angiogenesis. *Laboratory Invesigation,* Vol.75, No.4, pp.539–555, ISSN 0023-6837

Carmeliet P and Jain RK. (2000). Angiogenesis in cancer and other diseases. *Nature,* Vol.407, No.6810, pp.249-257, ISSN 0028-0836

Cermak T, Doyle EL, Christian M, Wang L, Zhang Y, Schmidt C, Baller JA, Somia NV, Bogdanove AJ and Voytas DF. (2011). Efficient design and assembly of custom TALEN and other TAL effector-based constructs for DNA targeting. *Nucleic Acid Research,* E-published ahead of print, ISSN 0305-1048

Childs S, Chen JN, Garrity DM and Fishman MC. (2002). Patterning of angiogenesis in the zebrafish embryo. *Development, Vol.*129, pp.973–982, ISSN 1011-6370

Clark KJ, Balciunas D, Pogoda HM, Ding Y, Westcot SE, Bedell VM, Greenwood TM, Urban MD, Skuster KJ, Petzold AM, Ni J, Nielsen AL, Patowary A, Scaria V, Sivasubbu S, Xu X, Hammerschmidt M and Ekker SC. (2011). In vivo protein trapping produces a functional expression codex of the vertebrate proteome. *Nature Methods,* Vol.8, No.6, pp.506-512, ISSN 1548-7091

Cunningham D, Humblet Y, Siena S, Khayat D, Bleiberg H, Santoro A, Bets D, Mueser M, Harstrick A, Verslype C, Chau I and Van Cutsem E. (2004). Cetuximab monotherapy and cetuximab plus irinotecan in irinotecan-refractory metastatic colorectal cancer, *New England Journal of Medicine,* Vol.351, No.4, pp.337–345, ISSN 0028-4793

Demetri GD, von Mehren M, Blanke CD, Van den Abbeele AD, Eisenberg B, Roberts PJ, Heinrich MC, Tuveson DA, Singer S, Janicek M, Fletcher JA, Silverman SG, Silberman SL, Capdeville R, Kiese B, Peng B, Dimitrijevic S, Druker BJ, Corless C, Fletcher CD and Joensuu H. (2002). Efficacy and safety of imatinib mesylate in advanced gastrointestinal stromal tumors. *New England Journal of Medicine,* Vol.347, No.7, pp.472-480, ISSN 0028-4793

Ekker SC. (2008). Zinc finger-based knockout punches for zebrafish genes. *Zebrafish,* Vo.5, No.2, pp.121-123, ISSN 1545-8547

Epstein RJ. (2007). VEGF signaling inhibitors: More pro-apoptotic than anti-angiogenic. *Cancer and Metastasis Reviews,* Vol.26, No.3-4, pp.443-452, ISSN 0167-7659

Foley JE, Maeder ML, Pearlberg J, Joung JK, Peterson RT and Yeh JR. (2009a). Targeted mutagenesis in zebrafish using customized zinc-finger nucleases. . *Nature Protocol,* Vol.4, No.12, pp.1855-1867, ISSN 1754-2189

Foley JE, Yeh JR, Maeder ML, Reyon D, Sander JD, Peterson RT and Joung JK. (2009b). Rapid mutation of endogenous zebrafish genes using zinc finger nucleases made by Oligomerized Pool ENgineering (OPEN). (2009b). *PLoS One,* Vol.4, No.2, e4384, ISSN 1932-6203

Folkman J. (2002). Role of angiogenesis in tumor growth and metastasis. *Seminars in Oncology,* Vol.29, No. 6, Supplement 16, pp.15-18, ISSN 0093-7754

Goishi K and Klagsbrun M. (2004). Vascular endothelial growth factor and its receptors in embryonic zebrafish blood vessel development. *Current Topics of Developmental Biology,* Vol.62, pp.127-152, ISSN 0070-2153

Graaf AO, de Witte T and Jansen JH. (2004). Inhibitor of apoptosis proteins: new therapeutic targets in hematological cancer? *Leukemia, Vol.*18, pp.1751-1759, ISSN 0887-6924

Gupta K, Kshirsagar S, Li W, Gui L, Ramakrishnan S, Gupta P, Law PY and Hebbel RP. (1999). VEGF prevents apoptosis of human microvascular endothelial cells via opposing effects on MAPK/ERK and SAPK/JNL signaling. *Experimental Cell Research,* Vol.247, No.2, pp.495-504, ISSN 0014-4827.

Habeck H, Odenthal J, Walderich B, Maischein HM, Tubingen 2000 screen consortium and Schulte-Merker S. (2002). Analysis of a Zebrafish VEGF Receptor Mutant Reveals Specific Disruption of Angiogenesis. *Current Biology,* Vol.12, No.16, pp.1405-1412, ISSN 0960-9822

Haldi M, Ton C, Seng WL and McGrath P. (2006). Human melanoma cells transplanted into zebrafish proliferates, migrates, produce melanin, from masses and stimulate angiogenesis in zebrafish. *Angiogenesis,* Vol.9, No.3, pp.139-151, ISSN 0969-6970

Hooper AT, Shmelkov SV, Gupta S, Milde T, Bambino K, Gillen K, Goetz M, Chavala S, Baljevic M, Murphy AJ, Valenzuela DM, Gale NW, Thurston G, Yancopoulos GD, Vahdat L,Evans T, and Rafii S. (2009). Angiomodulin is a specific marker of vasculature and regulates vascular endothelial growth factor-A–dependent neoangiogenesis. *Circulation Research,* Vol.105, No.2, pp :201–208, ISSN 0009-7300

Hudes G, Carducci M, Tomczak P, Dutcher J, Figlin R, Kapoor A, Staroslawska E, Sosman J, McDermott D, Bodrogi I, Kovacevic Z, Lesovoy V, Schmidt-Wolf IG, Barbarash O, Gokmen E, O'Toole T, Lustgarten S, Moore L and Motzer RJ. (2007). Temsirolimus, interferon alfa, or both for advanced renal-cell carcinoma. *New England Journal of Medicine,* Vol.356, No.22, pp.2271–2281, ISSN 0028-4793

Isogai S, Horiguchi M and Weinstein BM. (2001). The vascular anatomy of the developing zebrafish: an atlas of embryonic and early larval development. *Developmental Biology, Vol.*230, No.2, pp.278–301, ISSN 0012-1606

Jaffe EA, Nachman RL, Becker CG and Minick CR. (1973). Culture of human endothelial cells derived from umbilical veins. Identification by morphologic and immunologic criteria. *Journal of Clinical Investigation,* vol.52, No.11, pp.2745-2756, ISSN 0021-9738

Jin SW, Beis D, Mitchell T, Chen JN and Stainier DY. (2005). Cellular and molecular analyses of vascular tube and lumen formation in zebrafish. *Development,* Vol.132, pp.5199–5209, ISSN 1011-6370

Jung SP, Siegrist B, Wade MR, Anthoony CT and Woltering EA. (2001). Inhibition of human angiogenesis with heparin and hydrocortisone. *Angiogenesis,* Vol.4, No.3, pp.175-186, ISSN 0969-6970

Lawson ND and Weinstein BM. (2002a). Arteries and veins: Making difference with zebrafish. *Nature Reviews Genetics,* Vol.3, pp.674-682, ISSN 1471-0056

Lawson ND and Weinstein BM. (2002b). In vivo imaging of embryonic vascular development using transgenic zebrafish. *Developmental Biology,* Vol.248, No.2, pp.307-318, ISSN 0012-1606

Lawson ND, Mugford JW, Diamond BA and Weinstein BM. (2003). Phospholipase C gamma-1 is required downstream of vascular endothelial growth factor during arterial development. *Genes and Development,* Vol.17, No.11, pp.1346-51, ISSN 0890-9369

Lee LM, Seftor EA, Bonde G, Cornell RA and Hendrix MJ. (2005). The fate of human malignant melanoma cells transplanted into zebrafish embryos: assessment of migration and cell division in the absence of tumor formation. *Developmental Dynamics,* Vol.233, No.4, pp.1560-1570, ISSN 1097-0177

Lee SL, Rouhi P, Jensen LD, Zhang D, Hauptmann G, Ingham P and Cao Y. (2009). Hypoxia-induced pathological angiogenesis mediates tumor cell dissemination, invasion, and metastasis in zebrafish tumor model. *Proceedings of the National Academy of Science of the United States of America,* Vol.106, No.46, pp.19485-19490, ISSN 0027-8424

Leung T, Chen H, Stauffer AM, Giger KE, Sinha S, Horstick EJ, Humbert JE, Hansen CA and Robishaw JD. (2006). Zebrafish G protein gamma2 is required for VEGF signaling during angiogenesis. *Blood,* Vol.108, No.1, pp.160-166, ISSN 0006-4971

Liang D, Xu X, Chin AJ, Balasubramaniyan NV, Teo MA, Lam TJ, Weinberg ES and Ge R. (1998). Cloning and characterization of vascular endothelial growth factor (VEGF) from zebrafish, Danio rerio. *Biochimica et Biophysica Acta,* Vol.1397, No.1, pp.14-20, ISSN 0167-4781

Ma AC, Lin R, Chan PK, Leung JC, Chan LY, Meng A, Verfaillie CM, Liang R and Leung AY. (2007a). The role of survivin in angiogenesis during zebrafish embryonic development. BMC *Developmental Biology,* Vol.7, No.50. ISSN: 1471-213X

Ma AC, Liang R and Leung AY. (2007b). The role of phospholipase C gamma 1 in primitive hematopoiesis during zebrafish development. *Experimental Hematology,* Vol.35, No.3, pp.368-373, ISSN 0301-472X

Ma AC, Chung MI, Liang R and Leung AY. (2009). The role of survivin2 in primitive hematopoiesis during zebrafish development. *Leukemia,* Vol.23, No.4, pp.712-720, ISSN 0887-6924

Mesri M, Morales-Ruiz M, Ackermann EJ, Bennett CF, Pober JS, Sessa WC and Altieri DC. (2001). Suppression of vascular endothelial growth factor-mediated endothelial cell protection by survivin targeting. *American Journal of Pathology,* Vol.158, No.5, pp.1757-1765, ISSN 0002-9440

Miao Z, Luker KE, Summers BC, Berahovich R, Bhojani MS, Rehemtulla A, Kleer CG, Essner JJ, Nasevicius A, Luker GD, Howard MC and Schall TJ. (2007). CXCR7 (RDC1)

promotes breast and lung tumor growth in vivo and is expressed on tumor-associated vasculature. *Proceedings of the National Academy of Science of the United States of America*, Vol.104, No.40, pp.15735-15740, ISSN 0027-8424

Miller JC, Tan S, Qiao G, Barlow KA, Wang J, Xia DF, Meng X, Paschon DE, Leung E, Hinkley SJ, Dulay GP, Hua KL, Ankoudinova I, Cost GJ, Urnov FD, Zhang HS, Holmes MC, Zhang L, Gregory PD and Rebar EJ. (2011). A TALE nuclease architecture for efficient genome editing. *Nature Biotechnology*, Vol.29, No.2, pp.143-148, ISSN 1087-0156

Murphy EA, Shields DJ, Stoletov K, Dneprovskaia E, McElroy M, Greenberg JI, Lindquist J, Acevedo LM, Anand S, Majeti BK, Tsigelny I, Salsanha A, Waish B, Hoffman RM, Bouvet M, Klemke RL, Vogt PK, Arnold L, Wrasidlo W and Cheresh DA. (2010). Disruption of angiogenesis and tumor growth with an orally active drug that stabilizes the inactive state of PDGFRβ/BRAF. *Proceedings of the National Academy of Science of the United States of America*, Vol.107, No.9, pp.4299–4304, ISSN 0027-8424

Nicoli S, Ribatti D, Cotelli F and Presta M. (2007). Mammalian tumor xenograft induce neovascularization in zebrafish embryos. *Cancer Research*, Vol.67, No.7, pp.2927-2931, ISSN 1578-3445

Nicola S and Presta M. (2007). The zebrafish/tumor xenograft angiogenesis assay. *Nature Protocol*, Vol.2, No.11, pp.2918-2923, ISSN 1754-2189

Sander JD, Cade L, Khayter C, Reyon D, Peterson RT, Joung JK and Yeh JR. (2011). Efficient targeted gene modification in zebrafish using engineered TALE nucleases. *Nature Biotechnology*, in press, ISSN 1087-0156

Siekmann AF and Lawson ND. (2007). Notch signalling limits angiogenic cell behaviour in developing zebrafish arteries. *Nature*, Vol.445, pp.781-784, ISSN 0028-0836

Shepherd FA, Rodrigues Pereira J, Ciuleanu T, Tan EH, Hirsh V, Thongprasert S, Campos D, Maoleekoonpiroj S, Smylie M, Martins R, van Kooten M, Dediu M, Findlay B, Tu D,Johnston D, Bezjak A, Clark G, Santabárbara P and Seymour L. (2005). Erlotinib in previously treated non-small-cell lung cancer, *New England Journal of Medicine*, Vol.353, No.2, pp.123-132, ISSN 0028-4793

Staton CA, Reed MW and Brown NJ. (2009). A critical analysis of current in vitro and in vivo angiogenesis assays. *International Journal of Experimental Pathology*, Vol.90, No.3, pp.195-221, ISSN 1365-2613

Thijssen VL, Postel R, Brandwijk RJ, Dings RP, Nesmelova I, Satijn S, Verhofstad N, Nakabeppu Y, Baum LG, Bakkers J, Mayo KH, Poirier F and Griffioen AW. (2006). Galectin-1 is essential in tumor angiogenesis and is a target for antiangiogenesis therapy. *Proceedings of the National Academy of Science of the United States of America*, Vol.103, No.43, pp.15975-15980, ISSN 0027-8424

Tran J, Rak J, Sheehan C, Saibil SD, LaCasse E, Korneluk RG and Kerbel RS. (1999). Marked induction of the IAP family antiapoptotic proteins survivin and XIAP by VEGF in vascular endothelial cells. *Biochemical and Biophysical Research Communications,*Vol.264, No.3, pp.781-788, ISSN 0006-291X

Topczewska JM, Postovit LM, Margaryan NV, Sam A, Hess AR, Wheaton WW, Nickoloff BJ, Topczewski J and Hendrix MJ. (2006). Embryonic and tumorigenic pathways converge via nodal signaling: role in melanoma aggressiveness. *Nature Medicine*, Vol.12, No.8, pp.925-932: ISSN 1078-8956

Uren AG, Wong L, Pakusch M, Fowler KJ, Burrows FJ, Vaux DL, Choo KH. (2000). Survivin and the inner centromere protein INCENP show similar cell-cycle localization and gene knockout phenotype. *Current Biology*, Vol.10, No.21, pp.1319-28, ISSN 0960-9822

Van CE, Peeters M, Siena S, Humblet Y, Hendlisz A, B Neyns, Canon JL, Van Laethem JL, Maurel J, Richardson G, Wolf M and Amado RG. (2007). Open-label phase III trial of panitumumab plus best supportive care compared with best supportive care alone in patients with chemotherapy–refractory metastatic colorectal cancer. *Journal of Clinical Oncology*, Vol.25, No.13, pp.1658–1664, ISSN 1743-7563

Vlecken DH and Bagowski CP. (2009). LIMK1 and LIMK2 are important for metastatic behavior and tumor cell-induced angiogenesis of pancreatic cancer cells. *Zebrafish*, Vol.6, No.4, pp.433-439, ISSN 1545-8547

8

Therapeutic and Toxicological Inhibition of Vasculogenesis and Angiogenesis Mediated by Artesunate, a Compound with Both Antimalarial and Anticancer Efficacy

Qigui Li, Mark Hickman and Peter Weina
Division of Experimental Therapeutics, Walter Reed Army Institute of Research, Silver Spring, MD, USA

1. Introduction

Artemisinin (ART) and its derivatives, the lactonic sesquiterpenoid compounds, were discovered in China. A crude extract of the wormwood plant *Artemisia annua* (qinghao) was first used as an antipyretic 2000 years ago, and its specific effect on the fever of malaria was reported in the 16th century (Hsu, 2006). The active constituent of the extract was identified and purified in the 1970s, and named qinghaosu, or ART. Although ART proved effective in clinical trials in the 1980s, a number of semi-synthetic derivatives were developed to improve the drug's pharmacological properties and antimalarial potency (Li et al., 2007a).

ART and its active derivatives have been widely used as antimalarial drugs for more than 30 years, and they have also been shown recently to be effective in killing cancer cells. Artesunate (AS) and its bioactive metabolite, dihydroartemisinin (DHA), have been the topic of considerable research attention in recent years for both indications. The key structural feature in all of the ART-related molecules that mediates their antimalarial activity, and some of their anticancer activities, is an endoperoxide bridge. ART- induced apoptosis, or programmed parasite death, is a highly ordered form of parasite suicide affecting both mature and immature parasites. Apoptosis is widely believed to be the mechanism by which ART therapy rapidly kills malaria parasites. A number of research studies have shown that the mechanism of ART embryotoxicity appears to be associated with ART- driven inhibition of fetal hematopoiesis and vasculogenesis. Specifically, higher drug levels of ART have been shown to affect erythroblasts, endothelial cells and cardiovascular cells in the early embryo (Clark et al., 2004; 2008b, White et al., 2006).

Of the available derivatives, AS has the most favorable pharmacological profile for use in ART-based combination treatment of uncomplicated malaria and intravenous therapy of severe malaria (Li and Weina, 2010a). The presence of a hemisuccinate group in the molecule confers water solubility and relatively high oral bioavailability. In a clinical trial of oral and injectable AS (Batty et al, 1998a), the duration of the lag phase in the parasitemia curve was shown to be 1.92-2.81 hrs, which is much shorter than the lag phase of the other 4 ART drugs (4.03-8.89 hrs) suggesting the parasiticidal effect of AS is very rapid. In addition, the time to clear half the parasitemia (PC_{50}) after AS dosing was 3.18-8.48 hrs, which was much shorter than the PC_{50}s of the other ARTs which ranged from 10.05-19.08 hrs (Li et al, 2007b). AS is rapidly and quantitatively converted *in vivo* to the potent active metabolite, DHA, which was originally obtained by sodium borohydride reduction of ART, an endoperoxide-containing sesquiterpene lactone (Figure 1).

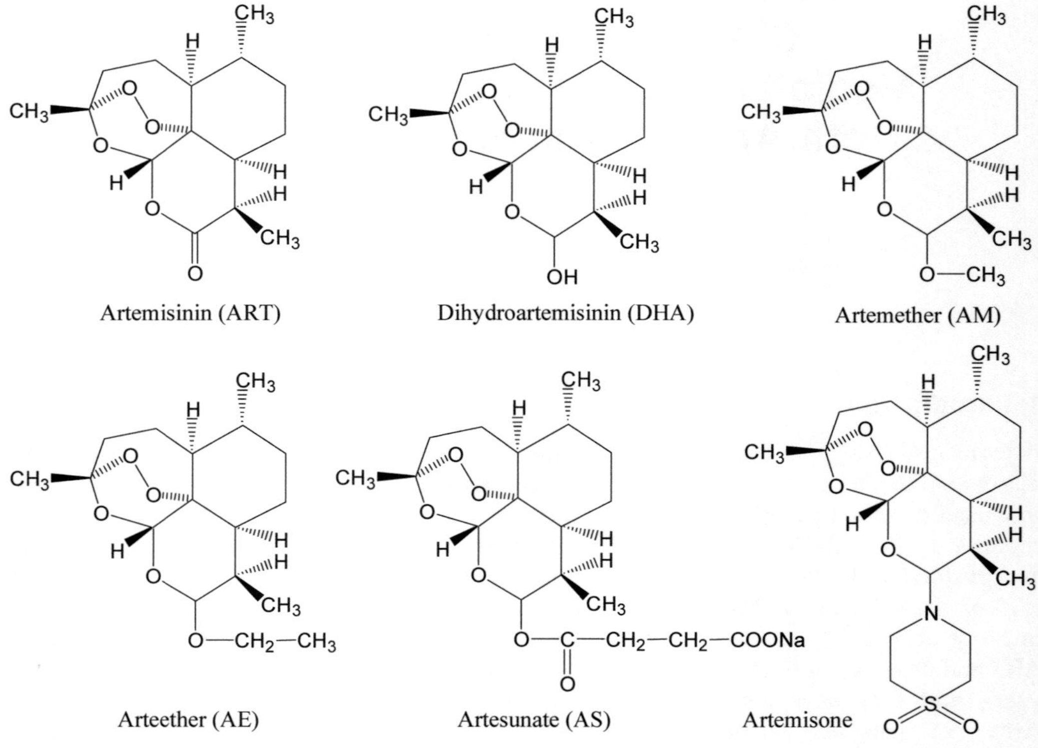

Fig. 1. Chemical structures of artemisinin (ART) and its five derivatives, dihydroartemisinin (DHA), artemether (AM), arteether (AE), artesunate (AS) and artemisone

The effectiveness of AS has been mostly attributed to its rapid and extensive hydrolysis to DHA (Batty et al., 1998b; Davis et al., 2001; Li et al., 1998; Navaratnam et al., 2000). However, due to its poor solubility in water or oils, DHA has only been formulated as an oral preparation and has been used primarily as a semisynthetic compound for derivatization to the oil soluble drugs, artemether and arteether, and the water soluble drug, AS. DHA has similar potency to AS (Li et al., 2007c) and is 3-5 fold more active and more toxic than the other ART derivatives (Li et al., 2002; McLean et al., 1998). It can completely inhibit parasite growth within 2-4 hours, and is the only ART derivative with activity against all asexual blood stage parasites (Skinner et al., 1996).
In recent years, the *in vitro* and *in vivo* anticancer activities of ART have been reported in a number of studies. ART has inhibitory effects on cancer cell growth and also inhibits angiogenesis. Several studies have revealed that ART inhibits the growth of many transformed cell lines and has a selective cytotoxic effect. In one study, ART was shown to be more toxic to cancer than normal cells. In this work, a synthetic compound composed of ART linked to holotransferrin showed enhanced potency and selectivity in killing human leukemia cells. The

cytotoxic effect of the ART-holotransferrin compound is likely due to the high concentration of transferrin receptors in cancer cells that resulted in increased influx of the ART-holotransferrin compound compared to normal cells. Finally, ART possesses an antiangiogenic activity. Angiogenesis, occurring through the proliferation and migration of endothelial cells, is a very important element of tumor development (Buommino et al., 2009; Nakase et al., 2007).

Treatment with AS or DHA can inhibit angiogenesis induced by human multiple myeloma RPMI8226 cells (Chen et al, 2010a;Wu et al, 2006). AS and DHA have been shown to inhibit the growth of Kaposi's sarcoma cells, a highly angiogenic multifocal tumor, and both drugs induced apoptosis in human umbilical vein endothelial cells (Chen et al., 2004a; Dell'Eva et al., 2004). AS and DHA also lowered vascular endotherial growth factor (VEGF) expression and VEGF receptor KDR (kinase insert domain containing receptor)/flk1 (fms-like tyrosine kinase) expression on tumor cells (Chen et al., 2004a, b). VEGF has been shown to be a potent angiogenic factor. It binds to VEGF receptors present on the surface of endothelial cells and activates various functions of angiogenesis.

More recently, the antiangiogenic activity of ARTs has been shown to result in embryotoxicity (Li & Weina, 2010b). Although not yet reported to be a problem in clinical use, embryotoxicity has been reported for this compound class in both *in vitro* and *in vivo* experimental models, in particular after AS and/or DHA treatment, which resulted in embryo death and developmental abnormalities in early pregnancy in different animal species. The embryotoxicity appears to be connected with defective angiogenesis and vasculogenesis in certain stages of embryo development. DHA has been shown in rat whole embryo cultures to primarily affect primitive red blood cells causing subsequent tissue damage and dysmorphogenesis. AS has also been found to be embryolethal and teratogenic in rats, suggesting that embryonic erythroblasts are the primary target of AS toxicity in the rat embryo after *in vivo* treatment, preceding embryolethality and organ malformations (Medhi et al., 2009).

In particular, cancer angiogenesis plays a key role in the growth, invasion, and metastasis of tumors. Therefore, AS or DHA induced inhibition of angiogenesis could be a promising therapeutic strategy for treatment of cancer. Other anticancer mechanisms induced by AS and DHA have been recognized recently that have guided various clinical cancer trials. Given the fact that AS and DHA have been shown to inhibit vasculogenesis, these drugs should be avoided in pregnant patients with malaria or cancers in order to prevent fatal embryotoxicity. Further research on the mechanism of efficacy could lead us to understand more clearly the possibilities inherent in therapeutic development of ARTs for malaria, cancer, and other indications. Further study of the effects of ART compounds on vascularization and angiogenesis may improve the usage of AS and DHA for treatment of malaria and cancer. In this chapter, a thorough review of the antivascular mechanisms of AS/DHA therapy will be provided along with an extended discussion of the downstream embryotoxicity and anti-tumor effects of AS/DHA therapy.

2. Embryotoxicity of AS/DHA caused by defective vasculogenesis/hematopoiesis

Preclinical studies in rodents have demonstrated that ARTs, especially injectable AS, can induce fetal death and congenital malformations at a low dose. AS induced embryotoxicity can be shown in those animals only within a narrow window of time in early embryogenesis. Further evidence has been presented that the mechanism by which embryotoxicity of AS/DHA occurs seems to be limited to fetal erythropoiesis and vasculogenesis/angiogenesis in the very earliest developing red blood cells. The effect of

AS/DHA on red cell precursors has been shown to cause severe anemia in embryos with higher drug peak concentrations (Clark et al., 2004; White et al., 2008).

2.1 AS/DHA induces severe embryotoxicity in animal species

Artemisinin-based combination therapies (ACTs) and injectable AS are currently recommended by WHO (2006a) as frontline antimalarial treatments for uncomplicated and severe malaria, respectively, with over 100 million courses administered annually. While ART-based therapies have been shown to be well tolerated and efficacious, embryotoxicity has been reported in a number of animal species in a variety of research studies. In this chapter, we will thoroughly discuss all aspects of the various research studies that have been conducted on the embryotoxic mechanisms of ARTs in rodents and monkeys. Animal studies are very valuable in showing possible risks to humans from drug compounds, and a number of studies on reproductive risk associated with ARTs have been conducted showing the potential for embryotoxicity in the first trimester of pregnancy. In general, ART and its derivatives are considered safe and effective in pregnant women who have been treated with ART compounds, including a small number treated in the first trimester, the most vulnerable period for ART-induced embryotoxicity. In clinical trials, the patients did not show any increases in miscarriage or stillbirth with evidence of abnormality. A follow–up of exposed babies did not reveal any delays in child developmental (Efferth & Kaina 2010).

Studies in rodents have demonstrated that ARTs can induce fetal death and malformations at high oral doses and low injectable dose levels (Dellicour et al., 2007). Embryotoxicity can be induced by ARTs only within a narrow time window in rodents during early embryogenesis. Red cell progenitors are produced during a very limited time period during embryogenesis so that a single exposure to ARTs can result in a significant rise in hematopoietic cell death (WHO, 2006b; White et al., 2008). Treatment with AS/DHA has been shown to lead to a loss of hematopoietic precursors which may result in embryo death. In those embryos that survived, malformations were observed. Limited data in primates suggest that ARTs may have a similar mechanism of action in monkeys where AS/DHA treatment leads to anemia and embryolethality, however, the monkeys required more than 12 days of treatment to induce such embryonic death (Clark et al., 2008a). No embryo malformations were observed in the primate studies but these were limited in scope. The significant difference between the time periods where embryos were vulnerable to AS/DHA induced embryolethality in rodents and monkeys suggests that the time window for ART induced embryolethality is much longer for primates and may well be much longer for humans.

Preclinical studies of the reproductive toxicity of ARTs in various animal species showed that the injectable AS formulation has the greatest potential for embryotoxicity (Table 1). Following intravenous, intramuscular, and subcutaneous administrations, injectable AS was shown to have an drug dose induces 50% fetus re-absorbed (FRD_{50}), the dose required for 50% of the fetuses to be resorbed, of less than 1.0 mg/kg , which is much lower than the therapeutic dose of AS, which is 2–4 mg/kg in humans. In contrast, those animal species treated with oral ARTs and intramuscular artemether were shown to have a much higher FRD_{50} of 6.1–51.0 mg/kg (Table 1)(Li et al., 2010b). The mechanism for development of severe embryotoxicity in animals after treatment with injectable AS was not known in 2006, and research on this subject has only been published in recent years.

In later studies, more data on the mechanism of AS-induced embryotoxicity was shown. A study by Efferth and Kaina (2010) suggested that AS-induced embryotoxicity could be due to the antivasculogenic and antihematopoietic effects of AS/DHA on the embryonic erythroblasts in the very earliest developing red blood cells. This study was inspired by anticancer studies conducted with AS (Efferth et al., 2001; 2006; Chen et al., 2003; 2004b).

Animal (drugs)	Dose duration	Dose regimens (daily)	Dosing route	No-observed-adverse-effect-level (NOAEL) on fetus resorption (mg/kg)				FRD_{100} (mg/kg)	FRD_{50} (95% CL) (mg/kg)
				Oral	IM	IV	SC		
Mice (AM)	GD 6-15	Multiple x 10	IM		5.4				11.3 (10.6 - 12.0)
(DHA)	GD 7	Single	SC				10		32.8 (27.7 – 38.9)
Rats (ART)	GD 1-6	Multiple x 6	Oral	5.6					11.5 (10.5 – 12.2)
(ART)	GD 7-13	Multiple x 7	Oral	7					≥ 35
(DHA)	GD 9.5, 10.5	Single	Oral	7.5					NA
(AM)	GD 6-15	Multiple x 10	Oral	2.5					14.4 (10.4 – 17.8)
(AS)	GD 6-17	Multiple x 12	Oral	5-7					7.74 (6.92 – 8.57)
(AS)	GD 10	Single	Oral					15.0	NA
(DHA)	GD 10	Single	Oral					11.1	NA
(AM)	GD10	Single	Oral					19.4	NA
(AE)	GD 10	Single	Oral					20.3	NA
(AS)	GD 11	Single	Oral					17.0	NA
(AS)	GD 6-15	Multiple x 10	SC				0.2		0.58 (0.55 – 0.61)*
(AM)	GD 6-15	Multiple x 10	IM		2.7				6.13 (4.52 – 8.26)
(AS)	GD 11	Single	IV			0.75		1.5	NA
(AS)	GD 6-13	Multiple x 13	IV, IM		0.5	0.4			0.60 - 0.61 (0.47-0.72)*
Hamster (DHA)	GD 7	Single	SC				4.2		6.06 (5.90 – 6.21)
(DHA)	GD 7	Single	Oral	20					51.0 (37.9 – 68.7)
(AS)	GD 5	Single	SC				0.35		1.0 (0.9 – 1.2)*
Guinea Pig (DHA)	GD 18	Single	IM		2.5				18.3 (13.9 – 24.2)
Rabbits (AM)	GD 7-18	Multiple x 12	IM		0.7				NA
(AS)	GD 7-19	Multiple x 13	Oral	5-7					NA
(DHA)	GD 9	Single	IM		5.0				7.57 (7.48 – 7.67)
Monkey (AS)	GD 20-50	Multiple x 12	Oral	4					≥ 12

FRD_{50} or $_{100}$ = drug dose induces 50% or 100% fetus re-absorbed; GD = gestation day
(The day of mating was defined as day 0 of gestation.)
* The severe toxic effects were detected in the animals treated with AS after single or multiple intramuscular, intravenous or subcutaneous injections. Values of ED_{50} are given as median (95% confidence limits). NA = not available.

Table 1. Embryotoxic effects (NOAEL and $FRD_{50 \text{ or } 100}$) of artemisinin (ART), dihydroartemisinin (DHA), artesunate (AS), artemether (AM) and arteether (AE) given intragastrically (Oral), intravenously (IV), intramuscularly (IM), and subcutaneously (SC) in pregnant mice, rats, hamster, guinea pig, rabbits, and monkeys (Li & Weina, 2010b).

2.2 AS/DHA therapy causes erythrocyte depletion and resulting embryotoxicity

The antihematopoietic, antivasculogenic, and antiangiogenic effects of artemisinins (ARTs) have been shown through *in vitro* and *in vivo* studies, which have been summarized in Table 2. This comprehensive list of publications provides a reference list of current work on AS-induced embryotoxicity.

Drugs	*in vitro* studies	Drugs	*in vivo* studies
ART	Increased levels of ROS and inhibition of angiogenesis in mouse embryonic stem cell-derived embryos	AS/DHA	Death and loss of primitive erythroblasts, reduction of maternal reticulocyte count, and anemia in embryos of rodents
ART	Down regulation of VEGF and HIF-1a in mouse embryonic cells, impairment of laminin organization, and impaired expression of MMP-1, 2, and 9.	AS	Embryonic death and fetal resorption during organogenesis in rats and monkeys
DHA	DHA effects on primitive RBCs lead to anemia, cell damage, and high concentrations of DHA inhabited vasculogenesis and angiogenesis in rodents	AS/AM/AE	Retardation of fetal growth among surviving fetuses, cardiotoxicity, heart and skeletal defects, delays in limb and tail development in rats
DHA	Reduction of primitive red blood cells in frog embryos	AS/AM/AE	Significant necrosis of embryonic livers in rats

AS = artesunate; DHA = dihydroART; ART = ART; ROS = reactive oxygen species; VEGF = vascular endothelial growth factor; HIF-1a = hypoxia-inducible factor 1a; MMP = matrix metalloproteinase;

Table 2. A summary of the research findings and possible mechanisms of artemisinin drugs in the embryotoxicity studies *in vitro* and *in vivo* (Clark et al., 2009; Efferth & Kaina 2010; Finaurini et al., 2010; Longo et al., 2006a, 2006b, 2008; Wartenberg et al., 2003; White et al., 2008)

2.2.1 Inhibitory effects of AS/DHA on hematopoiesis

AS is embryolethal and teratogenic in rats, with a very narrow window of sensitivity between days 10-14 of gestation (Clark et al., 2004; Li et al., 2009; White et al., 2006). Further studies with a single oral dose of 17 mg/kg AS on gestational day (GD) 10-11 demonstrated that a paling of the visceral yolk sacs was observed within 3-6 hr after treatment. Within 24 hr, marked paling was observed which persisted through GD 14. Histologically, embryonic erythroblasts were reduced; cells showed signs of necrosis within 24 hr, and the erythroblasts were maximally depleted by 48 hr (White et al., 2006). The depletion of embryonic erythroblasts was shown to be the root cause of prolonged and severe anemia in AS-induced developmental toxicity observed *in vitro* using whole embryo rat cultures (WEC) (Longo et al., 2006a).

To verify the primary target of DHA in WEC and to detect consequences induced by early damage on embryo development, pregnant female rats were orally treated on GD 9.5 and 10.5 with 7.5 or 15 mg/kg/day DHA. A parallel *in vitro* WEC study evaluated the role of oxidative damage and examined blood islands and primitive RBCs. Embryos were observed for yolk sac hematopoiesis (Wolffian blood island formation, vasculogenesis and hematopoiesis) at stages known to be affected by DHA exposure. In accordance with the WEC results, primitive RBCs from yolk sac hematopoiesis were shown to be the target of DHA *in vivo*. The resulting anemia led to cell damage, which depending on its degree, was either diffuse or focal. Embryonic response to acute anemia varied from complete recovery to malformation and death. The malformations were shown to occur only in litters with embryonic deaths. DHA has been shown to induce low glutathione levels in RBCs, indicating that oxidative stress may be involved in ART toxicity. These effects were shown to be extremely rapid, with altered RBCs seen as early as GD 10.

In early development, the first wave of embryonic erythropoiesis begins in the visceral yolk sac on GD 7-7.5 in the mouse (Baumann & Dragon, 2005; Palis & Yoder, 2001) corresponding to GD 8.5-9 in the rat. Clusters of progenitor cells (hemangioblasts) form blood islands and differentiate into primitive erythroblasts and vascular endothelial cells (Tavassoli, 1991). The primitive erythroblasts enter the embryonic circulation on GD 10 in the rat, at about the same time that the heart begins to beat. These are a self-sustaining population of nucleated cells that proliferate while in the circulating blood. The definitive embryonic erythroblasts begin entering the circulation at about GD 13 in the rat. They are formed in the liver from hematopoietic stem cells which originate in the visceral yolk sac and migrate to the liver (Palis and Yoder, 2001; Tavassoli, 1991). The marked depletion of embryonic erythroblasts after a single AS dose to rats on GD 10 or 11 (White et al., 2006) is due to the killing of the primitive erythroblast population. As the primitive erythroblast population is self-sustaining after GD 10, this population cannot be replaced after extensive depletion until definitive erythroblasts are introduced into the blood from the liver.

During the embryotoxicity of AS, the replacement of these erythroblasts may fail because the embryonic liver has also been shown to be a target for AS in rats. Abnormalities in liver shape and lobation were caused by all four ARTs tested (AS, DHA, artemether and arteether) when administered as a single dose on GD 10 (White et al., 2008; Clark et al., 2008b). Fetal liver necrosis was observed in this study, which could be the basis for the unusual liver shape variation that we observed in this study of the narrow window of AS embryotoxicity. Histologically, the livers of these animals showed marked necrosis involving both hepatocytes and developing hematopoietic cells on GD 13 following a single dose of 17 mg/kg AS on GD 10.5 or 11 (White et al., 2006). In addition, the hematopoietic cells in the adult and embryo have been shown to be the target for selective binding of radiolabeled AS (Clark, 2009).

2.2.2 Relevance of vasculogenesis and hematopoiesis to embryo development

In the vertebrate embryo, hematopoietic and vascular endothelial cells are the first cells in the visceral yolk sac to differentiate in response to induction of the mesoderm (Baron 2001). A common precursor cell, the hemangioblast, gives rise to both erythrocytes and endothelial cells within blood islands. Yolk sac or primitive hematopoiesis is restricted to the formation of nucleated erythrocytes that express embryonic hemoglobin (Wong et al., 1986) and macrophages (Cline & Moore, 1972). At about 12 days of gestation this extra-embryonic hematopoiesis gives way to intraembryonic "definitive" hematopoiesis, first in the fetal liver and later the bone marrow (BM) and spleen. Definitive hematopoiesis is the process whereby all types of blood cells are formed followed by their differentiation, including the enucleation of erythrocytes.

As embryonic development continues, the site for hematopoiesis changes to the fetal liver, and, as the animal matures, to the bone marrow, where hematopoiesis persists in the adult. During development of the yolk sac, hematopoiesis is intimately linked to the development of blood vessels. In fact, the ontogenic relationship between hematopoietic cells and the endothelial cells of the blood islands of the yolk sac was confirmed many years ago (Sabin, 1917). These observations suggest that vasculogenesis and hematopoiesis are part of the same process, in which formation of a blood vessel is accompanied by the simultaneous in situ production of blood cells within that vessel, a process known as hemo-vasculogenesis

(Sequeira Lopez et al., 2003). In this environment, the first hematopoietic structure is responsible for the production of the primitive erythrocytes and the first transient population of definitive erythrocytes. In parallel, angioblasts multiply and differentiate into endothelial cells. The endothelial cells form tubes and then a network of capillaries that eventually reaches the circulation of the embryo (Baumann & Dragon, 2005).

This widespread phenomenon occurs by hemovasculogenesis, the formation of blood vessels accompanied by the simultaneous generation of red blood cells. Erythroblasts develop within aggregates of endothelial cell precursors. When the lumen forms, the erythroblasts "bud" from endothelial cells into the forming vessel. The extensive hematopoietic capacity found in the embryo helps explain why, under pathological circumstances such as severe anemia, extramedullary hematopoiesis can occur in any adult tissue. Understanding the intrinsic ability of tissues to manufacture their own blood cells and vessels has the potential to advance the fields of organogenesis, regeneration, and tissue engineering (Sequeira Lopez et al., 2003).

Previous data confirm the rapid onset of action of DHA on primitive RBCs, as soon as they enter circulation. There is no clear explanation why primitive RBC's are susceptible to DHA (Longo et al., 2006a and 2006b). Like intraerythrocytic malaria parasites, primitive RBCs have high concentrations of iron and heme, which have been proposed as either activators or targets of ART compounds (Olliaro et al., 2001; Parapini et al., 2004). The depletion of embryonic erythroid cells is believed to occur as a consequence of AS/DHA inhibition of vasculogenesis. This hypothesis is supported by the fact that vasculogenesis and hematopoiesis are part of the same process, in which formation of a blood vessel is accompanied by the simultaneous in situ production of blood cells within that vessel (Baron, 2001; Baumann & Dragon, 2005; Sequeira Lopez et al., 2003). In addition, oral and injectable AS treatment has been shown to induce marked embryolethality and a low incidence of teratogenic effects, including cardiovascular defects (ventricular septal and great vessels defects), which significantly affected novel vessel formation (Clark et al., 2004, White et al., 2008; Ratajska et al., 2006a, 2006b).

2.2.3 Antivasculogenic and antiangiogenic effects of AS/DHA

Red blood cells and the cardiovascular system are the first embryonic organ systems to show overt differentiation. Together they constitute the principal support system of the growing embryo (Baumann & Dragon, 2005). Vessel development within the embryo occurs via two processes: vasculogenesis and angiogenesis (Rongish et al., 1994; Risau, 1995, 1997). Vasculogenesis is the formation in situ of coronary vessels from endothelial cell progenitors (angioblasts) or angioblast migration to areas of vessel formation and their subsequent differentiation into vascular channels. Angiogenesis is the development of vessels from preexisting ones by capillary sprouting, intussusceptive growth, and remodeling (Risau, 1997; Ratajska et al., 2006a, 2006b). The first morphological signs of vasculogenesis within an embryo are "blood islands," which consist of erythroblasts and premature endothelial cells (angioblasts). Blood islands are encountered within the yolk sac of GD 7.5–13 rat embryos. The first signs of vasculogenesis in heart development are blood island-like structures.

In a series of AS/DHA embryotoxicity studies, heart abnormalities (swollen or collapsed chambers) were observed within 24 hr in 25–60% of embryos and within 48 hr in 100% of embryos, correlating with histological signs of cardiac myopathy (thinned and underdeveloped heart walls and enlarged chambers) (White et al., 2006). Rats deficient for these genes had normal heart development through GD 12.5–13, dilated hearts with reduced trabeculation, histological evidence of a thinned compact zone, and embryonic death occurred by GD 11. In light of this information, White's data (2008) are consistent with the hypothesis that depletion of embryonic erythroblasts creates a hypoxic environment, limiting the availability of oxygen as a substrate for oxidative phosphorylation in the heart. As a result, the energy requirements for normal proliferation of heart tissue are not met, causing underdevelopment of the heart. This could then lead to impaired cardiac function and hemodynamic changes, resulting in ventricular septal defects and great vessel malformations (Clark et al., 2004), which could further impair cardiac function. The hypoxic conditions created by both anemia and impaired cardiac function could then lead to embryonic death (White et al., 2008).

New patterns of malformations not seen previously were observed in studies in which AS was administered orally at closely spaced doses during organogenesis in pregnant rats and rabbits (Clark et al., 2004). The malformations consisted of cardiovascular malformations (ventricular septal defects and various vessel defects) and a syndrome of skeletal defects including shortened and/or bent long bones and scapulae, misshapen ribs, cleft sternebrae, and incompletely ossified pelvic bones. In rats, malformations occurred only at embryolethal doses. The embryolethal effect occurred with a steep dose-response curve and was apparent as abortions in rabbits and post-implantation loss including total litter loss in both rats and rabbits. These developmental effects were observed largely in the absence of any apparent maternal toxicity (Clark et al., 2009).

Compared to rat embryos, the larvae of frogs treated with AS/DHA had no areas of necrosis but they shared similar heart defects. Heart defects were seen in both frog species treated with doses of DHA ≥ 0.1 μg/mL (abnormal heart looping, thin atrial and ventricular walls and underdeveloped trabeculae). The fact that cardiac defects are seen in Xenopus larvae in the absence of cell death offers an alternative explanation for the mode of action of ART. In rats these findings were attributed to cell death resulting from anemia and hypoxia (Longo et al., 2006a); here, frog larvae death may be secondary to anemia. Potentially larvae death may not be mediated by cell death but rather by altered intracardiac hemodynamics due to RBC degeneration, as speculated by White et al. (2006).

In embryotoxicity studies conducted with DHA administered at GD 9, the yolk sac was shown to be fully vascularized. However, at DHA concentrations ≥ 0.05 μg/mL, the visceral yolk sac was well vascularized but pale; yolk sac vessel formation and circulation appeared normal, but blood in the yolk sac was visibly paler than blood observed in the yolk sacs of control animals. This effect increased with higher DHA doses. At concentrations ≥ 0.5 μg/mL, the vasculature was also affected. Vessel diameter was reduced, small anastomotic vessels were not visible, and the number of circulating cells was further reduced. At DHA concentration of 1.0 μg/mL, yolk sac vasculature and circulating cells were markedly reduced, and at 2 μg/mL only a few poorly organized yolk sac vessels were present. At DHA concentrations ≥ 2 μg/mL, the heartbeat of the majority of the embryos was reduced and irregular.

These observations showed higher concentration and longer time exposure of AS/DHA inhibited vasculogenesis and angiogenesis (Longo et al., 2006a; 2006b; White et al., 2008). Therefore, the embryonic heart defects and killing of embryonic primitive erythroblasts after AS/DHA treatment significantly affected blood vessel development and the formation of a circulatory system. The sequence of defects noted began with the loss of primitive erythroblasts and ended with inhibition of heart vascularization (Finaurini et al., 2010; Kwee et al., 1995; Ratajska et al., 2006a; 2006b; Sequeira Lopez et al., 2003).

2.3 Possible antivascular mechanism associated with artemesinin-induced embryotoxicity

Current hypotheses on the pharmacological and toxicological mechanisms of ART action propose that the endoperoxide group of the ARTs functions as both the pharmacophore and toxicophore, and that chemical activation of these compounds is essential for activity. The antimalarial mode of action of the ARTs is thought to be related to activation of the endoperoxide bridge by heme-derived or chelatable iron during the erythrocytic stage of malaria, producing centered radicals via a well-characterized chemical pathway. Ultimately, it is these radicals that are the toxic species. The peroxide bridge is activated via the association of iron, in the form of Fe^{2+}, to either oxygen of the peroxide group, generating two distinct oxyl radicals (Mercer, 2009).

Evidence for the role of the mitochondria in both the pharmacological and toxicological mechanisms of action of the ARTs has been reported. The mitochondrion has long been recognized as a site of endoperoxide accumulation within plasmodium parasites, and this accumulation is co-incident with observed mitochondria damage (Maeno et al., 1993). Studies have also demonstrated that ARTs bind to active, not inactive, mitochondria in rat embryo erythroblasts (White et al., 2006; 2008). Other studies have further implicated mitochondria in the pharmacological and toxicological mechanism of action of ARTs. For example, researchers studying the ART mechanism of action using a yeast system published data to propose that the mitochondria play a dual role: the electron transport chain stimulates the effect of ART, most probably via activation of the peroxide group, and the mitochondria are subsequently damaged by locally generated free radicals (Li et al., 2005).

A recent study demonstrated that mitochondria are the main subcellular target of endoperoxides in primitive red blood cells in the Xenopus frog embryo teratogenesis model system (Longo et al., 2008). This study suggests that the mitochondria are a site of activation for DHA. This is an attractive premise as it can be used to explain the selectivity of AS/DHA between quiescent cells and rapidly proliferating cancer cells. In dividing cells, mitochondria are active in order to deliver sustained energy for continued growth. Furthermore, the presence of a high number of iron-sulfur containing enzymes, the redox activity of the electron transport chain and its role in the initiation of apoptosis are compatible with the hypothesized cytotoxic action of the ARTs via a one-electron reduction of the peroxide bridge to cytotoxic radical species. In addition, studies have demonstrated that endoperoxide activity is accompanied by the generation of oxidative stress, which is often associated with mitochondrial dysfunction (Disbrow et al., 2005). This rationale supports the role of mitochondria as a possible activating system and/or target of the ARTs and opens up an exciting new area for research in establishing the role of bioactivation and mechanism of action (Mercer, 2009).

2.4 Circumventing embryotoxicity in pregnant women treated with AS/DHA

Embryotoxicity, toxicokinetics, and tissue distribution studies after intravenous and intramuscular AS treatment of pregnant and non-pregnant animals have also been conducted (Li et al, 2008 & 2009). These data demonstrate that the severe embryotoxicity induced by injectable AS is due to a number of factors: 1) injectable AS treatment results in a much higher peak drug concentration than treatment with oral ARTs and intramuscular artemether; 2) DHA produced by hydrolysis of AS plays a key role in embryotoxicity; 3) Among all ARTs, AS has the highest conversion rate to DHA; 4) the conversion rate of AS to DHA has been shown to be significantly increased in pregnant animals; 5) the buildup of high peak concentrations of AS and DHA in the blood of pregnant rats has been shown to be significantly higher than those of non-pregnant animals; and 6) injectable AS treatment results in higher distribution of AS and DHA in feto-placental tissues in pregnant animals (Li et al., 2008).

2.4.1 Toxicity of AS/DHA occurs in a narrow time window during embryogenesis

Studies in rodents have demonstrated that ARTs can induce fetal death and congenital malformations at low dose levels, which can be induced in rodents only within a narrow window in early embryogenesis (GD 10-14). A recent study in cynomolgus monkeys found that AS treatment caused embryo death between GD 30 and 40. The no-observed-adverse-effect-level (NOAEL) was 4 mg/kg/day. No malformations were observed in four surviving fetuses in the 12 mg/kg/day group, but the sample size of this study was not adequate to conclude that AS is not teratogenic at that dose in monkeys. All three live embryos in the 30 mg/kg/day AS group dosed from GD 20 were removed by caesarean section on GD 26, 32 and 36 respectively, and these embryos showed marked reduction in erythroblasts. Since embryo death was observed only after more than 12 days of daily treatment at 12 mg/kg, the lack of developmental toxicity at a dose of 30 mg/kg/day indicates that a shorter treatment period decreases the potential for AS induced embryotoxicity in monkeys (Clark et al., 2008a).

Primitive erythroblasts develop in the visceral yolk sac and are released into the embryonic circulation on GD 10 in rats, at about the same time that the heart begins to beat. If the primitive erythroblasts are also the primary target of AS action in monkeys, then the most sensitive time window for embryotoxicity would be when those primitive erythroblasts predominate in the embryonic circulation. In the cynomolgus monkey, the heart starts beating at about GD 18. Although no data exist at this time to prove the timing of the switchover from primitive to definitive erythroblasts in monkeys, the erythroblasts visible in the sections of embryos from GD 26, 32, and 36 were > 90% nucleated, suggesting that they were probably primitive erythroblasts during GD 18 to 36. On GD 50, only 9% of blood cells were nucleated, indicating that the transition from primitive to definitive erythroblasts was nearly complete on GD 50 (Clark et al., 2008a).

The time window of AS/DHA sensitivity observed in animal studies would hypothetically correspond to humans during organogenesis. The earliest primitive erythrocytes are formed in the yolk sac starting at GD 18.5 (Clark et al., 2008a; Lensch & Daley, 2004). The onset of blood circulation coincides with the onset of the embryonic heartbeat, which probably occurs between GD 19 and GD 21 in humans, evidenced by the appearance of primitive erythrocytes in the cardiac cavity. The liver is the first organ to be colonized by the yolk sac and is the main site of definitive erythropoiesis from week 5 through week 24 of gestation (Segel & Palis, 2001). Primitive erythrocytes are the predominant circulating form in the first 8 to 10 weeks of gestation. Liver-derived definitive erythrocytes begin to enter the circulation by 8 weeks of gestation, but do not predominate until 11 to 12 weeks (Kelemen et al., 1979). All available studies agree that yolk sac hematopoiesis disappears completely after GD 60 (Lensch & Daley, 2004).

Therefore, the timing of the switchover from primitive to definitive erythroblasts is GD10-14 for rats, GD 18-50 for monkeys, and GD 16-60 for humans. Based on this information, if human embryos were sensitive to AS or DHA in the same way as rat and monkey embryos, then the most sensitive period for human development toxicity induced by ARTs would be predicted to begin with the onset of circulation in week 4 of gestation and end at approximately week 9 to 10 of gestation. At this time in gestation, the nucleated primitive erythroblasts have been largely replaced by non-nucleated definitive erythroblasts (Clark et al., 2008a). If primitive erythrocytes are formed over a longer period than that in rodents, then AS/DHA dosing for longer than 12 days may be required to produce a severe effect on the early blood cell population in primates or humans (Clark et al, 2008;WHO2006b).

2.4.2 Pharmacokinetic concerns of AS/DHA relating to embryotoxicity

Although no animal species exists that completely mimics man, non-human primates provide the best comparison to humans. With animal experiments only certain aspects of a highly complex system can be analyzed. In order to achieve this successfully, animal species and experimental set-up have to be chosen carefully to represent the human condition in as suitable a model as possible. The more the model deviates from the human condition the less predictive it will be. Today, more information is available on the pharmacokinetic and toxicokinetic properties of ARTs (Li & Weina, 2010b). This will help provide data on the embryotoxic/teratogenic doses of a substance or on their non-embryotoxic/teratogenic doses relevant to man. In addition, the relative duration of exposure to three day ACT for malaria in humans, with respect to the duration of organogenesis, may be too short to induce the severe embryotoxicity that is observed in animal species.

Another consideration when reviewing pharmacokinetic implications of AS/DHA therapy is the impact of pregnancy on drug metabolism. There are physiological changes in pregnancy that can cause a decrease in plasma drug concentrations and the area under the curve (AUCs), resulting in reduced efficacy (Dawes & Chowjenczyk, 2001). This is likely due to increased clearance, larger volume of distribution and perhaps altered absorption following oral administration. Clearly, oral dosages of these antimalarial drugs need to be adapted to maintain efficacy when given to pregnant patients and animals with malaria (Nosten et al., 2006). However, data obtained for the pharmacokinetic parameters for these antimalarial agents show no significant difference between pregnant and non-pregnant women and animal species after single intravenous or intramuscular injections (Li et al., 2008; Menendez 2006; Newton et al., 2000).

Preclinical studies of AS-induced embryotoxicity in pregnant rats has shown thta injectable AS administration resulted in severe toxicity to animals by routes of intraveous, intramuscular, and subcutaneous administration with doses higher than 1.0 mg/kg. However, animals treated with oral ARTs and intramuscular AM demonstrated that these ARTs were much safer than injectable AS with embryolethality demonstrated at doses ranging from 6.1–51.0 mg/kg (Table 1). Similar findings showed that treatment with a single dose of 17 mg/kg oral AS and 1.5 mg/kg intravenous AS administered on GD 11 both caused 100% embryolethality and are close to the threshold for that effect (10 mg/kg oral AS caused only 15% fetal resorption and 0.75 mg/kg intravenous AS caused 7%fetal resorption) (Clark et al., 2009; White et al., 2008). Toxicokinetic and tissue distribution data demonstrated that the severe embryotoxicity induced by injectable AS is due to the following six factors (Li et al., 2008).

1. Injectable AS can provide much higher peak concentrations (3–25 fold higher) than oral ARTs and intramuscular AM in animals (Li et al., 2008). *In vitro* results in other studies have shown that the drug exposure level and time are important to induce embryotoxicity (Longo et al., 2006a; 2006b; 2008). However, *in vivo* studies demonstrated that the drug exposure level is more important than drug exposure time because AS and DHA have very short half-lives (≤1 h) in animal species (Li et al., 2008).

2. AS is completely converted to DHA and is basically a prodrug of DHA. Also, DHA was shown to be more effective than AS in inhibition of angiogenesis and vasculogenesis *in vitro* (Longo et al., 2006a; 2006b; Chen et al., 2004b; White et al., 2006). In addition without DHA formation, the embryotoxicity of ARTs can be reduced by using artemisone, which has significantly less anti-angiogenic activity than DHA. Artemisone is a novel derivative of ART and is not metabolized to DHA (D'Alessandro et al., 2007; Schmuck et al., 2009).
3. The conversion rate of AS to DHA is the highest among all ARTs. The conversion rate of AS to DHA was shown to be 38.2–72.7% in comparison to that of AM and AE which show a conversion rate of 12.4–14.2% in animal species (Li et al., 2008).
4. In contrast to the data observed with single AS dosing, the conversion rate of AS to DHA was significantly increased in pregnant rats compared to non-pregnant animals following multiple injections. The concentrations of DHA generated in pregnant rats was 2.2-fold higher on day 1 and 4.5-fold higher on day 3 than that observed in non-pregnant animals, resulting in a total $AUC_{D1\text{-}3}$ of 15,049 ng·h/ml which is 3.7-fold higher in pregnant rats than the $AUC_{D1\text{-}3}$ of 4,015 ng·h/ml observed in non-pregnant rats. The ratios of AUC_{DHA}/AUC_{AS} were also shown to be 0.99–1.02 for pregnant rats and 0.42–0.48 for non-pregnant animals, indicating that the total exposure of pregnant rats to DHA during the whole period of treatment was much higher than in non-pregnant rats (Li et al., 2008).
5. The buildup of high peak concentrations of AS and DHA in the plasma of pregnant rats was significantly higher than those of non-pregnant animals after repeated dosing. In a study of the toxicokinetics (TK) of AS, the data revealed that the peak concentration (C_{max}) of AS (14,927-16,545 ng/ml) in pregnant rats was double the C_{max} of AS (5,037-8,668 ng/ml) in non-pregnant animals. Comparable to the C_{max} values, the mean AUC data of DHA showed values much higher in pregnant animals (3,681–4,821 ng·h/ml) than those observed in non-pregnant rats (1,049-1,636 ng·h/ml). The TK results also showed the mean AUC of DHA was significantly increased from day 1 (3,681 ng·h/ml) to 3 (4,821 ng·h/ml) in the pregnant rats, but remarkably decreased from day 1 (1,636 ng·h/ml) to Day 3 (1,049 ng·h/ml) in the non-pregnant animals (Li et al., 2008).
6. Injectable AS can also result in higher distribution of AS and DHA in the tissues of feto-placental tissues in pregnant animals after multiple administrations. A tissue distribution study of ^{14}C-AS showed that the total $AUC_{0\text{-}192h}$ of the radioactive labeled AS was 22,879 µg equivalents·h/g in all measured tissues of the pregnant rats, and 6.54% of the total radioactivity was present in all of the feto-placental tissues. During the 192 h treatment period, measured levels of radioactivity in the ovary, placenta, and uterus were 555, 367, and 216 µg equivalents·h/g, respectively. The values observed in feto-placental tissues were more than 2–4 fold higher than observed in blood (134 µg equivalents·h/ml) (Li et al., 2008).

The observed pharmacokinetics of antimalarials is altered in pregnancy after oral administration, and the drug plasma levels are decreased. However, previous data has shown that AS and DHA concentrations in the plasma and reproductive tissues of pregnant rats were significantly increased over the AS and DHA concentrations observed in non-pregnant animals after injectable AS treatment. The significant increase in blood ant tissue concentrations of AS and DHA may be related to the severe embryotoxicity observed after treatment of pregnant animals with injectable AS even in low dose regimens.

2.4.3 Current safety regimens for artemisinin therapy in pregnant women

There are three facts that support the assertion that oral ARTs are safe in pregnant women: 1) the pharmacokinetics of antimalarials is altered in pregnancy after oral administration, which can cause a decrease in drug exposure levels; 2) treatment with oral ARTs has been shown to result in low peak concentrations when compared to the peak concentrations observed after treatment with injectable ARTs as discussed above; and 3) data on clinical trials regarding the possible effects of ARTs on pregnancy have not shown any embryotoxic effects in humans for the past 25 years with oral ART monotherapy or oral ACTs.

Few studies in pregnant women have been published for ARTs or other antimalarials. For example, oral chloroquine prophylaxis treatment, oral mefloquine therapy, oral progaunil treatment as well as oral DHA therapy all show altered kinetics in pregnancy, and plasma levels of these drugs are significantly lower than those observed in non-pregnant patients with malaria (Li & Weina, 2010b). This is likely due to increased clearance, larger volume of distribution and perhaps altered absorption following oral administration. In comparison to non-pregnant Thai women, the C_{max} and AUC of DHA values were 4.2 and 1.8 fold, lower in pregnant patients (McGready et al., 2006; Ward et al., 2007). A similar observation has also been found in animal studies of oral administration of AS (Clark et al., 2004). Clearly, oral dosage of these antimalarials needs to be adapted to maintain efficacy when given to pregnant patients and animals with malaria (Nosten et al., 2006). In this case, treatment with oral drugs appears safe due to the decreased drug exposure and fast elimination in pregnant women.

There is now a reasonable body of evidence for safety from most of the clinical trials published from 1989 to 2009 in nearly 1,837 pregnant women exposed to an ART agent or ACT with 176 pregnant patients in the first trimester. There were no clinically significant adverse effects of the drug treatment, nor any adverse outcome of the pregnancies, nor any adverse outcomes related to development (neurological and physical) of the infants, including 44 infants exposed during the first trimester (Li & Weina 2010b). Recent data published by the WHO (2006b) provided data on ART exposure in pregnancy from ongoing studies in Thailand, Zambia and Bangladesh. In Thailand, a study was recently conducted on 1,530 first trimester exposures to a range of antimalarial medicines including 170 pregnant women treated with ARTs. The highest risk of abortion in pregnant women with *P. falciparum* malaria treated with any antimalarial was associated with the number of episodes of infection and the number of times the women had to be treated in the first trimester. In addition, fever, hyperparasitemia and older maternal age were significant positive risk factors for an abortion in the first trimester, whereas antimalarial drug treatments were not significantly related.

The WHO concluded that there is insufficient evidence at present to warrant a change in the current WHO policy recommendations on the use of ACTs for the treatment of malaria in pregnancy. Current WHO Guidelines recommend that in uncomplicated malaria, ACTs should be used in the second and third trimester, but ACTs should only be used in the first trimester if they are the only effective treatments available (WHO 2006a). These recommendations are still valid based on the data presented in this chapter. However, the medicine of choice for initial treatment in the first trimester of pregnancy varies because of differences in drug sensitivities in different regions. The immediate use of ARTs is justified in situations where the first treatment fails because of the dangers of repeated malaria infections during later pregnancy. In the future, ACTs may be used to treat pregnant women in all trimesters after review of further safety studies to evaluate the risk of embryotoxicity.

3. Anticancer effect of artemisinins (ARTs) via an antiangiogenic mechanism

ART and its bioactive derivatives (AS, DHA, artemether and arteether) exhibit potent anticancer effects in a variety of human cancer cell model systems (Figure 1). The pleitropic response in cancer cells includes: 1) growth inhibition by cell cycle arrest, 2) apoptosis, 3) inhibition of angiogenesis, 4) disruption of cell migration, and 5) modulation of nuclear receptor responsiveness. These effects of ARTs result from perturbations of many cellular signaling pathways.

3.1 *In vitro* and *in vivo* research on anticancer effects of ARTs

3.1.1 Anticancer properties of ARTs

Molecular, cellular and physiological studies have demonstrated that, depending on the tissue type and experimental system, ART and its derivatives arrest cell growth, induce an apoptotic response, alter hormone responsive properties and/or inhibit angiogenesis of human cancer cells. The Developmental Therapeutics Program of the National Cancer Institute (NCI), USA, which analyzed the activity of AS on 55 human cancer cell lines (IC_{50} values shown between 0.512 and 124.295 mM, depending on the cancer cell line), showed that AS has strong anticancer activity against leukemia and colon cancer cell lines, and has intermediate effects on melanomas, breast, ovarian, prostate, central nervous system, and renal cancer cell lines (Efferth et al., 2001, 2006).

Moreover, the highly stable ARTs and ART-derived trioxane dimers were shown to inhibit growth and selectively kill several human cancer cell lines without inducing cytotoxic effects on normal neighboring cells. One proposed mechanism by which ART targets cancer cells is cleavage of the endoperoxide bridge by the relatively high concentrations of iron in cancer cells, resulting in generation of free radicals such as reactive oxygen species (ROS) and subsequent oxidative damage as well as iron depletion in the cells. This mechanism resembles the action of ART in malarial parasites. In addition to possessing higher iron influx via transferrin receptors, cancer cells are also sensitive to oxygen radicals because of a relative deficiency in antioxidant enzymes. A significant positive correlation can be made between AS sensitivity and transferrin receptor levels as well as between AS sensitivity and expression of ATP binding cassette transporter 6.

Expression profiling of several classes of tumor cells revealed that ART treatment caused selective expression changes of many more oncogenes and tumor suppressor genes than genes responsible for iron metabolism, which suggests that the anticancer properties of ARTs cannot be explained simply by the global toxic effects of oxidative damage. ARTs have also been observed to attenuate multidrug resistance in cancer patients, an effect due in part to the inhibition of glutathione S-transferase activity. ART and its bioactive derivatives elicit their anticancer effects by concurrently activating, inhibiting and/or attenuating multiple complementary cell signaling pathways, which have been described in a variety of human cancer cell systems as well as in athymic mouse xenograft models. The ART compounds exert common as well as distinct cellular effects depending on the phenotype and tissue origin of the examined human cancer cells. (Firestone & Sundar 2009)

3.1.2 *In vitro* anticancer effect of ART and its derivatives

While most of the investigations on the anticancer activities of ARTs have been performed with cell lines *in vitro*, there are a few reports in the literature showing activity *in vivo* against xenograft tumors, e.g., breast tumors, ovarian cancer, Kaposi sarcoma, fibrosarcoma, or liver cancer. The *in vitro* data in the literature supports the hypothesis that ART derivatives kill or inhibit the growth of many types of cancer cell lines, including drug-resistant cell lines, suggesting that ART could become the basis of a new class of anticancer drugs. In addition, the co-administration of holotransferrin and other iron sources with ARTs has been shown to increase the potency of ARTs in killing cancer cells.

Artemisinin (ART)

ART was tested using a drug-sensitive H69 human small-cell lung carcinoma (SCLC) cell line and also by using multi-drug-resistant (H69VP) SCLC cells pretreated with holotransferrin. The cytotoxicity of ART on H69VP cells (IC_{50} = 24 nM) was ten-fold lower than for H69 cells (IC_{50} = 2.3 nM). Pretreatment with 880 nM holotransferrin did not alter the cytotoxicity of ART on H69 cells, but significantly enhanced the effect on H69VP cells (IC_{50} = 5.4 nM) (Sadava et al., 2002).

A recent study demonstrated that ART induced cell growth arrest in A375M malignant melanoma tumor cells, and also affected the viability of A375P cutaneous melanoma tumor cells with both cytotoxic and growth inhibitory effects, while ART was not effective in inhibiting growth of other tumor cell lines (MCF7 and MKN). In addition, ART affected the migratory ability of A375M cells by reducing metalloproteinase 2 (MMP-2) productions and down-regulating $\alpha v\beta 3$ integrin expression. These findings introduce a potential of ART as a chemotherapeutic agent in melanoma treatment (Buommino et al., 2009).

Dihydroartemisinin (DHA)

DHA selectively killed Molt-4 lymphoblastoid cells when co-incubated with holotransferrin, while the same treatment was significantly less toxic to normal human lymphocytes. The drug combination of DHA and holotransferrin was approximately 100 times more effective on Molt-4 cells than normal lymphocytes (LC_{50s} of Molt-4 and normal lymphocytes were 2.6 μM and 230 μM, respectively). Incubation with DHA alone was found to be less effective than in combination with holotransferrin, indicating that intracellular iron plays a role in the cytotoxic effect (Lai & Singh, 1995).

HTB 27 cells, a radiation-resistant human breast cancer cell line, were killed effectively (reduced to 2% of original concentration) after 16 hr of treatment with DHA (200 μM) and holotransferrin (12 μM). However HTB 125 cells, a normal breast cell line, were not significantly affected by the same treatment. Also, when breast cancer cells were treated with only DHA (200 μM) (without holotransferrin), the cytotoxicity observed was significantly lower (Singh & Lai, 2001).

DHA is also cytotoxic to human glioma cells (U373MG), and the cytotoxicity is markedly enhanced by the addition of holotransferrin (Kim et al., 2006). In addition, radiation-induced expression of the endogenous antioxidant enzyme glutathione-S-transferase was found to be suppressed by DHA (Kim et al., 2006).

After treatment with DHA *in vitro*, the rates of proliferative inhibition of pancreatic cancer cells BxPC-3 and AsPC-1 were 76.2% and 79.5% respectively. The rates of apoptosis were increased to 55.5% and 40.0%, respectively, ($P < 0.01$ when compared with controls) (Chen et al., 2009).

DHA was shown to exhibit significant anticancer activity against the renal epithelial LLC cell line. DHA also induced apoptosis of LLC cells and influenced the expression of the vascular endothelial growth factor (VEGF) receptor KDR/flk-1. Furthermore, in both tumor xenografts, a greater degree of growth inhibition was achieved when DHA and chemotherapeutics were used in combination. The affect of DHA combined with chemotherapy on LLC tumor metastasis was significant (Zhou et al., 2010).

Artesunate (AS)

AS has been shown to inhibit the growth of Kaposi's sarcoma cells, a highly angiogenic multifocal tumor, and the degree of cell growth inhibition correlated with the induction of apoptosis. AS also inhibited the growth of normal human umbilical endothelial cells and of KS-IMM cells that were established from a Kaposi's sarcoma lesion obtained from a renal transplant patient. The inhibition of cell growth correlated with the induction of apoptosis in KS-IMM cells. Apoptosis was not observed in normal endothelial cells, which showed drastically increased cell doubling times upon AS treatment (Dell'Eva et al., 2004).
Fe(II)-glycine sulfate and transferrin enhanced the cytotoxicity (10.3-fold) of free AS, AS microencapsulated in maltosyl-ß- cyclodextrin, and ARTs towards CCRF-CEM leukemia and U373 astrocytoma cells (Efferth et al., 2004). Treatment with AS at more than 2.5 μM for 48 h inhibited the proliferation of human vein endothelial cell (HUVEC) in a concentration dependent manner using an MTT (3-(4,5-dimethylthiazol-2-yl)-2,5-diphenyltetrazolium bromide) based growth proliferation assay ($p < 0.05$). The IC_{50} value was 20.7 μM and HUVEC cells were also shown to be inhibited 88.7% by 80 μM AS (Chen et al., 2004b).
The inhibitory effect of AS on in vitro angiogenesis was tested on aortic cells cultured on a fibrin gel. AS was shown to effectively suppress the stimulating angiogenic ability of chronic myeloid leukemia cells (line K562) when the K562 cells were pretreated for 48 h with AS in a time-dependent manner (days 3-14). AS treatment was also found to decrease the VEGF level in chronic myeloma K562 cells, even at a lower concentration (2 μmol/l, $P < 0.01$). (Zhou et al., 2007).
AS at low concentration was shown to significantly decrease VEGF and Ang-1 secretion by human multiple myeloma cells (line RPMI8226, $P < 0.05$), which correlated well with the reduction of angiogenesis induced by the myeloma RPMI8226 cells. This study also showed that AS downregulated the expression of VEGF and Ang-1 in RPMI8226 cells and reduced the activation of extracellular signal regulated kinase 1 (ERK1) as well. Therefore, AS can block ERK1/2 activation, downregulate VEGF and Ang-1 expression and inhibit angiogenesis induced by human multiple myeloma RPMI8226 cells. Combined with our previous published data, results from this study indicate that AS possesses potential anti-myeloma activity (Chen et al., 2010a).
AS has been shown to decrease the secretion of VEGF and IL-8 from TNFα- or hypoxia-stimulated rheumatoid arthritis fibroblast-like synoviocyte (line RA FLS) in a dose-dependent manner. AS inhibited TNFα- or hypoxia-induced nuclear expression and translocation of HIF-1α. AS also prevented Akt phosphorylation, but there was no evidence that phosphorylation of p38 and ERK was averted. TNFα- or hypoxia-induced secretion of VEGF and IL-8 and expression of HIF-1α were hampered by treatment with the PI3 kinase inhibitor LY294002, suggesting that inhibition of PI3 kinase/Akt activation might inhibit VEGF, IL-8 secretion, and HIF-1α expression induced by TNFα or hypoxia. Therefore, AS has been shown to inhibit angiogenic factor expression in RA FLS, and this latest study provides new evidence that, as a low-cost agent, AS may have therapeutic potential for rheumatoid arthritis (He et al., 2011).

3.1.3 *In vivo* anticancer effect of ART and its derivatives

There are a small number of papers dealing with the *in vivo* anticancer activity of ARTs which may provide insight into the potential activity of ARTs *in vivo*.

Artemisinin (ART)

A study was conducted to determine the potential of ART to prevent the development of breast cancer in rats treated with 7, 12-dimethylbenz[a]anthracene (DMBA), a carcinogen known to induce multiple breast tumors. In 43% of DMBA-treated rats fed ART for 40 weeks, breast cancer tumor development was prevented, while almost all the rat fed normal food developed tumors within that time. Breast tumors of ART-fed rats were also significantly fewer and smaller in size compared with those tumors found in control animals (Lai & Singh, 2006).

Dihydroartemisinin (DHA)

DHA and ferrous sulfate have been shown to inhibit the growth of implanted fibrosarcoma tumors in rats. The growth rate of the tumors was retarded (30% less than control group) by daily oral administration of ferrous sulfate (20 mg/kg/day) followed by DHA (2–5 mg/kg/day) and no significant tumor growth inhibition was observed in the animals given either DHA or ferrous sulfate alone (Moore et al., 1995).

DHA was shown to inhibit ovarian cancer cell growth when administered alone or in combination with carboplatin, presumably through a caspase mediated apoptotic pathway. These effects were observed *in vivo* in ovarian A2780 and OVCAR-3 xenograft tumor models. DHA was shown to exhibit significant anticancer activity against ovarian cancer cells *in vivo*, with minimal toxicity to non-tumourigenic human OSE cells, indicating that DHA and ferrous sulfate may be promising therapeutic agents for ovarian cancer, either used alone or in combination with conventional chemotherapy (Chen et al, 2009).

DHA has been shown to inhibit the growth of pancreatic xenograft tumors in nude mice. The proliferation index and apoptosis index found in this study were 49.1% and 50.2% respectively in the treatment group treated with 50 mg/kg of DHA, while the proliferation index and apoptosis index of the control group was 72.1% and 9.4% respectively ($P < 0.01$). A Western blot assay conducted in the course of this study indicated that DHA up-regulated expression of the proliferation-associated protein p21(WAF1) and down-regulated expression of PCNA, increased expression of apoptosis-associated protein Bax, and decreased expression of Bcl-2 and activated caspase-9 in BxPC-3 cells. DHA was shown to exert its anti-tumor activity in pancreatic cancer both *in vitro* and *in vivo* by proliferation inhibition and apoptosis induction. The data supports the hypothesis that DHA has potential to be used as an anti-tumor drug in pancreatic cancer (Chen et al., 2009; 2010b).

Artesunate (AS)

AS has been studied in variety of tumor models as a potential antitumor drug. In one study of vascularization, a critical element of tumor metastasis, AS was shown to strongly reduce angiogenesis *in vivo* by inhibiting vascularization in Matrigel plugs injected subcutaneously into syngenic mice. This data suggests that AS represents a promising candidate drug for the treatment of the highly angiogenic Kaposi's sarcoma. As a low-cost drug, it might be of particular interest for use in areas of the world where Kaposi's sarcoma is highly prevalent. (Dell'Eva et al., 2004).

In a second study of the efficacy of AS, as an anticancer agent, tumor growth in rats given AS subcutaneously at a dose of 50 mg/kg/day and at a dose of 100 mg/kg/day for 15 days was reduced by 41%, in the 50 mg/kg treatment group and 62% in the 100 mg/kg treatment group. The density of micro-vessels which was used as a measure of angiogenic activity in the tumors of animals treated with 100 mg/kg of AS daily was at least four times lower than in the control group (Chen et al., 2004b).

In a third study, AS was also found to inhibit angiogenesis *in vivo*. The antiangiogenic activity of AS *in vivo* was evaluated in nude mice implanted with a human ovarian cancer HO-8910 cell line. The specific AS activity that inhibited angiogenesis in the ovarian tumors was determined through immunohistochemical staining for microvessel formation (CD31), VEGF and the VEGF receptor KDR/flk-1. Tumor growth was noted to be decreased and the density of the tumor microvessels was reduced following AS treatment with no apparent toxicity to the animals. ART also remarkably lowered VEGF expression in tumor cells and the expression of KDR/flk-1 in endothelial cells as well as in tumor cells (Chen et al., 2004a, 2004b).

In a fourth study, the anticancer activity of AS was correlated with the inhibition of activity in the Wnt/beta-catenin signaling pathway. *In vivo*, AS treatment resulted in a significant decrease in the rate of growth of colorectal tumor xenografts. Bioluminescent imaging also revealed that AS decreased the physiological activity of tumor xenografts and delayed spontaneous liver metastases. These antitumor effects were related to the translocation of beta-catenin to the cell membrane and the inhibition of the unrestricted activation of the Wnt/beta-catenin pathway, which was confirmed by the immunohistochemical staining of tumor tissues. These results support the use of AS for treatment of colorectal cancer and also outline a mechanism of action of AS against colorectal cancer cells (Li et al, 2007).

The antiangiogenic effect of AS was further evaluated *in vivo* in the chicken chorioallantoic membrane (CAM) neovascularization model. The results showed that stimulating angiogenic activity was decreased in response to the treatment of myeloblastic K562 cells with ART and tumor growth was inhibited when K562 cells were pretreated with ART in a dose-dependent manner (3-12 μmol/l). Furthermore, we analyzed the level of VEGF expression by Western blot and also assayed VEGF mRNA by RT-PCR in K562 cells. The experiments showed that ART could inhibit VEGF expression, and the inhibition correlated well with the level of VEGF secreted in the culture medium. These findings suggest that AS may have potential as a treatment for chronic myelogenous leukemia (CML) or as an adjunct to standard chemotherapeutic regimens (Zhou et al., 2007).

In a further study, AS inhibited the growth of ret-tumor cells and induced their apoptosis in a concentration-dependent manner (0.1-200 μmol/l). In addition, we assessed the effects of AS treatment on the immune system of treated and control animals through flow cytometric measurement quantitating different immune cell populations. No significant differences in the numbers of CD4 and CD8 T cells, T regulatory or suppressor cells, or NK cells were observed in the ret-transgenic mice and nontransgenic C57BL/6 littermates treated for 2 weeks with a daily dose of 1 mg AS. These results indicate that the cytostatic and apoptotic effects of AS are not diminished by concomitant immune suppression (Ramacher et al., 2009).

Other studies have been conducted on the successful treatment of human cancers with ART derivatives. These studies encourage further investigation of the use of ART in human cancer cases under well controlled clinical studies (Berger et al., 2005; Singh & Panwar, 2006).

3.2 Mechanistic perspectives on the antiangiogenic activities of ARTs

Angiogenesis and vasculogenesis refer to the growth of blood vessels. Angiogenesis is the growth most often associated with repair of damaged vessels or the growth of smaller blood vessels, while vasculogenesis is the process by which the primary blood system is being created or changed. Vasculogenesis occurs during the very early developmental stages of an organism when the blood vessel pathways are created. Angiogenesis, while a similar process, does not depend on the same set of genes as vasculogenesis, and this process is activated instead in the presence of an injury to a blood vessel. In the last three decades, considerable research has been reported that supports the hypothesis that tumor growth and metastasis require angiogenesis. Angiogenesis, the proliferation and migration of endothelial cells resulting in the formation of new blood vessels, is an important process for the progression of tumors (Figure 2). ARTs have been shown in a number of published papers to have antiangiogenic effects.

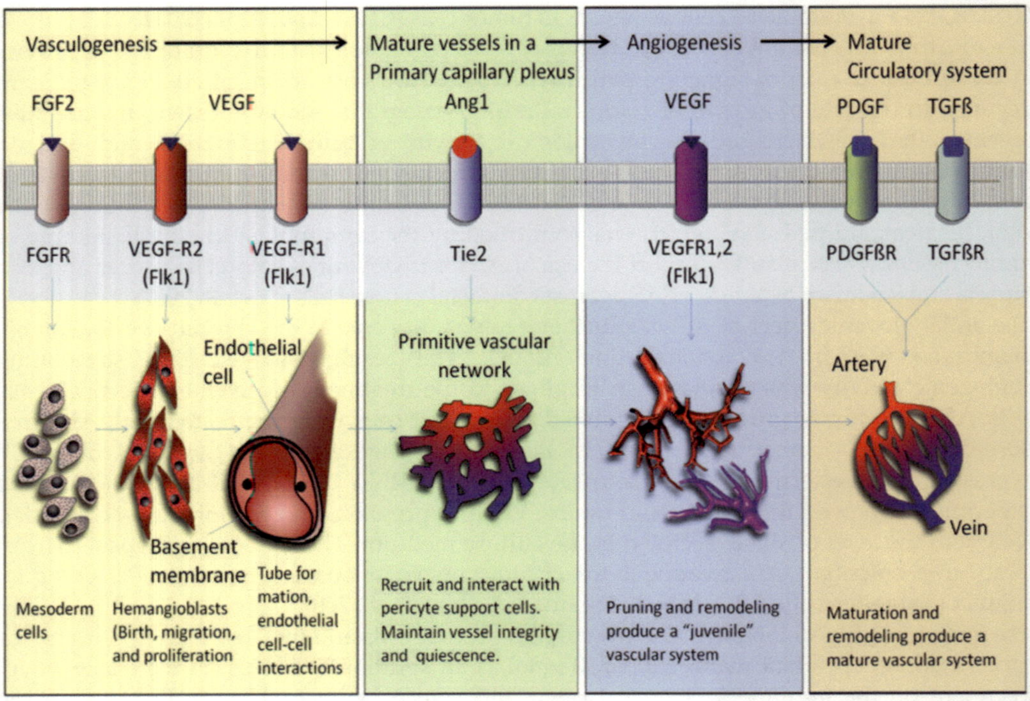

Fig. 2. The modes of vasculogenesis and angiogenesis. Vasculogenesis occurs during the very early developmental stages of an organism when the blood vessel pathways are created. Angiogenesis, while a similar process, does not depend on the same set of genes as vasculogenesis, and this process is activated instead in the presence of an injury to a blood vessel. Angiogenesis finishes the circulatory connections begun by vasculogenesis and builds arteries and veins from the capillaries. In this diagram, the major paracrine factors involved in each step are shown boxed, and their receptors (on the vessel-forming cells) are shown beneath them. (Modified from Hanahan, 1997)

3.2.1 Inhibition of vasculogenesis and angiogenesis leads to embryotoxicity

Given the potent effects of ART and its derivatives on inhibition of angiogenesis, it is perhaps not surprising that these compounds have been reported to be embryotoxic in rodents. In several reports, DHA was shown to cause significant embryotoxicity accompanied by developmental defects in the neural tube, branchial arches, somites and caudal region in rat embryos *in vitro*. This finding has great significance for potential *in vivo* effects as DHA has been shown to cross embryonic membranes, and the embryonic yolk sac has also been shown to be highly susceptible to ART compounds (Longo et al., 2006a; 2006b; White et al., 2008).

Previous data has shown the rapid onset of action of AS and DHA on primitive RBCs as soon as they enter embryonic circulation. There is no clear explanation as to why primitive RBCs are susceptible to DHA (Longo et al., 2006a, 2006b). Like intraerythrocytic malaria parasites, primitive RBCs have high concentrations of iron and heme, which have been proposed as either activators or targets of ART compounds (Olliaro et al., 2001; Parapini et al., 2004). The depletion of embryonic erythroid cells by ART compounds likely occurs as a consequence of the inhibition of vasculogenesis. This is a plausible hypothesis because the processes of vasculogenesis and hematopoiesis are actually strongly related. Formation of a blood vessel is accompanied by the simultaneous in situ production of blood cells within that vessel (Baron 2001; Baumann & Dragon, 2005; Sequeira Lopez et al., 2003). One additional study that supports this hypothesis involved the effects of AS on embryo development. In this study, oral and injectable AS were shown to induce marked embryo lethality accompanied by a low incidence of teratogenic effects, including cardiovascular defects (ventricular septal and great vessels defects), which significantly affected novel vessel formation (Clark et al., 2004, White et al., 2008; Ratajska et al., 2006a, 2006b).

3.2.2 Anti-VEGF of ARTs plays a key role during normal and pathological angiogenesis

Angiogenesis is promoted by numerous factors including cytokines such as VEGF, bFGF, PDGF and others. It is negatively regulated by angiostatin, endostatin, thrombospondin, TIMPs and other factors. The factors that are produced in tumor cells as well as in surrounding stromal cells act in a balance to promote either proangiogenic or antiangiogenic processes. Among the cytokines for regulating angiogenesis, VEGF and angiopoietin-1 (Ang-1) have specific modulating effects on the growth of vascular endothelial cells, and they play a key role in the process of angiogenesis (Thurston, 2002).

VEGF is a homodimeric 34-42 kDa, heparin-binding glycoprotein with potent angiogenic, mitogenic and vascular permeability-enhancing activities specific for endothelial cells. Two receptor tyrosine kinases have been described as putative VEGF receptors, Flt-1 and KDR. Flt-1 (fms-like tyrosine kinase), and KDR (kinase-insert-domain-containing receptor) proteins have been shown to bind VEGF with high affinity.

In vitro, VEGF is a potent endothelial cell mitogen. In cultured endothelial cells, VEGF has been shown to activate phospholipase C and induce rapid increases of free cytosolic Ca^{2+}. VEGF has also been shown to stimulate the release of von Willebrand factor from endothelial cells and induce expression of tissue factor activity in endothelial cells as well as in monocytes. VEGF has also been shown to be involved in the chemotaxis of monocytes and osteoblasts. *In vivo*, VEGF can induce angiogenesis as well as increase microvascular permeability. As a vascular permeability factor, VEGF acts directly on the endothelium and does not degranulate mast cells. It promotes extravasation of plasma fibrinogen, leading to fibrin deposition which alters the tumor extracellular matrix. The modified extracellular matrix subsequently promotes the migration of macrophages, fibroblasts and endothelial cells. Based on its *in vitro* and *in vivo* properties, VEGF is believed to play important roles in inflammation and also in normal and pathological aspects of angiogenesis, a process that is associated with wound healing, embryonic development, growth, and metastasis of solid tumors. Elevated levels of VEGF have been reported in synovial fluids of rheumatoid arthritis patients and in sera from cancer patients.

Over the last three decades, a growing body of evidence has developed on the role of angiogenesis in tumor growth and metastases of tumors (Firestone & Sundar, 2009).

Angiogenesis can be divided into a series of temporally regulated responses, including induction of proteases, migration of endothelial cells, cell proliferation and differentiation. This is a highly complex process, in which a number of cytokines and growth factors released by endothelial cells, tumor cells and matrix cells are involved. The expression of VEGF has been suggested to be related to some fundamental features of solid tumors, such as the growth rate, the density of tumor microvessels, and the development of tumor metastases

3.2.3 Antiangiogenic mechanisms of ARTs

Pathological angiogenesis, the formation of new blood vessels from pre-existing ones in tumors, is essential for supplying tumors with oxygen and nutrients and critical for the spread of metastatic cells throughout the body. Inhibitors of angiogenesis that block angiogenic signals have been developed, and antiangiogenic therapy strategies have been shown to be valuable adjuncts to cytostatic and cytotoxic chemotherapy (Efferth 2005).

3.2.3.1 Effect of ARTs on angiogenesis-related genes

Establishment of a network of vasculature in a tumor is a critical event for tumor growth and survival. This process is accomplished by a complex sequence of temporal events involving vasculogenic secretions from tumor cells, restructuring of the extracellular matrix using matrix metalloproteinases and formation of new vasculature. Because angiogenesis involves tissue restructuring, genes that regulate angiogenesis, such as chemokine receptors, can also affect tumor metastasis (Wu et al., 2009). In a study conducted with an NCI panel of 60 tumor cell lines, treatment of these cells with ART and related compounds resulted in altered expression of genes implicated in angiogenesis suggesting antiangiogenic activity (Anfosso et al., 2006).

In this study, microarray analysis of mRNA expression of 30 out of 89 angiogenesis-related genes correlated significantly with the cellular response to several ARTs. Among this panel of genes were many fundamental angiogenic regulators such as vascular endothelial growth factor C (*VEGFC*), fibroblast growth factor-2 (*FGF2*), matrix metalloproteinase 9 (*MMP9*), thrombospondin-1 (*THBS1*), hypoxia-inducing factor-α (*HIF1a*), angiogenin (*ANG*) and others. By means of hierarchical cluster analysis, expression profiles were identified that demonstrated significant cellular responses to AS, arteether, artemether, and dihydroartemisinylester stereoisomer 1. A borderline significance was observed after treatment with dihydroartemisinylester stereoisomer 2 and ART (Efferth 2005). The sensitivity and resistance of these tumor cells correlated with the mRNA expression of angiogenesis-related genes. This suggests that that the anti-tumor effects of ARTs are likely due to their role in inhibiting tumor angiogenesis (Anfosso et al., 2006).

3.2.3.2 ART treatment leads to decreases in expression levels of HIF-1a

Tumor hypoxia activates the transcription factor hypoxia inducible factor-1α (HIF-1α). This adaptation increases tumor angiogenesis to support the survival of poorly nourished cancer cells. Hypoxic tumors are resistant to radiation and many anti-cancer agents. HIF-1α is activated during angiostatic therapy, and HIF-1α has also been shown to up-regulate the expression of transferrin receptors. Since ART is selectively toxic to iron-loaded cells, radio and drug-resistant tumors might be selectively susceptible to attack by a treatment strategy consisting of iron-loading and ART treatment (Efferth 2005).

These findings are consistent with previous findings (Wartenberg et al., 2003) that noted ART-dependent decreases in expression levels of HIF-1a. HIF-1a is known to be a transcriptional activator of VEGF, and it plays a crucial role in neo-vasculogenesis in hypoxic tissues. ART treatment of leukemic and glioma cells *in vitro* at a concentration of 12 mM was shown in another study to inhibit angiogenesis. This ART driven angiogenesis inhibition was shown to involve suppression of VEGF and HIF-1a expression at the transcriptional level. (Huang et al., 2008; Zhou et al., 2007). Loss of HIF-1a and VEGF expression after ART treatment appears to be dependent on production of ROS because co-treatment with free-radical scavengers such as vitamin E and mannitol reversed the effects of ART (Wartenberg et al., 2003).

3.2.3.3 Anti-VEGF activities of ARTs

1. ART decreases expression of VEGF and alters VEGF receptor binding

ART and DHA have been shown to significantly inhibit angiogenesis in a dose-dependent manner as demonstrated by measurement of the proliferation, migration and tube formation of human umbilical vein endothelial (HUVE) cells (Chen et al., 2003). DHA was shown to markedly reduce VEGF binding to its receptors on the surface of HUVE cells and reduced the expression levels of two major VEGF receptors, Flt-1 and KDR/flk-1, on HUVE cells. Chicken chorioallantoic membrane (CAM) neovascularization was significantly inhibited by DHA (Chen et al., 2004a). The inhibitory effect of ART on HUVE cell proliferation was stronger than the effect of ART on HO-8910 cancer cells, NIH-3T3 fibroblast cells or human endometrial cells (Chen et al., 2004b). ART derivatives also inhibited HUVE cell tube formation and exhibited antiangiogenic effects (Oh et al., 2004).

In addition to affecting expression of the VEGFs, ART and its derivatives have been shown to target the VEGF receptors. In an ovarian cancer xenograft model, treatment with 50 mM AS resulted in the inhibition of microvessel formation, and immunohistochemical staining revealed that AS treated xenografts displayed significantly reduced levels of CD31 (a neovasculogenesis marker) and the VEGF receptor KDR. AS also inhibited VEGF-induced migration and differentiation of cultured human umbilical vascular endothelial cells (Chen et al., 2009).

2. Torilin, a related sesquiterpene, inhibits blood vessel formation

It is interesting to note that torilin, another sesquiterpene (derived from the fruits of *Torilis japonica)*, has also been shown to be a potent antiangiogenic factor which also inhibits blood vessel formation by disrupting VEGFA expression. A similar finding was also shown by using DHA (Kim et al., 2000; 2006). Hence, the ability of ART to inhibit angiogenesis may be due to its chemical nature as a sesquiterpene. Another compelling finding is that other phytosesquiterpene lactones, such as costunolide from *Saussurea lappa*, can inhibit KDR signaling (Jeong et al., 2002). Comparisons with other sesquiterpenes may shed more light on the unique features of the anticancer actions of ART, and potentially lead to better angiostatic drug design

3. ARTs down-regulate expressions of HIF-1a and VEGF

Wartenberg et al. (2003) investigated the anti-angiogenic effects of ART on mouse embryonic stem cell-derived embryoid bodies, which are a model system for early post implantation embryos which differentiate well into capillaries. ART dose-dependently inhibited angiogenesis in embryoid bodies and raised the level of intracellular reactive oxygen species. Furthermore, ART treatment was shown over the time course of embryoid body differentiation to impair organization of the extracellular matrix laminin component and altered expression patterns of matrix metalloproteinases 1, 2, and 9. Analysis of mRNA expression in embryoid bodies showed that ART treatment resulted in the down-regulation-of HIF-1α and VEGF, both of which control endothelial cell growth.

4. ART inhibits chicken chorioallantoic membrane (CAM) angiogenesis

By utilizing the chicken CAM culture technique, it is possible to detect the microangium-like structures formed by *in vitro* cultivated arterial rings. Through this method, AS has been shown to also have antiangiogenic effects. AS treatment significantly inhibited chicken CAM angiogenesis, proliferation and differentiation of human microvascular dermal endothelial cells in a dose-dependent manner and reduced Flt-1 and KDR/flk-1 expression (Huan-Huan et al., 2004). AS was shown to strongly reduce angiogenesis *in vivo* as shown by changes in vascularization of Matrigel plugs injected subcutaneously into syngenic mice (Dell'Eva et al., 2004). AS has also been shown to retard the growth of human ovarian cancer HO-8910 xenografts in nude mice. In this study, microvessel density was reduced following AS treatment with no apparent animal toxicity. In addition, AS treatment also markedly lowered VEGF expression in tumor cells and KDR/flk-1 expression in endothelial cells as well as tumor cells (Chen et al., 2004a).

Through a human umbilical vein endothelial cell (HUVEC) injury migration experiment, AS has been shown to inhibit the multiplication, migration and cannulation of endothelial cells, and AS was shown to effectively suppress the genesis and growth of tumor vessels. The tumor angiogenesis and growth inhibitory effect of ART was also shown by Chen, et al. (2004a), and results of their study showed that ART could inhibit the production of VEGF and its receptor, KDR/flk-1, in tumor cells, and AS was also shown to induce cellular apoptosis in oophoroma, a rare ovarian tumor. In experimental studies using CAM and aortic ring non-serum cultures, the secretion of VEGF was monitored using ELISA testing. AS treatment of CAM cultures at a concentration as low as 2 mmol/L was shown to reduce the level of VEGF, effectively inhibiting angiogenesis in co-cultured chronic myelocytic leukemia K562 cells (Lee et al., 2006; Zhou et al., 2007). In summary, these experimental studies have provided a wealth of evidence to support the hypothesis that ART treatment can effectively inhibit leukemia cell proliferation and inhibit angiogenesis of solid tumor cells. The mechanisms of this anticancer activity include direct inhibition of tumor cell multiplication, induction of apoptosis, the inhibition of angiogenesis through suppression of VEGF secretion, and inhibition of VEGF receptor expression.

3.3 Anticancer case reports and clinical trials of ARTs in humans

Clinical evidence has accumulated showing that artemisinin-derived drugs have promise for treatment of laryngeal carcinomas, uveal melanomas and pituitary macroadenomas. ART compounds are also in phase I-II trials against breast, colorectal and non-small cell lung cancers (Table 3).

Artemisinins	Cancer targets	Clinical studies	Protocols & References
Artemisinin	Colorectal cancer	Clinical trial, Phase I	ISRCTN05203252, 2011 UK
Artesunate	Non-small cell lung cancer	Clinical trial Phase I-II	Zhang et al., 2008 CHINA
	Metastatic uveal melanoma	Case report	Berger et al., 2005 GERMANY
	Laryngeal carcinoma	Case report	Singh & Verma, 2002 INDIA
	Metastatic breast cancer	Clinical Trial, Phase I-II	NCT00764036 2008 GERMANY
Artemether	Pituitary macroadenoma	Case report	Singh& Panwar 2006 INDIA

All clinical trials listed here are completed.

Table 3. Anticancer effects of artemisinin (ART), artesunate (AS), and artemether (AM) in case reports of treatments and clinical trials (Ghantous et al., 2010)

3.3.1 Case reports

1. Metastatic uveal melanomas treated with AS

Berger et al. reported on the first long-term treatment of two cancer patients with AS in combination with standard chemotherapy. These patients with metastatic uveal melanoma were treated on a compassionate-use basis, after standard chemotherapy alone was ineffective in stopping tumor growth. The therapy regimen was well tolerated with no additional side effects other than those caused by standard chemotherapy alone. One patient experienced a temporary response after the addition of AS to Fotemustine while the disease was progressing under therapy with Fotemustine alone. The second patient first experienced a stabilization of the disease after the addition of AS to Dacarbazine, followed by objective regressions of splenic and lung metastases. This patient is still alive 47 months after first diagnosis with stage IV uveal melanoma, a diagnosis with a median survival of 2-5 months.

Despite the small number of treated patients, AS may be a promising adjuvant drug for the treatment of melanoma and possibly other tumors in combination with standard chemotherapy. AS is well tolerated, and the lack of serious side effects will facilitate prospective randomized trials in the near future. From *in vitro* studies already conducted (Efferth et al., 2004), it is further conceivable that loading tumor cells with bivalent iron, by simply providing Fe^{2+} in tablet form, might increase the susceptibility of cancer cells to AS treatment. It is tempting to speculate that, in the case of the second patient previously discussed, the addition of Fe^{2+} had an actual clinical impact and resulted in an improved response to therapy (Berger et al., 2005).

2. Laryngeal carcinoma treated with AS

AS injections and tablets were used in one study to treat a laryngeal squamous cell carcinoma patient over a period of nine months. The tumor was significantly reduced in size by 70% after two months of treatment. Overall, the AS treatment of the patient was beneficial in prolonging and improving quality of life. Without treatment, laryngeal cancer patients die within an average of 12 months. The patient lived for nearly one year and eight months until his death due to pneumonia.

The observations that the patient regained his voice, appetite, and weight after a short term treatment with AS, and the fact that the tumor was significantly reduced in size without any apparent adverse side effects suggests that AS treatment could be an effective and economical alternative treatment for cancer, especially in cases of late cancer detection where available treatments are limited. Since this case report was published, several patients with different types of cancers have begun treatment with artemisinin and its analogs with promising results. AS therapy has potential to prevent and treat a wide range of cancers given its efficacy, low cost, and due to the common mechanisms of action demonstrated against various cancer cells (Singh & Verma, 2002).

3. Pituitary macroadenoma treated with artemether

Artemether, an ART analogue, was used to treat a 75-year old male patient with pituitary macroadenoma. This patient presented with vision, hearing, and locomotion-related problems as a consequence of his disease. Artemether was administered orally to the patient over a period of 12 months. Although the tumor remained consistent in size, CT scans showed a reduction in tumor density, and clinically, the related symptoms and signs improved significantly as therapy progressed. Overall, the artemether treatment was beneficial in improving the patient's quality of life. Artemether and other artemisinin analogs appear to have promise for treatment of this type of cancer (Singh and Panwar, 2006).

3.3.2 Clinical trials of ARTs as anticancer agents

1. Phase I study of oral AS to treat colorectal cancer (Completed)

The primary objective of this study was to determine the effects of oral AS in inducing apoptosis in patients awaiting surgical treatment of colorectal adenocarcinoma. The secondary objective of this study was to establish the tolerability of oral AS for the treatment of colorectal cancer. Subjects were randomized to receive either 200 mg AS or placebo orally once daily for 14 days while awaiting surgery for definitive surgical treatment of colorectal adenocarcinoma. A significant difference in the proportion of colorectal adenocarcinoma cells exhibiting apoptosis was noted between the two treatment groups (placebo and AS), assessed at the time of surgery after two weeks of drug treatment. No result was publicly issued (Protocol Number: ISRCTN05203252).

2. Phase II study of AS treatment as an adjunct to treat non-small cell lung cancer (Completed)

This study was designed to compare the efficacy and toxicity of AS treatment combined with NP (a chemotherapy regimen of vinorelbine and cisplatin) and NP alone in the treatment of advanced non-small cell lung cancer (NSCLC). One hundred and twenty cases of advanced NSCLC were randomly divided into an NP chemotherapy group and a combined AS with NP therapy group. Patients in the control group were treated with the NP regimen of vinorelbine and cisplatin. Patients in the trial group were treated with the NP regimen supplemented with intravenous AS injections (120 mg, once-a-day intravenous injection, from the 1st day to 8th day, for 8 days). At least two 21-day-cycles of treatment were performed. There were no significant differences in the short-term survival rates, mean survival times and the 1-year survival rates between the trial group and the control group, which were 44 weeks and 45 weeks, respectively. The disease controlled rate of the trial group (88.2%) was significantly higher than that of the control group (72.7%) ($P < 0.05$), and the trial group's time to disease progression (24 weeks) was significantly longer than that of the control group (20 weeks). No significant difference was found in toxicity between the two treatment groups. Therefore. AS combined with NP can increase the disease controlled rate and prolong the time to progression of patients with advanced NSCLC without significant side effects (Zhang et al., 2008).

3. Phase I study with metastatic breast cancer (Completed)

The purpose of this study was to evaluate the tolerability of an adjunctive therapy with AS for a period of 4 weeks in patients over the age of 18 years with advanced metastatic breast cancer, which was defined as a histologically or cytologically confirmed. Women of childbearing potential were tested to rule out pregnancy prior to their treatment. Relevant neurological symptoms, adverse events, and the relation between adverse events and the use of AS, as an adjunct, saliva cortisol profile, overall response rate, clinical benefit, and assessment of patients' expectations will be monitored as study endpoints. No result of this study has yet been publicly issued (Protocol Number: NCT00764036).

4. Therapeutic implications of ARTs due to alternative vascularization mechanisms

Until recently, normal and abnormal processes of vascularization (vasculogenesis and angiogenesis) were considered to be based on a limited number of known mechanisms. Recent advances have been made in identifying a number of novel alternate processes involved in vasculogenesis and angiogenesis. If these new findings of alternate mechanisms are confirmed, cancer therapy strategies may also be affected

4.1 The role of the visceral yolk sac endoderm in primitive erythropoiesis

The role of the visceral yolk sac endoderm in the control of primitive erythropoiesis and vasculogenesis remains a subject of debate. During mouse embryogenesis, the first hematopoietic and endothelial cells form in blood islands located between layers of visceral endoderm and mesoderm in the yolk sac. One study assessed the consequences of the absence of a visceral endoderm layer on blood cell and vessel formation using embryoid bodies derived from mouse embryonic stem (ES) cells deficient in GATA-4, a transcription factor expressed in the yolk sac endoderm.

When differentiated *in vitro*, these mutant embryoid bodies did not develop an external visceral endoderm layer. GATA-4 deficient embryoid bodies (GATA 4-1 ES cells), grown either in suspension culture or attached to a substratum, were shown to be defective in primitive hematopoiesis and vasculogenesis as evidenced by a lack of recognizable blood islands, vascular channels, and a reduction in the expression of primitive erythrocyte markers. Expression of the endothelial cell transcripts for Flk-1, Fit-1, and platelet-endothelial cell adhesion molecule (PECAM) was not affected in the mutant embryoid bodies. Gata4-1-ES cells retained the capacity to differentiate into primitive erythroblasts and endothelial cells when cultured in methylcellulose or Matrigel. Analysis of chimeric mice, generated by injecting Gata4-l-ES cells into 8-cell stage embryos of ROSA26 transgenic animals, showed that Gata4-l-ES cells can form blood islands and vessels when juxtaposed to visceral endoderm *in vivo*. The authors of this study concluded that the visceral endoderm is not essential for the differentiation of primitive erythrocytes or endothelial cells, but this cell layer plays an important role in the formation and organization of yolk sac blood islands and vessels (Bielinska et al., 1996).

4.2 Origin of the first definitive erythropoiesis

Although primitive and definitive blood cells arise at separate locations in advanced stage embryos, some experimental evidence suggests that cell migration may occur between the blood-forming compartments. Thus, the origin of stem cells for multi-lineage hematopoiesis has been a controversial issue in the field. Studies from amniotes have linked the first stem cell activity to the aorta-gonad-mesonephros (AGM) region, whereas others suggest that the yolk sac is the true source of hematopoietic stem cells.

The oldest hypothesis is based on the thought that all hematopoietic stem cells originate from the yolk sac. The most relevant supporting evidence for this hypothesis is based on the observation that host chick bodies grafted on to a donor yolk sac contain cells from the yolk sac in their hematopoietic organs. Additional work conducted more recently has focused on the use of molecular tools to characterize the underlying events that initiate erythropoiesis in vertebrate embryos. Several key genes have been identified that are necessary for primitive and subsequent definitive erythropoiesis, which differs in several aspects from primitive erythropoiesis (Baumann and Dragon, 2005). This data is informative, but it is also clear that more physiological data are needed to understand in detail the function of embryonic hemoglobin and primitive RBCs. These reports offer an interesting perspective for future study to answer two questions: 1) what are the molecular determinants for the initiation of erythropoiesis? and 2) what are the physiological functions of early erythroid cells?

4.3 Erythropoiesis in the embryonic heart

Another possible explanation of early erythropoiesis is in situ differentiation from progenitor cells that migrate to the embryonic heart at the onset of vascularization. The embryonic heart has been postulated to be a hematopoietic organ in previous reports supporting the hypothesis that hematopoiesis within the embryo is strictly limited to the areas of vasculogenesis. However, a separate study on this issue showed the absence of hematopoietic stem cells in the embryonic heart by both transmission electron microscopy (TEM) and also through immunohistochemical staining with antibodies to hematopoietic stem cell (HSC) antigens. Investigators performing this study also could not find any evidence for the presence of blood islands exhibiting a pattern of cellular assembly similar to a yolk sac blood island. This study suggests that the embryonic heart supplies only new erythroblasts owing to their proliferative capacity within the primitive vascular vesicles at the time before coronary vessels are connected to the aorta (Ratajska et al., 2006b). It is doubtful that the embryonic heart possesses a hematopoietic activity since this activity is always associated with production of a wealth of descendent cells. Since formation of blood island-like structures occurs throughout prenatal life (Rongish et al., 1994), it is possible that red blood cells (nucleated or enucleated) enter the embryonic heart also at later stages of development (Ratajska et al., 2006b).

4.4 Glioblastoma vascularization formed by vasculogenic mimicry

EL Hallani et al. (2010) described a new mechanism of alternative glioblastoma vascularization and opened a new perspective for an antivascular treatment strategy. Glioblastomas are the most frequent and malignant primary brain tumors in adults and have a poor prognosis despite surgery and conventional radio-chemotherapy. Histologically, glioblastomas are highly angiogenic and are characterized by microvascular proliferations (Louis et al., 2007). Antivascular endothelial growth factor therapy has demonstrated significant efficacy in treatment of glioblastomas with nearly 50% of treated patients responding to therapy, but it is still possible for these tumors to acquire antiangiogenic resistance (Kreisl et al., 2009). It is known that alternative vascularization mechanisms may occur in brain tumors, such as co-opting of existing vessels, angioblast vasculogenesis, intussusceptive microvascular growth and vasculogenic mimicry. The term vasculogenic mimicry describes the formation of fluid-conducting channels by highly invasive and genetically dysregulated tumor cells. Two distinctive types of vasculogenic mimicry have been reported in tumors, vascular mimicry of the patterned matrix type and vascular mimicry of the tubular type.

Vasculogenic mimicry of the patterned matrix type results in the ability of tumor cells to express endothelium-associated genes that are also involved in embryonic vasculogenesis. Such plastic properties could be associated with cancer stem cells, a subpopulation of undifferentiated tumor cells that present with a marked capacity for proliferation, self-renewal, multiple lineage differentiation and tumor initiation. This finding provides a better understanding of the process of tumor vascularization involving cancer stem-cell plasticity, and it has important implications in determining a proper treatment strategy. The evaluation of the overall contribution of such tumor cell-formed vessels to glioblastoma blood flow should be based on the sensitivity of gliomas to current antiangiogenic therapies using quantitative methods with appropriate sampling. Also, understanding the influence of the microenvironment in determining the vascular fate of glioblastoma cells may provide new perspectives on tumor cell plasticity that could be exploited for novel strategies in cancer differentiation therapy (El Hallani et al., 2010).

4.5 Vascularization mechanism in cancer pathology

Before discussing the different ways a tumor is vascularized, we should emphasize that these mechanisms are not mutually exclusive; in fact, in most cases they are interlinked, being involved concurrently in physiological as well as in pathological angiogenesis. Although the molecular regulation of endothelial sprouting has been extensively studied

and reviewed in the literature, the morphogenic and molecular events associated with alternative cancer vascularization mechanisms are less understood. Cancer cells are not generally controlled by normal regulatory mechanisms, but tumor growth is highly dependent on the supply of oxygen, nutrients, and host-derived regulators. It is now established that tumor vasculature is not necessarily derived from endothelial cell sprouting. Cancer tissue can acquire vasculature by a variety of mechanisms to include co-opting pre-existing vessels, intussusceptive microvascular growth, postnatal vasculogenesis, glomeruloid angiogenesis, or vasculogenic mimicry. The best-known molecular pathway driving tumor vascularization is the hypoxia-adaptation mechanism. Other pathways involving a broad and diverse spectrum of genetic aberrations, however, are associated with the development of the "angiogenic phenotype." Based on this knowledge, novel forms of antivascular modalities have been developed in the past decade.
When applying these targeted therapies, the stage of tumor progression, the type of vascularization of the given cancer tissue, and the molecular machinery behind the vascularization process all need to be considered. A further challenge is finding the most appropriate combinations of antivascular therapies and standard radio- and chemotherapies. The most promising therapeutic plan of action will involve the integration of our recent knowledge in this field into a rational strategy to for developing effective clinical modalities using antivascular therapy for cancer (Döme et al., 2007).

4.6 Genetic effects of ARTs contribute to sensitivity of cancer cells to chemotherapy

Endothelial cells involved in vasculogenesis and angiogenesis are key targets in cancer therapy. Recent evidence suggests that tumor cells can express some genes typically expressed by endothelial cells and form extracellular matrix–rich tubular networks, a phenomenon known as vasculogenic mimicry. Schaft et al. (2004) examined the effects of three angiogenesis inhibitors on vasculogenic mimicry in human melanoma MUM-2B and C8161 cells and compared them with their effects in human endothelial HMEC-1 and HUVEC cells. Their data reveals biologically significant differences in the responses of endothelial cells and aggressive melanoma cells that are engaged in vasculogenic mimicry to select angiogenesis inhibitors. Because vasculogenic mimicry has been reported in several other tumor models, including breast, prostatic, ovarian, and lung carcinoma (Hendrix et al. 2003), these findings may contribute to the development of new antivascular therapeutic agents that target both angiogenesis and tumor cell vasculogenic mimicry.
Similar analyses have identified angiogenesis-related genes that are differentially expressed in AS-sensitive and resistant cell lines (Anfosso et al., 2006). The sensitivity of cells to AS therapy was shown to correlate with cell viability, growth and an angiogenic phenotype. Resistance to AS treatment to inhibit growth would also thus extend to an antiangiogenic response of an AS-resistant tumor cell in its microenvironment. It is therefore probable that these genes associated with AS resistance also determine the antiangiogenic response of the cell lines when treated with AS. Anfosso et al. (2006) have shown that a panel of genes that correlate with the cellular response to AS contains many fundamental angiogenic regulators, such as the vascular endothelial growth factors, which stimulate proliferation and migration of endothelial cells, a fundamental step in vessel formation. Three human genes encode for vascular endothelial growth factors (VEGFA, VEGFB, and VEGFC). The investigators decided to include in the cluster analysis only those genes whose mRNA expression correlated with GI_{50} values (the concentration needed to inhibit the growth of treated cells to half that of untreated cells) of at least four ARTs. After this truncation of the gene panel, only VEGF-C remained as an angiogenic regulator among the 30 genes in the cluster analysis panel.

Through knockout studies in mice, a number of genes participating in yolk sac hematopoiesis and vasculogenesis have been identified. Some of these gene disruptions affect only hematopoiesis, while other gene disruptions were shown to disturb vascular development, and still others were shown to affect both processes. Additional factors influencing yolk sac vasculogenesis and hematopoiesis are likely to emerge in the coming years. Gata4-1 embryoid bodies will provide a useful visceral endoderm free system in which to study the effects of growth or differentiation factors normally produced by the visceral endoderm, including substances that affect primitive hematopoiesis and vasculogenesis (Bielinska et al., 1996).
The antiangiogenic activities of both ART and AS have been investigated by a number of researchers. ART has been shown to downregulate vascular endothelial growth factor (VEGF) expression, an effect that was reversed upon co-treatment with the free radical scavengers mannitol and vitamin E. This indicates that ART may act in an antiangiogenic manner via generation of reactive oxygen species. AS and DHA have been shown to reduce the expression of the two major VEGF receptors, Flt-1 and KDR/flk-1, as determined by immune histochemistry in the chicken chorioallantoic membrane neovascularization model, in HUVE cells , and in nude mice injected with the human ovarian cancer line HO-8910, respectively. The results of these authors and others suggest that the antiangiogenic effect induced by ARTs might occur by induction of cellular apoptosis and inhibition of expression of VEGF receptors (Chen et al., 2004a; Oh et al., 2004; Wartenberg et al., 2003).

5. Further development of ARTs as antiangiogenic cancer agents

Cancer angiogenesis has been confirmed by measurement of high proliferation indices for endothelial cells, not only in rapidly growing animal tumors, but also in human tumors. The rationale for developing antiangiogenic strategies for cancer therapy was based on the fact that physiological angiogenesis only occurs in a limited number of situations, such as wound healing and the menstrual cycle. This suggests there is an opportunity for developing highly tumor-specific antiangiogenic applications which utilize drugs such as the ARTs which have demonstrated antiangiogenic efficacy with little toxicity.

5.1 Prevention and therapy strategies of ARTs as anticancer agents

The tumor vasculature is an attractive target for cancer therapy because of its accessibility to blood-borne anticancer agents and the reliance of most tumor cells on an intact vascular supply for their survival. Therapeutic targeting of the tumor vasculature can be divided into two approaches, an antiangiogenic approach and an antivascular approach. Antiangiogenic approaches are focused on disrupting the processes involved in the outgrowth of new blood vessels from pre-existing ones, while antivascular approaches are targeted to affect the established tumor vasculature. Individual agents may possess both antiangiogenic and antivascular properties. However, a practical distinction between the two approaches can be made based on the dosing strategies employed. In order to prevent angiogenesis, a chronic dosing schedule is appropriate, whereas single dose or split dose treatments are more effective for antivascular activity, which is targeted to rapidly shut-down blood flow in established tumor blood vessels.
Today the angiosuppressive strategy is the most developed, containing a variety of agents. The first class of angiosuppressive agents developed targets the primary angiogenic cytokine in cancer, VEGF, by monoclonal antibodies, which act to trap VEGF (so called VGF trap agents) or antisense antibodies directed at VEGF (VEGF-antisense agents). The second approach is to

target VEGF receptors through the use of monoclonal antibodies. Interestingly, anti-receptor antibody therapy is in the early phase of development, and most of the available agents are small molecular VEGF receptor signal transduction inhibitors. Since VEGF is not the only pro-angiogenic cytokine produced by cancers, it will likely be necessary to develop other anti-angiogenic agents , but these targets and the appropriate agent to block either a novel cytokine or its receptor are unknown today (Tímár & Döme, 2008).

In contrast to the antiangiogenesis approach, antivascular strategies aim to cause a rapid and extensive shut-down of the established tumor vasculature, leading to secondary tumor cell death. Cell death following blood flow shut-down, induced by clamping or ligation of the tumor-supplying blood vessels, is characterized by an early and extensive tumor cell necrosis (Tozer, 2003). Therefore, this pattern of cell death following treatment is indicative of vascular-mediated cytotoxicity. There is potential for specific targeting of the tumor vasculature based on selective expression of proteins on tumor endothelial cells. Recent development of techniques for the isolation of tumor-derived endothelial cells and gene expression has led to the identification of a number of gene transcripts which are specifically elevated in tumor-associated endothelium. Antivascular approaches under investigation include integrin-binding peptides conjugated to anticancer drugs, antibodies targeted to endothelial-specific proteins, and gene therapy approaches (Tozer, 2003).

5.2 Combination strategies to enhance efficacy of ARTs as anticancer agents

There is growing evidence supporting the use of ART and its derivatives in cancer therapy. ARTs are a class of compounds that are first-line treatment options for malaria. They also have potent antiproliferative, antimetastatic and antiangiogenic activity, which makes them potential anticancer drugs (Liu et al., 2011). Scientists investigating the cancer-fighting properties of AS have found early evidence that combining it with an existing cancer drug has the potential to make each drug more effective than when used alone. There is currently limited published data exploring the value of ART as a combination partner in treatment regimens. These studies have used simple approaches to studying drug–drug interactions, and as a consequence, their conclusions are still open to debate. The idea of combining drugs in therapeutic regimens is to achieve an overall effect that is greater than the sum of the individual effects of each agent (Liu, 2008).

Drug combinations that involve ART have been reported *in vitro*, which show value in this approach, both as a sensitizing agent to chemotherapy in solid tumors (Hou et al., 2008; Sieber et al., 2009), and as a synergistic partner with doxorubicin in leukemia (Efferth et al., 2007). Incubation of cancer cells with DHA alone was found to be less effective than in combination with holotransferrin, indicating that intracellular iron plays a role in the cytotoxic effects of DHA (Lai & Singh, 1995). In addition to conventional chemotherapies, ART was also combined with the immune modulatory drug LEN (Galustian & Dalgleish, 2009). These in vitro studies demonstrated the effects of ART on the cell cycle, and the studies showed restoration of cytotoxicity in an ART-resistant cell by adopting a pulsed-schedule of combination treatment. The mechanism underlying the combinatorial interaction, and indeed the mechanism of ART action in cancer per se is still not fully elucidated; however, those studies are ongoing and currently form the basis of further studies (Liu et al., 2011).

Many antiangiogenic and antivascular agents are now in clinical trials for the treatment of cancer. It is conceivable that loading tumor cells with bivalent iron by simply providing Fe^{2+} in tablet form might increase the susceptibility of cancer cells to the action of AS. It is tempting to speculate that, in the case of the second patient in the Berger study the addition of Fe^{2+} had an actual clinical impact and resulted in an improved response to therapy (Berger et al., 2005). Continued research in this area is encouraged by the recent success of a Phase II clinical trial of

AS combined with NP chemotherapy in treatment of advanced non-small cell lung cancer. The disease controlled rate of the trial group of AS plus NP chemotherapy (88.2%) was significantly higher than that of the NP chemotherapy alone group (72.7%), and the trial group's time to progression (24 weeks) was significantly longer than that of the NP chemotherapy alone group (20 weeks). AS combined with NP chemotherapy can increase the short-term survival rate of patients with advanced non-small cell lung cancer and prolong the time to progression without extra side effects (Zhang et al., 2008). The diversity in the targets of ART supports the possibility that it could be used in combination with other agents.

5.3 Toxicity avoidance strategies when employing ARTs

At high concentrations, ARTs appear to be active against cancer *in vivo*. However, the use of ARTs at high concentrations or for long drug exposure times has substantial risk of severe toxicities, both embryotoxicity and neurotoxicity. Animal data have shown that high concentrations of AS and DHA can induce embryotoxicity, and the longer exposure times associated with therapy using oil-soluble ARTs, such as artemether, will produce fatal neurotoxicity (Li et al., 2007a). To prevent embryotoxicity in pregnant women with malaria, current WHO policy recommendations on the use of ARTs in uncomplicated malaria state that ARTs should be used only in the second and third trimester, limiting the use of ARTS in the first trimester to cases where it is the only effective treatment available (WHO 2006b).
Studies with laboratory animals have demonstrated fatal neurotoxicity associated with intramuscular administration of artemether (AM) and arteether (AE) or oral administration of artelinic acid (AL) These effects suggest that the exposure time of artemisinins was extended in these studies due to the accumulation of drug in the bloodstream, and this accumulation, in turn, resulted in neurotoxicity. In one study (Li and Hickman, 2011), the drug exposure time with a neurotoxic outcome (neurotoxic exposure time) was evaluated as a predictor of neurotoxicity *in vivo*. The neurotoxic exposure time represents a total time spent above the lowest observed neurotoxic effect levels (LONEL) in plasma. The dose of AE required to induce minimal neurotoxicity requires a 2-3 fold longer exposure time in rhesus monkeys (179.5 hr) than in rats (67.1 hr) and dogs (113.2 hr) when using a daily dose of 6-12.5 mg/kg for 7-28 days, indicating that the safe dosing duration in monkeys should be longer than 7 days under this exposure. Oral AL treatment required much longer LONEL levels (8-fold longer) than intramuscular AE to induce neurotoxicity, suggesting that water-soluble artemisinins appear to be much safer than oil-soluble artemisinins. Due to the lower doses (2-4 mg/kg) used with current artemisinins and the more rare use of AE in treating humans, the exposure time is much shorter in humans. Therefore, the current regimen of 3-5 days dosing duration should be quite safe. Advances in our knowledge of artemisinin-induced neurotoxicity can help refine the treatment regimens used to treat malaria with oral ARTs as well as injectable AS products to avoid the risk of neurotoxicity. Although the water-soluble artemisinins, like AS, appear to be much safer, further study is needed in when employing ARTs as anticancer agents (Li & Hickman, 2011).

5.4 Strategies to utilize ART derivatives as anticancer agents

As mentioned above, AS is completely converted to DHA and is best described as a prodrug of DHA. Also, DHA was shown to be more effective than AS in inhibition of angiogenesis and vasculogenesis *in vitro* (Longo et al., 2006a; 2006b; Chen et al., 2004; White et al., 2006). In addition, , the embryotoxicity and neurotoxicity of artemisinins can be reduced by using artemisone, which is a novel derivative of artemisinin that is not metabolized to DHA (Figure 1) (D'Alessandro et al., 2007; Schmuck et al., 2009).

Artemisone is a novel amino alkyl ART that has recently entered Phase II clinical trials (D'Alessandro et al., 2007). The compound was rationally designed to have reduced lipophilicity in order to impede transport to the brain and embryo. In addition, the inclusion of a thiomorpholine 1,1-dioxide group at the C10 position blocks the conversion of artemisone to the more lipophilic DHA. This structural modification does not affect anti-parasitic activity but reduces neurotoxicity and embryotoxicity, as assessed in primary neuronal brain stem cell cultures from fetal rats and in vivo in female rats (Schmuck et al., 2009). The retention of artemisone antimalarial activity infers that chemical activation of the peroxide bridge to a toxic parasiticidal chemical species remains unchanged, but recent literature also suggests that artemisone has a direct cytotoxic activity without activation of the endoperoxide bridge. In fact, two subsequent studies have provided conflicting results concerning the dependence of the pharmacological activity of artemisone on iron-activation of the endoperoxide group.
Interestingly, in an in vitro study by D'Alessandro et al, the anti-angiogenic effects of artemisone were reduced compared with DHA, and it was suggested that this reduction may limit the potential of artemisone to cause embryotoxicity mediated by defective angiogenesis and vasculogenesis during embryo development (D'Alessandro et al., 2007). Together these studies suggest that, while artemisone was designed to optimize safety by physicochemical means, the structural changes induced to create artemisone may also affect the intracellular chemical and molecular pathways which underlie toxicity, perhaps via reduced or alternative mechanisms of bio-activation and/or reduced cellular accumulation, when compared with the traditional ARTs. Therefore, artemisone represents an exciting novel compound in which increased anti-parasitic activity is combined with a reduced potential to cause both embryotoxicity and neurotoxicity.
Increased knowledge of the molecular mechanisms of ART-derived drugs and recent developments in novel ART applications demonstrates that further pharmacokinetic and pharmacodynamic analyses of novel ART derivatives are needed to understand why these compounds differ in efficacy and toxicity. This information will prove useful for the rationale design of more-effective ART-based molecules for use as anticancer agents. New derivatives of ARTs may act not only as treatment drugs, but also may have potential as potent cancer preventative agents due to their inhibition of tumor promotion and progression.

6. Conclusion

AS and its bioactive metabolite, DHA, have been the topic of considerable research study in recent years. Both drugs have been used to effectively treat infections with different forms of malarial parasites including multidrug-resistant strains. The key structural feature in all of the artemisinin (ART)-related molecules that mediates their antimalarial activity, and some of their anticancer activities, is an endoperoxide bridge. ARTs have been shown to induce apoptosis, a highly ordered form of parasite suicide, affecting both mature and immature parasites. Apoptosis is widely believed to be the mechanism by which ART therapy rapidly kills malaria parasites. However, severe embryotoxicity in a number of animal species has been reported after treatment with AS and DHA. A number of research studies have shown that the mechanism of ART embryotoxicity appears to be associated with ART- driven inhibition of fetal hematopoiesis and vasculogenesis. Specifically, higher drug levels of AS and DHA have been shown to affect erythroblasts, endothelial cells and cardiovascular cells in the early embryo. The inhibition of angiogenesis induced by ART-derived drugs has also been shown to be a mechanism of anticancer activity *in vitro* and *in vivo*. In particular, cancer angiogenesis plays a key role in the growth, invasion, and metastasis of tumors. ARTs-induced inhibition of angiogenesis could be a promising therapeutic strategy for treatment of cancer. Other anticancer mechanisms induced by ARTs have been recognized recently that have guided various clinical trials in anticancer therapy. Since new and alternative vascularization mechanisms have been found, further research on the mechanism of efficacy and toxicity could lead us to understand more deeply the possibilities inherent in therapeutic development of ARTs for malaria, cancer, and other indications. The new therapeutic strategies for use of ARTs should be also considered to avoid problems associated with reproductive toxicity and neurotoxicity.

Taken together, the ARTs and the derivatives of ARTs have been shown to have potent antivasculogenic and antiangiogenic effects in tumor cells as well as in healthy embryos in animals and cultures. These observations have many implications in terms of cancer therapy and prevention as well as avoidance of drug toxicity associated with inhibition of vasculogenesis and angiogenesis.

7. References

D'Alessandro, S., Gelati, M., Basilico, N., Parati, EA., Haynes, R.K.,, Taramelli, D. (2007) Differential effects on angiogenesis of two antimalarial compounds, dihydroartemisinin and artemisone: implications for embryotoxicity. Toxicology 241, 66–74.

Anfosso, L., Efferth, T., Albini, A., Pfeffer, U. (2006) Microarray expression profiles of angiogenesis-related genes predict tumor cell response to artemisinins. Pharmacogenomics J. 6, 269-278.

Baron, M. (2001) Induction of embryonic hematopoietic and endothelial stem/progenitor cells by hedgehog-mediated signals. Differentiation 68; 175–185.

Batty, K.T., Thu, L.T., Davis, T.M., Ilett, K.F., Mai, T.X., Hung, N.C., Tien, N.P., Powell, S.M., Thien, H.V., Binh, T.Q., Kim, N.V. (1998a) A pharmacokinetic and pharmacodynamic study of intravenous vs oral artesunate in uncomplicated falciparum malaria. Br. J. Clin. Pharmacol. 45, 123-129.

Batty, K.T., Le, A.T., Ilett, K.F., Nguyen, P.T., Powell, S.M., Nguyen, C.H., Truong, X.M., Vuong, V.C., Huynh, V.T., Tran, Q.B., Nguyen, V.M., Davis, T.M. (1998b) A pharmacokinetic and pharmacodynamic study of artesunate for vivax malaria. Am. J. Trop. Med. Hyg. 59, 823-827.

Baumann, R., Dragon, S. (2005) Erythropoiesis and red cell function in vertebrate embryos. Eur. J. Clin. Invest. 35 Suppl 3, 2-12.

Berger, T.G., Dieckmann, D., Efferth, T., Schultz, E.S., Funk, J.O., Baur, A., Schuler, G. (2005) Artesunate in the treatment of metastatic uveal melanoma--first experiences. Oncol. Rep. 14, 1599-1603.

Bielinska, M., Narita, N., Heikinheimo, M., Porter, S.B., Wilson, D.B. (1996) Erythropoiesis and vasculogenesis in embryoid bodies lacking visceral yolk sac endoderm. Blood. 88, 3720-3730.

Buommino, E., Baroni, A., Canozo, N., Petrazzuolo, M., Nicoletti, R., Vozza, A., Tufano, M.A. (2009) Artemisinin reduces human melanoma cell migration by down-regulating alpha V beta 3 integrin and reducing metalloproteinase 2 production. Invest, New Drugs. 27, 412-418.

Chen, H., Sun, B., Pan, S.H., Li, J., Xue, D.B., Meng, Q.H., Jiang, H.C. (2009) Study on anticancer effect of dihydroartemisinin on pancreatic cancer]. Zhonghua Wai Ke Za Zhi. 47, 1002-1005.

Chen, H., Shi, L., Yang, X., Li, S., Guo, X., Pan, L. (2010a) Artesunate inhibiting angiogenesis induced by human myeloma RPMI8226 cells. Int. J. Hematol. 92, 587-597.

Chen, H., Sun, B., Wang, S., Pan, S., Gao, Y., Bai, X., Xue, D. (2010b) Growth inhibitory effects of dihydroartemisinin on pancreatic cancer cells: involvement of cell cycle arrest and inactivation of nuclear factor-kappaB. J. Cancer Res. Clin. Oncol. 136, 897-903.

Chen, H.H., Zhou, H.J., Fang, X. (2003) Inhibition of human cancer cell line growth and human umbilical vein endothelial cell angiogenesis by artemisinin derivatives in vitro. Pharmacol. Res. 48, 231–236.

Chen, H.H., Zhou, H.J., Wang, W.Q., Wu, G.D. (2004a) Antimalarial dihydroartemisinin also inhibits angiogenesis. Cancer Chemother. Pharmacol. 53, 423-432.

Chen, H.H., Zhou, H.J., Wu, G.D., Lou, X.E. (2004b) Inhibitory effects of artesunate on angiogenesis and on expressions of vascular endothelial growth factor and VEGF receptor KDR/flk-1. Pharmacology 71, 1–9.

Chen, T., Li, M., Zhang, R., Wang, H. (2009) Dihydroartemisinin induces apoptosis and sensitizes human ovarian cancer cells to carboplatin therapy. J. Cell Mol. Med. 13, 1358-1370.

Clark, R.L., White, T.E., Clode, S.A., Gaunt, I., Winstanley, P., Ward, S.A. (2004) Developmental toxicity of artesunate and an artesunate combination in the rat and rabbit. Birth Defects Res. B Dev. Reprod. Toxicol. 71, 380–394.

Clark, R.L., Arima, A., Makori, N., Nakata, Y., Bernard, F., Gristwood, W., Harrell, A., White, T.E., Wier, P.J. (2008a) Artesunate: developmental toxicity and toxicokinetics in monkeys. Birth Defects Res. B Dev. Reprod. Toxicol. 83, 418–434.

Clark, R.L., Lerman, S.A., Cox, E.M., Gristwood, W.E., White, T.E. (2008b) Developmental toxicity of artesunate in the rat: comparison to other artemisinins, comparison of embryotoxicity and kinetics by oral and intravenous routes, and relationship to maternal reticulocyte count. Birth Defects Res B Dev Reprod Toxicol. 83, 397-406.

Clark, R.L. (2009) Embryotoxicity of the artemisinin antimalarials and potential consequences for use in women in the first trimester. Reprod Toxicol. 28, 285-296.

Cline, M.J., Moore, M.A. (1972) Embryonic origin of the mouse macrophage. Blood 39, 842–849.

Davis, T.M., Phuong, H.L., Ilett, K.F., Hung, N.C., Batty, K.T., Phuong, V.D., Powell, S.M., Thien, H.V., Binh, T.Q. (2001) Pharmacokinetics and pharmacodynamics of intravenous artesunate in severe falciparum malaria. Antimicrob. Agents Chemother. 45, 181-186.

Dawes, M., Chowienczyk, P.J. (2001) Drugs in pregnancy. Pharmacokinetics in pregnancy. Best Pract. Res. Clin. Obstet. Gynaecol. 15, 819–826.

Dell'Eva, R., Pfeffer, U., Vené, R., Anfosso, L., Forlani, A., Albini, A., Efferth, T. (2004) Inhibition of angiogenesis in vivo and growth of Kaposi's sarcoma xenograft tumors by the anti-malarial artesunate. Biochem. Pharmacol. 68, 2359–2366.

Dellicour, S., Hall, S.; Chandramohan, D.; Greenwood, B. (2007) The safety of artemisinins during pregnancy: a pressing question. Malar. J. 6, 15.

Disbrow, G.L., Baege, A.C., Kierpiec, K.A., Yuan, H., Centeno, J.A., Thibodeaux, C.A., Hartmann, D., Schlegel, R. (2005) Dihydroartemisinin is cytotoxic to papillomavirus-expressing epithelial cells in vitro and in vivo. Cancer Res. 65, 10854-10861.

Döme, B., Hendrix, M.J., Paku, S., Tóvári, J., Tímár, J. (2007) Alternative vascularization mechanisms in cancer: Pathology and therapeutic implications. Am. J. Pathol. 170, 1-15.

Efferth, T., Dunstan, H., Sauerbrey, A., Miyachi, H., Chitambar, C.R. (2001) The anti-malarial artesunate is also active against cancer. Int. J. Oncol. 18, 767–773.

Efferth, T., Benakis, A., Romero, M.R., Tomicic, M., Rauh, R., Steinbach, D., Häfer, R., Stamminger, T., Oesch, F., Kaina, B., Marschall, M. (2004) Enhancement of cytotoxicity of artemisinins toward cancer cells by ferrous iron. Free Radic. Biol. Med. 37, 998-1009.

Efferth, T. (2005) Mechanistic perspectives for 1,2,4-trioxanes in anti-cancer therapy. Drug Resist Updat. 8, 85-97.

Efferth, T. (2006) Molecular pharmacology and pharmacogenomics of artemisinin and its derivatives in cancer cells. Curr. Drug Targets. 7, 407–421.

Efferth, T., Giaisi, M., Merling, A., Krammer, P.H., Li-Weber, M. (2007) Artesunate induces ROS-mediated apoptosis in doxorubicin-resistant T leukemia cells. PLoS One. 2, e693.

Efferth, T., Kaina, B. (2010) Toxicity of the antimalarial artemisinin and its derivatives. Crit Rev Toxicol. 40, 405-421.

El Hallani, S., Boisselier, B., Peglion, F., Rousseau, A., Colin, C., Idbaih, A., Marie, Y., Mokhtari, K., Thomas, J.L., Eichmann, A., Delattre, J.Y., Maniotis, A.J., Sanson, M. (2010) A new alternative mechanism in glioblastoma vascularization: tubular vasculogenic mimicry. Brain. 133, 973-982.

Firestone, G.L., Sundar, S.N. (2009) Anticancer activities of artemisinin and its bioactive derivatives. Expert Rev Mol Med. 11, e32.

Finaurini, S., Ronzoni, L., Colancecco, A., Cattaneo, A., Cappellini, M.D., Ward, S.A., Taramelli, D. (2010) Selective toxicity of dihydroartemisinin on human CD34+ erythroid cell differentiation. Toxicology. 276, 128-134.

Galustian, C., Dalgleish, A. (2009) Lenalidomide: a novel anticancer drug with multiple modalities. Expert Opin. Pharmacother. 10, 125-133.

Ghantous, A., Gali-Muhtasib, H., Vuorela, H., Saliba, N.A, (2010) Darwiche N. What made sesquiterpene lactones reach cancer clinical trials? Drug Discov. Today. 15, 668-678.

Hanahan, D. (1997) Signaling vascular morphogenesis and maintenance. Science. 277, 48–50.

He, Y., Fan, J., Lin, H., Yang, X., Ye, Y., Liang, L., Zhan, Z., Dong, X., Sun, L., Xu, H. (2011) The anti-malaria agent artesunate inhibits expression of vascular endothelial growth factor and hypoxia-inducible factor-1α in human rheumatoid arthritis fibroblast-like synoviocyte. Rheumatol. Int. 31, 53-60.

Hendrix, M.J., Seftor, E.A., Hess, A.R., Seftor, R.E. (2003) Vasculogenic mimicry and tumour-cell plasticity: lessons from melanoma. Nat. Rev. Cancer. 3, 411-421.

Hou, J., Wang, D., Zhang, R., Wang, H. (2008) Experimental therapy of hepatoma with artemisinin and its derivatives: in vitro and in vivo activity, chemosensitization, and mechanisms of action. Clin Cancer Res. 14, 5519-5530.

Hsu, E. (2006) The history of qinghao in the Chinese materia medica. Trans. R. Soc. Trop. Med. Hyg. 100, 505-508.

Huan-Huan, C., Li-Li, Y., Shang-Bin, L. (2004) Artesunate reduces chicken chorioallantoic membrane neovascularisation and exhibits antiangiogenic and apoptotic activity on human microvascular dermal endothelial cell. Cancer Lett. 211, 163–173.

Huang, X.J., Li, C.T., Zhang, W.P., Lu, Y.B., Fang, S.H., Wei, E.Q. (2008) Dihydroartemisinin potentiates the cytotoxic effect of temozolomide in rat C6 glioma cells. Pharmacology 82, 1-9.

Jeong, S.J., Itokawa, T., Shibuya, M., Kuwano, M., Ono, M., Higuchi, R., Miyamoto, T. (2002) Costunolide, a sesquiterpene lactone from Saussurea lappa, inhibits the VEGFR KDR/Flk-1 signaling pathway. Cancer Letters. 187, 129-133.

Kelemen, E., Calvo, W., Fliedner, T. (1979) Atlas of human hemopoietic development. Springer–Verlag: Berlin, Germany, p. 21.

Kim, M.S., Lee, Y.M., Moon, E.J., Kim, S.E., Lee, J.J., Kim, K.W. (2000) Anti-angiogenic activity of torilin, a sesquiterpene compound isolated from Torilis japonica. Int. J. Cancer 87, 269-275

Kim, S.J., Kim, M.S., Lee, J.W., Lee, C.H., Yoo, H., Shin, S.H., Park, M.J., Lee, S.H. (2006) Dihydroartemisinin enhances radiosensitivity of human glioma cells in vitro. J. Cancer Re.s Clin. Oncol. 132, 129-135.

Kreisl, T.N., Kim, L., Moore, K., Duic, P., Royce, C., Stroud, I., Garren, N., Mackey, M., Butman, J.A., Camphausen, K., Park, J., Albert, P.S., Fine, H.A. (2009) Phase II trial of single-agent bevacizumab followed by bevacizumab plus irinotecan at tumor progression in recurrent glioblastoma. J. Clin. Oncol. 27, 740-745.

Kwee, L., Baldwin, H.S., Shen, H.M., Stewart, C.L., Buck, C., Buck, C.A., Labow, M.A. (1995) Defective development of the embryonic and extraembryonic circulatory systems in vascular cell adhesion molecule (VCAM-1) deficient mice. Development. 121, 489-503.

Lai, H., Singh, N.P. (1995) Selective cancer cell cytotoxicity from exposure to dihydroartemisinin and holotransferrin. Cancer Lett. 91, 41-46.

Lai, H., Singh, N.P. (2006) Oral artemisinin prevents and delays the development of 7,12-dimethylbenz[a]anthracene (DMBA)-induced breast cancer in the rat. Cancer Lett. 231, 43-48.

Lee, J., Zhou, H.J., Wu, X.H. (2006) Dihydroartemisinin downregulates vascular endothelial growth factor expression and induces apoptosis in chronic myeloid leukemia K562 cells. Cancer Chemother. Pharmacol. 57, 213-220.

Lensch, M.W., Daley, G.Q. (2004) Origins of mammalian hematopoiesis: in vivo paradigms and in vitro models. Curr. Top. Dev. Biol. 60, 127–196.

Li, L.N., Zhang, H.D., Yuan, S.J., Tian, Z.Y., Wang, L., Sun, Z.X. (2007) Artesunate attenuates the growth of human colorectal carcinoma and inhibits hyperactive Wnt/beta-catenin pathway. Int. J. Cancer. 121, 1360-1365.

Li, Q.G., Peggins, J.O., Fleckenstein, L.L., Masonic, K., Heiffer, M.H., Brewer, T.G. (1998) The pharmacokinetics and bioavailability of dihydroartemisinin, arteether, artemether, artesunic acid and artelinic acid in rats. J Pharm Pharmacol. 50, 173-182.

Li, Q., Mog, S.R., Si, Y.Z., Kyle, D.E., Gettayacamin, M., Milhous, W.K. (2002) Neurotoxicity and efficacy of arteether related to its exposure times and exposure levels in rodents. Am J Trop Med Hyg. 66; 516-525.

Li, Q., Milhous, W.K., Weina, P. Eds. (2007a) Antimalarial in Malaria Therapy. Nova Science Publishers Inc, New York; 1st edition. pp.1-133.

Li, Q., Weina, P., Milhous, W. (2007b) Pharmacokinetic and pharmacodynamic profiles of rapid-acting artemisinins in the antimalarial therapy. Current Drug Therapy. 2, 210-223.

Li, Q., Gerena, L., Xie, L., Zhang, J., Kyle, D., Milhous, W. (2007c) Development and validation of flow cytometric measurement for parasitemia in cultures of P. falciparum vitally stained with YOYO-1. Cytometry A. 71, 297-307.

Li, Q., Si, Y., Smith, K.S., Zeng, Q., Weina, P.J. (2008) Embryotoxicity of artesunate in animal species related to drug tissue distribution and toxicokinetic profiles. Birth Defects Res. B Dev. Reprod. Toxicol. 83, 435–445.

Li, Q., Si, Y.Z., Xie, L.H., Zhang, J., Weina, P. (2009) Severe embryolethality of artesunate related to pharmacokinetics following intravenous and intramuscular doses in pregnant rats. Birth Defects Res. B Dev. Reprod. Toxicol. 86, 385–393.

Li, Q., Weina, P. (2010a) Artesunate: the best drug in the treatments of severe and complicated malaria. Pharmaceuticals. 3, 2322-2332

Li, Q., Weina, P. (2010b) Severe embryotoxicity of artemisinin derivatives in experimental animals, but possibly safe in pregnant women. Molecules. 15, 40-57.

Li, Q., Hickman, M. (2011) Toxicokinetic and toxicodynamic (TK/TD) evaluation to determine and predict the neurotoxicity of artemisinins. Toxicology. 279, 1-9.

Li, W., Mo, W., Shen, D., Sun, L., Wang, J., Lu, S., Gitschier, J.M., Zhou, B. (2005) Yeast model uncovers dual roles of mitochondria in action of artemisinin. PLoS Genet. 1, e36.

Liu, W.M. (2008) Enhancing the cytotoxic activity of novel targeted therapies--is there a role for a combinatorial approach? Curr. Clin. Pharmacol. 3, 108-117

Liu, W.M., Gravett, A.M., Dalgleish, A.G. (2011) The antimalarial agent artesunate possesses anticancer properties that can be enhanced by combination strategies. Int. J. Cancer. 128, 1471-1480.

Longo, M., Zanoncelli, S., Manera, D., Brughera, M., Colombo, P., Lansen, J., Mazué, G., Gomes, M., Taylor, W.R., Olliaro, P. (2006a) Effects of the antimalarial drug dihydroartemisinin (DHA) on rat embryos in vitro. Reprod. Toxicol. 21, 83–93.

Longo, M., Zanoncelli, S., Torre, P.D., Riflettuto, M., Cocco, F., Pesenti, M., Giusti, A., Colombo, P., Brughera, M., Mazué, G., Navaratman, V., Gomes, M., Olliaro, P. (2006b) In vivo and in vitro investigations of the effects of the antimalarial drug dihydroartemisinin (DHA) on rat embryos. Reprod. Toxicol. 22, 797–810.

Longo, M., Zanoncelli, S., Torre P.D., Rosa, F., Giusti, A., Colombo, P., Brughera, M., Mazué, G., Olliaro, P. (2008) Investigations of the effects of the antimalarial drug dihydroartemisinin (DHA) using the Frog Embryo Teratogenesis Assay–Xenopus (FETAX). Reprod. Toxicol. 25, 433–441.

Louis, D.N., Ohgaki, H., Wiestler, O.D., Cavenee, W.K., Burger, P.C., Jouvet, A., Scheithauer, B.W., Kleihues, P. (2007) The 2007 WHO classification of tumours of the central nervous system. Acta Neuropathol. 114, 97-109.

Maeno, Y., Toyoshima, T., Fujioka, H., Ito, Y., Meshnick, S.R., Benakis, A., Milhous, W.K., Aikawa, M. (1993) Morphologic effects of artemisinin in Plasmodium falciparum. Am. J. Trop. Med. Hyg. 49, 485-491.

McGready, R., Stepniewska, K., Ward, S.A., Cho, T., Gilveray, G., Looareesuwan, S., White, N.J., Nosten, F. (2006) Pharmacokinetics of dihydroartemisinin following oral artesunate treatment of pregnant women with acute uncomplicated falciparum malaria. Eur. J. Clin. Pharmacol. 62, 367–371.

McLean, W.G., Ward, S.A. (1998) In vitro neurotoxicity of artemisinin derivatives. Med Trop (Mars). 58(3 Suppl), 28-31.

Medhi, B., Patyar, S., Rao, R.S., Byrav, D.S.P., Prakash, A. (2009) Pharmacokinetic and toxicological profile of artemisinin compounds: an update. Pharmacology. 84, 323-332.

Menendez, C. (2006) Malaria during pregnancy. Curr. Mol. Med. 6, 269–273.

Mercer, A.E. (2009) The role of bioactivation in the pharmacology and toxicology of the artemisinin-based antimalarials. Curr. Opin. Drug Discov. Devel. 12, 125-132.

Meshnick, S.R. (2002) Artemisinin: mechanisms of action, resistance and toxicity. Int. J. Parasitol. 32, 1655–1660.

Moore, J.C., Lai, H., Li, J.R., Ren, R.L., McDougall, J.A., Singh, N.P., Chou, C.K. (1995) Oral administration of dihydroartemisinin and ferrous sulfate retarded implanted fibrosarcoma growth in the rat. Cancer Lett. 98, 83–87.

Nakase, I., Lai, H., Singh, N.P., Sasaki, T. (2007) Anticancer properties of artemisinin derivatives and their targeted delivery by transferrin conjugation. Int. J. Pharm 354, 28–33

Navaratnam, V., Mansor, S.M., Sit, N.W., Grace, J., Li, Q.G., Olliaro, P. (2000) Pharmacokinetics of artemisinin-type compounds. Clin. Pharmacokinet. 39, 255-270.

Newton, P., Suputtamongkol, Y., Teja–Isavadharm, P., Pukrittayakamee, S., Navaratnam, V., Bates, I., White, N. (2000) Antimalarial bioavailability and disposition of artesunate in acute falciparum malaria. Antimicrob. Agents Chemother. 44, 972–977.

Nosten, F., McGready, R., d'Alessandro, U., Bonell, A., Verhoeff, F., Menendez, C., Mutabingwa, T., Brabin, B. (2006) Antimalarial Drugs in Pregnancy: a review. Currt. Drug Saf. 1, 1–15.

Oh, S., Jeong, I.H., Ahn, C.M., Shin, W.S., Lee, S. (2004) Synthesis and antiangiogenic activity of thioacetal artemisinin derivatives. Bioorg. Med. Chem. 12, 3783–3790.

Olliaro, P.L., Haynes, R.K., Meunier, B,, Yuthavong, Y. (2001) Possible modes of action of the artemisinin-type compounds. Trends Parasitol. 17, 122–126.

Palis, J., Yoder, M.C. (2001) Yolk-sac hematopoiesis: the first blood cells of mouse and man. Exp. Hematol. 29, 927–936.

Parapini, S., Basilico, N., Mondani, M., Olliaro, P., Taramelli, D., Monti, D. (2004) Evidence that haem iron in the malaria parasite is not needed for the antimalarial effects of artemisinin. FEBS Lett. 575, 91–94.

Ramacher, M., Umansky, V., Efferth, T. (2009) Effect of artesunate on immune cells in ret-transgenic mouse melanoma model. Anticancer. Drugs. 20, 910-917.

Ratajska, A., Czarnowska, E. (2006a) Vasculogenesis of the embryonic heart: contribution of nucleated red blood cells to early vascular structures. Cardiovasc. Hematol. Disord. Drug Targets. 6, 219-225.

Ratajska, A., Czarnowska, E., Kołodzińska, A., Kluzek, W., Leśniak, W. (2006b) Vasculogenesis of the embryonic heart: origin of blood island-like structures. Anat. Rec. A Discov. Mol. Cell Evol. Biol. 288, 223-232

Risau, W. (1995) Differentiation of endothelium. FASEB J. 9, 926-933.

Risau, W. (1997) Mechanisms of angiogenesis. Nature. 386, 671-674.

Rongish, B.J., Torry, R.J., Tucker, D.C., Tomanek, R.J. (1994) Neovascularization of embryonic rat hearts cultured in oculo closely mimics in utero coronary vessel development. J. Vasc. Res. 31, 205-215.

Sadava, D., Phillips, T., Lin, C., Kane, S.E. (2002) Transferrin overcomes drug resistance to artemisinin in human small-cell lung carcinoma cells. Cancer Lett. 179, 151-156.

Sabin, F.R. (1917) Origin and development of the primitive vessels of the chick and the pig. Contrib. Embryol. 6; 61–124.

van der Schaft, D.W., Seftor, R.E., Seftor, E.A., Hess, A.R., Gruman, L.M., Kirschmann, D.A., Yokoyama, Y., Griffioen, A.W., Hendrix, M.J. (2004) Effects of angiogenesis inhibitors on vascular network formation by human endothelial and melanoma cells. J. Natl. Cancer Inst. 96, 1473-1477.

Schmuck, G., Klaus, A.M., Krötlinger, F., Langewische, F.W. (2009) Developmental and reproductive toxicity studies on artemisone. Birth Defects Res. B Dev. Reprod Toxicol. 86, 131-143.

Segel, G., Palis, J. (2001) Hematology of the Newborn. In: Williams hematology: Beutler, E., Lichtman, M., Coller, B., Kipps, T., Seligsohn, U., editors. McGraw–Hill: New York, NY, USA, p. 77.

Sequeira Lopez, M.L., Chernavvsky, D.R., Nomasa, T., Wall, L., Yanagisawa, M., Gomez, R.A. (2003) The embryo makes red blood cell progenitors in every tissue simultaneously with blood vessel morphogenesis. Am. J. Physiol. Regul. Integr. Comp. Physiol. 284, R1126-1137.

Sieber, S., Gdynia, G., Roth, W., Bonavida, B., Efferth, T. (2009) Combination treatment of malignant B cells using the anti-CD20 antibody rituximab and the anti-malarial artesunate. Int. J. Oncol. 35, 149-158.

Singh, N.P., Lai, H. (2001) Selective toxicity of dihydroartemisinin and holotransferrin toward human breast cancer cells. Life Sci. 70, 49-56.

Singh, N.P., Verma, K.B. (2002) Case report of a laryngeal squamous cell carcinoma treated with artesunate. Arch Oncol. 10, 279-280.

Singh, N.P., Panwar, V.K. (2006) Case report of a pituitary macroadenoma treated with artemether. Integr. Cancer Ther. 5, 391-394.

Skinner, T.S., Manning, L.S., Johnston, W.A., Davis, T.M. (1996) In vitro stage-specific sensitivity of Plasmodium falciparum to quinine and artemisinin drugs. Int. J. Parasit. 26, 519-525.

Tavassoli, M.(1991) Embryonic and fetal hemopoiesis: an overview. Blood Cells. 17, 269–281.

Thurston, G. (2002) Complementary actions of VEGF and angiopoietin-1 on blood vessel growth and leakage. J. Anat. 200, 575-580.

Tímár, J., Döme, B. (2008) Antiangiogenic drugs and tyrosine kinases. Anticancer Agents Med Chem. 8, 462-469.

Tozer, G.M. (2003) Measuring tumour vascular response to antivascular and antiangiogenic drugs. Br. J. Radiol. 76 Spec No 1, S23-35

Ward, S.A., Sevene, E.J., Hastings, I.M., Nosten, F., McGready, R. (2007) Antimalarial drugs and pregnancy: safety, pharmacokinetics, and pharmacovigilance. Lancet Infect. Dis. 7, 136–144.

Wartenberg, M., Wolf, S., Budde, P., Grünheck, F., Acker, H., Hescheler, J., Wartenberg, G., Sauer, H. (2003) The antimalaria agent artemisinin exerts antiangiogenic effects in mouse embryonic stem cell-derived embryoid bodies. Lab. Invest. 83, 1647-1655.

White, T.E., Bushdid, P.B., Ritter, S., Laffan, S.B., Clark, R.L. (2006) Artesunate-induced depletion of embryonic erythroblasts precedes embryolethality and teratogenicity in vivo. Birth Defects Res. B Dev. Reprod. Toxicol. 77, 413–429.

White, T.E., Clark, R.L. (2008) Sensitive periods for developmental toxicity of orally administered artesunate in the rat. Birth Defects Res. B Dev. Reprod. Toxicol. 83, 407–417.

WHO. (2006a) Guidelines for the Treatment of Malaria: World Health Organization: Geneva, Switzerland.

WHO. (2006b) Assessment of the safety of artemisinin compounds in pregnancy. In The Special Programme for Research and Training Diseases (TDR) and The Global Malaria Programme of the World Health Organization; World Health Organization: Geneva, Switzerland.

Wong, P.M., Chung, S.W., Chui, D.H., Eaves, C.J. (1986) Properties of the earliest clonogenic hemopoietic precursors to appear in the developing murine yolk sac. Proc. Natl. Acad. Sci. USA. 83, 3851–3854.

Wu, X.H., Zhou, H.J., Lee, J. (2006) Dihydroartemisinin inhibits angiogenesis induced by multiple myeloma RPMI8226 cells under hypoxic conditions via downregulation of vascular endothelial growth factor expression and suppression of vascular endothelial growth factor secretion. Anticancer. Drugs. 17, 839-848.

Wu, X., Lee, V.C., Chevalier, E., Hwang, S.T. (2009) Chemokine receptors as targets for cancer therapy. Curr. Pharm. Des. 15, 742-757.

Zhang, Z.Y., Yu, S.Q., Miao, L.Y., Huang, X.Y., Zhang, X.P., Zhu, Y.P., Xia, X.H., Li, D.Q. (2008)Artesunate combined with vinorelbine plus cisplatin in treatment of advanced non-small cell lung cancer: a randomized controlled trial. Zhong Xi Yi Jie He Xue Bao. 6, 134-138.

Zhou, H.J., Wang, W.Q., Wu, G.D., Lee, J., Li, A. (2007) Artesunate inhibits angiogenesis and downregulates vascular endothelial growth factor expression in chronic myeloid leukemia K562 cells. Vascul. Pharmacol. 47, 131-138.

Zhou, H.J., Zhang, J.L., Li, A., Wang, Z., Lou, X.E. (2010) Dihydroartemisinin improves the efficiency of chemotherapeutics in lung carcinomas in vivo and inhibits murine Lewis lung carcinoma cell line growth in vitro. Cancer Chemother. Pharmacol. 66, 21-29.

Part 4

Regenerative Medicine

9

The Mechanics of Blood Vessel Growth

Rui D. M. Travasso
Centro de Física Computacional, Departamento de Física, Universidade de Coimbra, Centro de Oftalmologia e Ciências da Visão, Instituto Biomédico de Investigação da Luz e Imagem (IBILI), Faculdade de Medicina, Universidade de Coimbra, Centro de Física da Matéria Condensada, Universidade de Lisboa Portugal

1. Introduction

Blood vessel growth is pivotal in various processes in health and disease; examples are embryogenesis, inflammation, wound healing, cardiac ischemia, diabetic retinopathy, and tumor growth. The latter, in particular, has been the subject of extensive studies due to the high mortality rates associated with oncologic diseases. However, and despite the continuous efforts by the scientific community, both the genomic characterization of tumors (Maley et al., 2006; Wood et al., 2007) and the main physical mechanisms driving their development (Araújo & McElwain, 2004) are currently a matter of debate. These efforts have been greatly enriched through an interdisciplinary approach. Physics, Mathematics and computer simulation and modeling have currently a key role in the research of tumor growth in general and vessel development in particular. The approach of mathematicians and physicists provides remarkable new ways of looking into Biology: starting the modeling from basic principles, the fundamentals of the problem can be tested and understood.

The relevance of blood vessel growth for tumor development is well documented (Figg & Folkman, 2008). In the early stages of development, the growth of a solid tumor is limited in size due to cell apoptosis at its core by lack of nutrients. In simple terms, the acquisition of nutrients at the boundary is not able to meet the needs of the inner cells. This, in addition to a problem of confinement of the inner cells (the fast growth does not allow them to migrate) produces the so called core necrosis inside the tumor. When this stationary non-threatening stage is reached, malignant tumors adapt to the environment and undergo an active search for the nutrients they need to survive and proliferate. This can be achieved by releasing factors, such the Vascular Endothelial Growth Factor (VEGF), which drive nearby vessels to extend new branches in the direction of the tumor, through a process called angiogenesis, providing it with nutrients (Figg & Folkman, 2008). Hence, understanding angiogenesis is essential to the potential control of the blood delivered to a neoplasic tissue in order to prevent and contain its development and metastatic colonies. In fact, though hyper-vascularization is not a requirement for a tumor to metastasize (Mateus et al., 2009), the cells of a densely vascularized tumor have a much higher facility in entering the blood circulation.

During the last decade cancer therapies based on anti-angiogenic factors have been a focus of interest. However, this type of treatment has not given the expected results (Mayer, 2004) and recently, the concept of normalization of tumor vasculature has been proposed (Jain, 2005), where it is suggested that certain anti-angiogenic agents can transiently normalize the abnormal tumor vasculature, to make more efficient the delivery of drugs (provided by chemotherapy) and the delivery of oxygen (thus enhancing the efficiency of radiation therapy). Therefore, a better understanding of vessel growth and remodeling will have an positive impact in the design of cancer treatments.

Pathological angiogenesis is central to various other diseases besides tumor growth. In fact, it is implicated in more than 70 disorders, and according to the Angiogenesis Foundation, the lives of at least 1 billion people worldwide could be improved with therapies targeting angiogenesis (Adair & Montani, 2010). Depending on the disorder type, angiogenesis might be either excessive or deficient, and therefore different pathologies will require different approaches to actively normalize the vasculature of the diseased tissue.

Processes related to vessel growth are extremely complex, typically involving hundreds of proteins and receptors in a well balanced cross-talk. Any modeling attempt of these systems involves forcefully a simplification by considering only some of the proteins and mechanisms present. There is a generalized agreement within the community with respect to which are the main biological mechanisms driving angiogenesis, nevertheless different teams of researchers opt for choosing different modeling strategies, and therefore the implementation of these mechanisms is far from being consensual.

To make matters worse, angiogenesis and vascular remodeling have an intrinsic multi-scale nature, and the final morphology of a vascular network depends on phenomena which occur at the cell level (e.g. the activation and subsequent sprouting of new branches) (Gerhardt et al., 2003) as well as on the large scale collective movements of the cells (which are a function of endothelial cell proliferation and the tissue mechanical properties) (Friedl, 2004; Friedl & Wolf, 2003; Painter, 2009). The majority of the computational works on this topic are devoted to sprouting angiogenesis, and in this case the multi-scale nature of this process led different research groups to address the topic through either the macroscopic or the microscopic perspective.

The first simulations were done 20 years ago using diffusion equations, and many others followed the same strategy (reviewed in Mantzaris et al. (2004)). These models describe the system macroscopically, through average endothelial cell densities. Some of these works are able to delimitate a capillary by considering the points where the concentration of endothelial cells is higher, but do not evidence branching and do not predict the resulting capillary network, or the areas where vessels are more fragile.

In the beginning of the nineties microscopic cell based models appeared in the context of angiogenesis (Bauer et al., 2007; Bentley et al., 2008; Chaplain et al., 2006; Markus et al., 1999; Owen et al., 2009). The large number of different cells in the tissue and the many processes in which they participate are a major stumbling block to cell based models. These models incorporate an extremely large number of rules and parameters, while being hard to control, because of their high sensitivity to small modifications. This is of importance, since many of the required parameters are a true challenge to measure experimentally, and have to be postulated.

Recently, hybrid models that integrate continuous and discrete descriptions of angiogenesis have come to light (Milde et al., 2008; Travasso et al., 2011a). In these models the capillary cells are described as a tissue, not as individual cells. This allows for a fast integration of the equations and a relatively low number of model parameters. Capillary tip cells, however, are modeled through an agent based component due to their distinct phenotype and relevance in the chemotactic migration mechanism of capillary sprouts (Gerhardt et al., 2003). Being multi-scale at their core, hybrid models are able to include processes occurring at the cellular and tissue levels, thus originating vascular patterns qualitatively similar to the ones observed *in vivo* (Travasso et al., 2011a).

In spite of important advances in the modeling field, the large majority of sprouting angiogenesis mathematical models do not yet include the mechanical properties of tissues and capillaries, and are not able to predict how these properties determine vessel growth (Waters et al., 2011). While far from trivial, the endothelial cells' response to mechanical signals is at the core of the dynamics of capillary growth. In fact in the biomedical engineering community it has been noticed that "because angiogenesis occurs in a mechanically dynamic environment, future investigations should aim at understanding how cells integrate chemical and mechanical signals so that a rational approach to controlling angiogenesis will become possible" (Shiu et al., 2005). Still in Shiu et al. (2005) the authors call for computational models that correctly integrate this mechanical aspect into angiogenesis simulations.

Strikingly, mathematical models of the processes of intussusceptive angiogenesis and vessel remodeling have included mechanical forces from the start. In particular, some of the models describing these processes integrate directly the experimentally measured biological responses of capillaries to different stimuli, such as varying the capillary wall shear stress, through a rule-based model (Pries et al., 2005). This approach has recently been used to support the hypothesis of a new signaling mechanism present in capillary development (Pries et al., 2010).

In this chapter we will explore the mechanics of vessel growth and remodeling by focusing in the modeling strategies used in the community. We start by describing the influence of mechanical forces in endothelial cells and their relevance in angiogenesis and vascular remodeling. Next we focus on the modeling tools that have been used to describe the processes related to vessel growth and remodeling that are able to integrate the mechanical response of endothelial cells and of the vascular tissue. We finally conclude by calling for a collaborative effort between Material and Biomedical scientists to address the effect of these mechanisms in vessel growth, remodeling and maturation.

2. Mechanical influence in vessel growth and remodeling

2.1 Endothelial cells and the extracellular matrix

Cells have a cytoskeleton which can actively extend and alter, thus exerting forces in their surroundings (Alberts et al., 2002; Bray, 2001). In the various strategies cells adopt to move, they take advantage of their ability of changing shape and altering their micro-environment (Friedl, 2004; Friedl & Wolf, 2003). In the same way as they can exert forces in the extracellular matrix (ECM) and also produce proteins that are able to degrade and remodel the ECM (Painter, 2009), the forces exerted upon the cells are also able to influence their phenotype by changing their gene expression. Endothelial cells are no exception: their protein levels as well as the characteristics of the vessels they belong to strongly depend on forces exerted by the ECM and the blood flow.

Endothelial cells sense mechanical forces using membrane proteins such as integrins, which link the cells to the ECM, or E-cadherins, which link to other endothelial cells. The E-cadherins, for example, being directly attached to the cell's cytoskeleton, thus playing an active role in the regulation of the cell's size, trigger signaling pathways some of which regulate the proliferation rate of the cell (Nelson et al., 2004). In more detail, in regions of low cell density, the cell E-cadherins signaling through RhoA leads to a higher proliferation rate and lower adhesion to the ECM *in vitro*. The E-cadherin mediated proliferation control is influenced by the mechanical tension to which the cell is exposed (Nelson et al., 2004). A tension dependent proliferation rate should be present in mathematical models of angiogenesis and remodeling since it is shown theoretically and experimentally the relevance of such process for the final vascular morphology (Gerhardt & Betsholtz, 2005; Travasso et al., 2011a). This dependence is straightforward to include in a discrete model which includes every endothelial cell (Merks et al., 2008), however, in continuous and hybrid models the inclusion of these effects has been proven to be challenging.

Measurement of the forces exerted on 2D and 3D environments by a single cell have showed a complex scenario of stresses depending on the cell type, matrix properties and previous matrix remodeling events (Kraning-Rush et al., 2011).

By exerting force in the ECM, endothelial cell are able to re-orient the ECM fibers thus altering the mechanical properties of their micro-environment. Endothelial cells migrate along these restructured fibers (Korff & Agustin, 1999). Through this mechanism two endothelial cells can interact mechanically via the forces they exert in the ECM without being in contact (Califano & Reinhart-King, 2009). These forces can be measured experimentally and are suggested as being the initiators of the movement of approximation between endothelial cells in a 2D matrix. The inclusion of these "long-range" mechanical interactions, which result from the cell's action upon the ECM, is an important ingredient of many models that describe the observed formation of a network structure when endothelial cells grow on a flat substrate (Murray, 2003).

Recently it has been found clear evidence of a signaling pathway triggered mechanically that is able to control the number of receptors of vascular endothelial growth factor, VEGFR2, at the cell membrane (Mammoto et al., 2009). VEGF, is the main factor driving sprouting angiogenesis *in vivo*, having a three-fold role at the cell scale: (i) to trigger the permeability of the capillaries and the subsequent activation of the tip cell phenotype, (ii) to promote migration of tip cells in the direction of its gradient, and (iii) to promote the proliferation and survival of the stalk endothelial cells. An alteration of the number of VEGFR2 in the endothelial cells has an large impact in the resulting vessel network.

Mechanical effects are therefore determinant for endothelial cell functioning, and in processes of vessel network growth such as vasculogenesis or sprouting angiogenesis, the mechanical interplay between the endothelial cells movement and the surrounding tissue is extremely relevant to the resulting network morphology. These effects have to be included in current models of angiogenesis, though a better quantitative understanding of the forces and motion of sprouts in 3D is needed.

2.2 Blood flow

A major player in exerting stresses in vessels is blood flow which has a pivotal role as a remodeling agent of vasculature. The process of intussusceptive angiogenesis, a fast branching process where the formation of new blood vessels results from the insertion and extension of transluminar pillars, can be triggered by alterations in blood flow (Djonov et al., 2002; Filipovic et al., 2009; Styp-Rekowska et al., 2011). Also the procedure of creating a hierarchical vasculature formed by vessels with different characteristics (arteries, arterioles, capillaries, venules, veins) results from an interplay of genetic and mechanical processes regulated to a large extent by blood flow.

Endothelial cells change their gene expression as a function of the flow pressure and shear stress, type of flow (laminar or turbulent) as well as the blood composition (hematocrit, oxygen pressure, etc). Also, the shear stress is able to align endothelial cells in the flow direction, thus influencing the vessel's mechanical properties (Allen et al., 2011; Styp-Rekowska et al., 2011). Due to the large importance of the influence of shear stress on gene expression there are currently a variety of assays with the aim of studying protein transcription for different types of flow (Nash & Egginton, 2006).

It is suggested that an important regulatory function of blood flow is the stabilization of the vasculature. In fact shear stress has been shown *in vitro* to up-regulate anti-angiogenic factors such as the proteinase ADAMTS1 (Hohberg, et al.) and down-regulate pro-angiogenic factors such as the Forkhead box protein O1A, Foxo-1 (Chlench et al., 2007). Alterations in blood flow have consequences to vessel stability, and for example, a localized low shear stress region at bifurcations may lead to intussusceptive angiogenesis, while a generalized low shear stress leads to vessel destabilization and regression (Styp-Rekowska et al., 2011). Sprouting angiogenesis has also been suggested to be modulated by blood flow shear stress, with sprouting in 3D collagen matrices being observed for increasing flow above the endothelial cell culture (Kang et al., 2008).

In vessel remodeling is also relevant the role of pericytes and smooth muscle cells in controlling lumen size and vessel wall thickness (Jacobsen et al., 2009; Pries et al., 2005; 2009). In fact, these cells can alter their (and the vessel's) mechanical properties depending on their activation state and on the chemical and mechanical stimuli in their micro-environment, through the process of tone-driven remodeling (VanBavel et al., 2006).

The mechanical mechanisms driving vascular remodeling, intussusceptive angiogenesis and sprouting angiogenesis are different. In the next section we will explore how the current mathematical modeling approaches in the literature of these three topics describe the influence of the mechanical forces in each process. We start, however, by analyzing the modeling strategies used to address the mechanics of vascular stability.

3. Modeling mechanical processes in vessels development

3.1 Vascular stability: stresses in blood vessels

Blood vessels in physiological conditions are under varied types of mechanical stresses. The interior layer of the vessel constituted by endothelial cells is in direct contact with the blood flow and is exposed to the blood pressure and to the flow produced wall shear stress (see Figure 1). The wall shear stress is the main remodeling agent in vascular systems (Jacobsen et al., 2009). Blood vessels also exhibit a stretch in the longitudinal direction which ranges between 1.4 and 1.6 (Learoyd & Taylor, 1966). This stretch is the result of a longitudinal stress imposed by the tissue and its absence may lead to vessel malformations (Goriely & Vandiver, 2010). On the other hand, the circumferential stress is related to the vascular pressure but also to the structure and properties of the vascular wall, which provides blood vessels with high residual stresses. These residual stresses are closely related to vascular remodeling (Fung, 1991).

Due to the large axial stretch and residual stresses in arteries, a study of the mechanical properties of vessels cannot be done using elementary mechanics, since these large displacements require the use of non-linear continuum mechanics. Models of this type of vessel mechanical properties have to consider the different layers of arteries, since their layered structure is responsible for the large residual stresses (Holzapfel et al., 2000). These models do not take in consideration the genetic response of the vessel cells and do not describe vascular remodeling, however, the use non-linear continuum mechanics can provide important insights about the stability of single vessels and vessel networks.

The area of non-linear elastic modeling of vessels is very active (Fung, 1991; Holzapfel et al., 2000; Holzapfel & Weizsäcker, 1998; Ogden, 2003; Rachev & Hayashi, 1999), and to exemplify the methods used by this community, we will look into detail to the work of Goriely & Vandiver (2010). These authors have extended the model in Holzapfel et al. (2000) to consider vessel growth. In the formalism used, the deformation gradient tensor $\mathbf{F}(\mathbf{X}, t)$ relating the transformation from an initial unstressed reference state $\mathcal{B}_0$ (with a material point

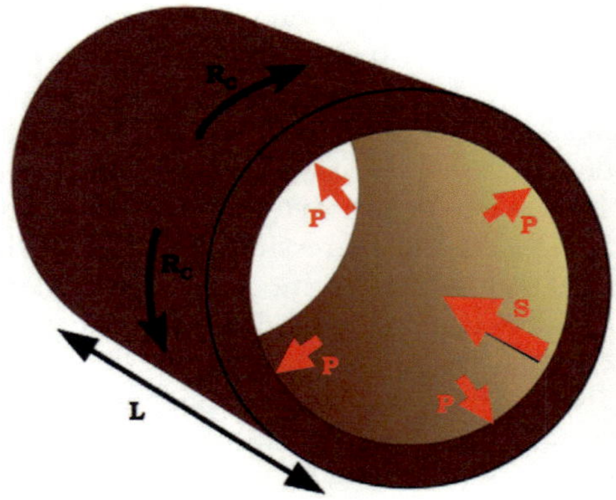

Fig. 1. Forces related to the vessel wall. Arrows in red represent forces exerted by the blood flow on the endothelial layer: pressure forces normal to the interior of the vessel (**P**) and the shear stress of the flow, in the flow direction (**S**). Arrows in black represent forces that, though influenced by the blood flow, may have a different origin: longitudinal forces (**L**) and circumferential stresses ($\mathbf{R_C}$). Figure based on Jacobsen et al. (2009) with permission of Elsevier B. V.

given by a position vector **X**) to the current state $\mathcal{B}_f$ (at time t) is the result of a local growth step defined by the tensor **G** and an elastic process **A**. The local growth transformation originates conceptually a virtual discontinuous stress-free configuration $\mathcal{V}$, which, through the elastic process **A**, leads finally to the stressed continuous current configuration $\mathcal{B}_f$ (see Figure 2):

$$\mathbf{F}(\mathbf{X},t) = \mathbf{A}(\mathbf{X},t) \cdot \mathbf{G}(\mathbf{X},t) \,. \tag{1}$$

In the final step, the interior blood pressure **P** is included as a boundary condition in order to obtain the correct stresses in the vessel as a function of the flow pressure. The wall shear stress is not considered.

The experiments of cutting an artery and measuring the opening angle (see conformation $\mathcal{B}_1$ in Figure 2) allow the quantification of the residual stresses in the current conformation $\mathcal{B}_f$. In Goriely & Vandiver (2010) this analysis is done using the parameters measured experimentally for a rabbit carotid artery. Having obtained the residual stresses, the authors calculate the value of the stresses in the system as a function of the pressure. The total stress is much lower in the system with residual stress than in a hypothetic vessel without residual stresses. This is the traditional function associated with residual stresses in Biology and Engineering: to decrease the stress the system undergoes when subjected to pressure forces (Fung, 1991).

Afterwards the authors study the behavior of the pressure in function of the axial stretch observed for different external loads. They observe that for higher external loads, the stretch becomes approximately independent of the interior pressure, thus providing a biological function for the high stretches in arteries.

Finally the authors preform a stability analysis where they observe that a increase in pressure or a decrease in the external load leads to a buckling instability. They suggest that the remodeling of the artery after the instability may lead to permanent tortuosity, though this step is out of the scope of this modeling approach. Permanent vessel tortuosity is a hallmark

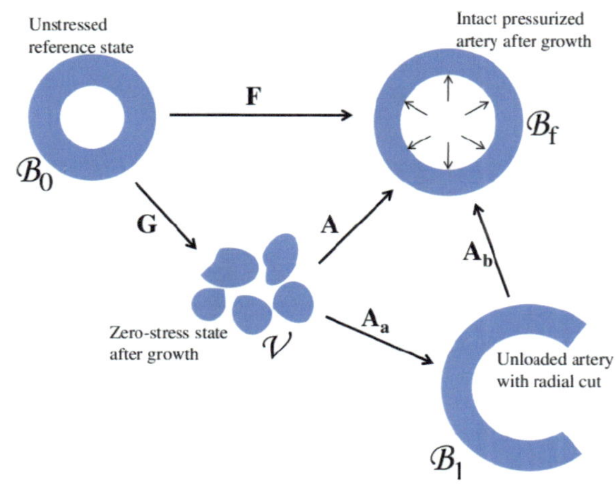

Fig. 2. Schematic representation of the decomposition of the deformation tensor **F** into growth tensor **G** and elastic deformation tensor **A**. In the presence of a radial cut, the boundary conditions are different and the elastic deformation tensor $\mathbf{A_a}$ will also be different. In both conformations $\mathcal{B}_f$ and $\mathcal{B}_1$ residual stresses are present. Figure from Goriely & Vandiver (2010) with permission of Oxford University Press.

of various pathological scenarios such as proliferative diabetic retinopathy and also may lead to stroke, vertigo or permanent tinnitus.

Models using non-linear elasticity such as the one presented above provide a detailed analysis of the mechanical forces in vessels. These models are rather complex and though do not include the biological driven alteration of the mechanical properties of the tissues, they are still extremely useful in laying down the conditions needed for vessel stability. These models could be used to tackle important questions such as: how would the vessel stability be influenced as a function of the tissue mechanical properties?, how is the external load applied *in vivo*?, what are the required geometries of bifurcations and the corresponding vessel lengths in order for a network in a particular tissue to be stable?

3.2 Vessel remodeling

Using the previously discussed models, the stresses could in principle be calculated and used to predict how the cells respond to alterations in the mechanical cues of the environment. Hence, mathematical models have been developed that are able to calculate the mechanical adaptation of the system and draw important conclusions related to relevant biological mechanisms regulating this process. These models are based in experimental observations, for example on the data of how does a vessel diameter changes in response to an increase in the wall shear stress, and aim at describing the progressive change in vessel morphology and the consequent development of a hierarchical structure in a vessel network.

Vessels can alter independently their lumen diameter (by a process called *remodeling*) and their wall area (*trophic* response, see Figure 3) by responding to mechanical and physiological cues in their micro-environment. These alterations may be the result of cell rearrangement (smooth muscle cells may rearrange themselves, leading to a change in lumen diameter while keeping the same wall area, i.e. leading to eutrophic remodeling), or smooth muscle cells or endothelial cells may undergo extension, contraction, proliferation or apoptosis, leading to

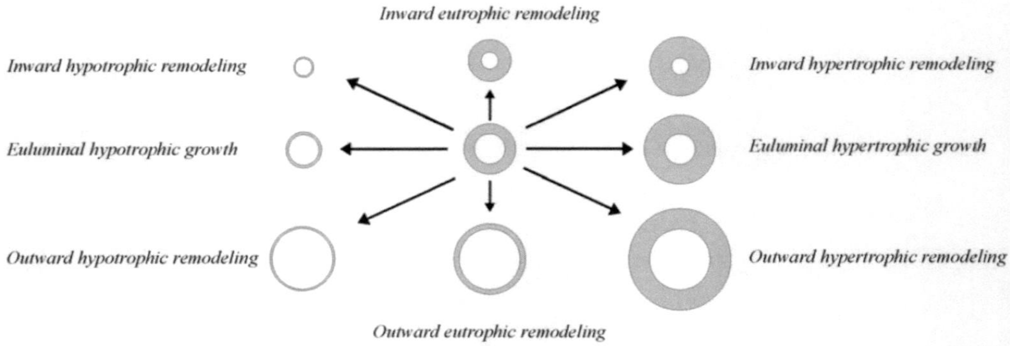

Fig. 3. Possible models of remodeling (lumen diameter change) and trophic response (change of vessel wall area). Figure based on Mulvany (1999) with permission of Oxford University Press.

alterations both in lumen size and wall area. Essentially, the micro-environmental cues are transduced at cell level leading to complex signaling pathways and a consequent alteration of the cell's properties and/or gene expression. These signaling pathways are theme of intense investigation nowadays, and most of their mechanisms are not yet known. The solution adopted by many models of vessel remodeling is either using dependences obtained from *in vitro* and *in vivo* experiments or using educated guesses about these dependences (Jacobsen et al., 2009).
The influence of the ECM is not explored in the current models of vessel remodeling (Jacobsen et al., 2009; Waters et al., 2011): the ECM has been interpreted as serving as support for the vessels, while the major mechanical role is played by the blood flow, the stresses acting upon the vessels, and the tissue nutrient requirement. Moreover, most models use a rather simplified description of both flow and vessel elasticity (typically using the Kirchhoff laws and the Poiseuille flow profile, with some models considering the Fåhræus-Lindqvist effect, to obtain blood flow, pressure and shear stresses; and being still far from the non-linear elastic description introduced previously), and because of the lack of knowledge about the cell response to the mechanical stimuli *in vivo*, a careful calculation of the stresses in the system would not bring an increase in the precision of the results of the code.
Nevertheless, in spite of this lack of biochemical knowledge, mathematical models have been very important in providing evidence for new mechanisms relative to cell-cell communication (Pries et al., 2009; 2010; Pries & Secomb, 2008). The model described in Pries & Secomb (2008), and also used in complex multi-scale simulations of vascular dynamics (Owen et al., 2009; Perfahl et al., 2011), takes into account both mechanical and metabolical stimuli relevant to vessel dynamics. It focuses on lumen dynamics, not considering alterations in the vessel wall area. Essentially, the diameter D of a particular vessel is given by

$$\frac{1}{D}\frac{\partial D}{\partial t} = k_h(S_t + k_p S_p) + k_m(S_m + k_c S_c) - k_s\,, \tag{2}$$

where k_h, k_p, k_m, and k_c are constants, S_t, S_p, S_m, and S_c are the different stimuli for the vessel to grow and k_s represents the tendency of the vessel to shrink if no stimuli are present. The first two stimuli represent the tendency for the vessel to become wider with increasing pressure and wall shear stress. The stimulus S_m represents the response to the concentration of a metabolite present in the blood flow which is included in the current at a rate proportional to the lack of oxygenation of the tissue at that particular point. When entering the blood stream, the metabolite flows with the current triggering the response of increasing vessel thickness if there is little oxygenation. Pries & Secomb (2008) show that the model is only able to provide reasonable results, if there is a counter-flow signaling mechanism, through a chemokine conducted upstream along the endothelial cells of the vessel. The last stimulus, S_c, represents the response of the diameter to this last signaling mechanism.

With this model, Pries et al. (2010) address the situation of the existence of shunts connecting arterial to venous flow in tumor vasculature. Pries et al. (2010) show that the presence of S_c is sufficient for the shunt formation to be controlled. In the presence of this signaling mechanism when the shunt is formed, there is a lowering of the irrigation downwards in the vascular tree, and the signal for a vessel remodeling is sent upstream. This will lead to a thicker equilibrium artery diameter, but not to a thick shunt. Besides, since the shunt is not providing oxygenation to the tissue it may regress due to the k_s term of the model. The authors suggest that in a tumor this mechanism is altered giving rise to a non functional vessel network with a higher density of vascular shunts.

The same model is used in Pries et al. (2009) to show that a network with vascular shunts and whose vessels do not organize hierarchically is obtained after running the model on a normal vasculature but using the parameters that stabilize a tumor vasculature. On the other hand, a tumor vasculature may be "normalized", i.e. present a hierarchical structure, by carrying out remodeling with the parameters of a healthy tissue.

Hence the authors suggest that malformations in the tumor vasculature might be the result of deficient remodeling. Therefore the biochemical mechanisms involved in vascular remodeling may be a valid target for anti-angiogenic therapy.

While most of the recently published work in vascular network remodeling *in silico* is based on models which compute the different stimuli and simulate lumen dynamics, there are other models in the literature that go further, by focusing as well on the description of the vessel wall dynamics (Jacobsen et al., 2003). On the other hand, other researchers adopt a rather different strategy and use rule-based cellular automata (Peirce et al., 2004) to predict the evolution of the network.

Modeling vessel remodeling, even under the simplified setting up discussed in this section, can suggest mechanisms that can be pivotal in vessel remodeling in pathological scenarios and that are worthwhile to investigate. However, integrating more precise descriptions of the mechanics in these models would require more experimental work leading to the understanding of how the different cells respond to the different mechanical factors.

3.3 Intussusceptive angiogenesis

Angiogenesis occurs when new vessels have to be created in order to vascularize a growing tissue. In tissues with a little number of vessels, through the process of sprouting angiogenesis new capillaries sprout from existing vessels. Sprouting angiogenesis is a slow process that is dependent on the migration of endothelial cells and also on their proliferation, and occurs extensively in embryo growth and in retinas of new-born mice, for example.

On the other hand, in situations where a vasculature already exists, intussusceptive angiogenesis occurs with the aim of increasing local vessel density. In this process vessels divide in two through the insertion and extension of a transluminar pillar (see Figure 4). This type of angiogenesis occurs in inflammation and in tumor growth. It is fast and does not depend on proliferation. The resulting thinner vasculature is afterwards target of remodeling in a maturation process (as described previously).

Mechanical forces are at the onset of intussusceptive angiogenesis, which is enhanced with an increase of the flow velocity (Djonov et al., 2002). Blood flow simulations in the geometries

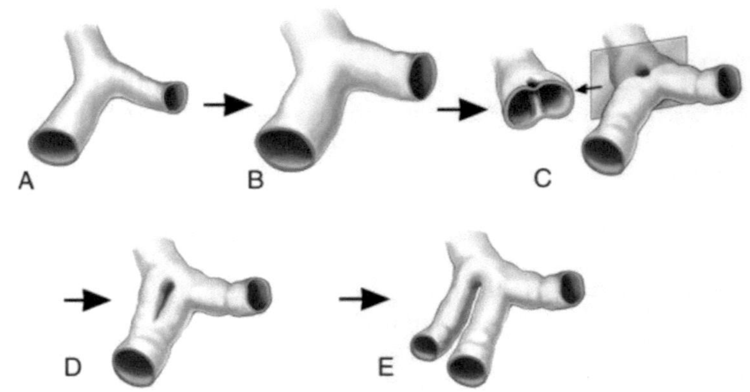

Fig. 4. Intussusceptive angiogenesis: from formation of pillar until the branching of a new vessel. Figure from Filipovic et al. (2009) with permission of Elsevier B. V.

of a bifurcation have identified the location of the new pillars with the regions of low shear stress (Styp-Rekowska et al., 2011). In Figure 5A the wall shear stress is plotted in a bifurcation of two vessels (Filipovic et al., 2009). It is clearly visible a ring of low stress just before the bifurcation apex. It is in this region where the pillar will be formed.

In Figure 5B it is observed that when the pillar is formed, the high stresses are located on the sides of the pillar, closer to the lateral vessel walls, while there is a "dead zone" of very low stress between the pillar and the bifurcation apex. The growing of the pillar comes from this anisotropic distribution of stresses around it, and can extend in different directions depending on the relative flow of the two out vessels (Filipovic et al., 2009).

The main mechanisms responsible for the formation of the pillar are still unknown. It is suggested that there is a softening of the capillary wall allowing it to bend inwards in the region of low shear stress, until the two walls merge and form the pillar (Djonov et al., 2002). This softening is blamed on the regression of the fibers that provide rigidity to the vessel. However more mathematical and experimental studies should be done to unravel the mechanics of pillar formation.

Simulations of the process of pillar evolution are very challenging because of the interplay between continuum mechanics, flow and biological mechanisms, many of which are not yet known. Recently Szczerba et al. (2009) have implemented a level-set model of pillar evolution. Their model integrates the blood flow, simulated through Navier-Stokes equation together with the incompressibility condition and a shear dependent viscosity $\eta = m\dot{\gamma}^{n-1}$, where m and n are system parameters and $\dot{\gamma}$ is the shear rate. The concentration of various proteins in the blood can also be tracked through a diffusion-convection-reaction equation:

$$\partial_t c + \mathbf{u} \cdot \nabla c = D\nabla^2 c + R_c \, , \tag{3}$$

where c is the concentration of the protein advected in the blood flow with velocity $\mathbf{u}$ and diffusion constant D. R_c is a reaction term describing the reactions in which the protein participates.

The remodeling agents considered are the measured shear stress on the capillary wall, the concentration of pro- and anti-angiogenic factors (modeled by equation (3)) and the wall surface tension (giving rise to a velocity proportional to the local curvature in the direction of straightening up the vessel locally). The velocity of the wall is a function of the value of

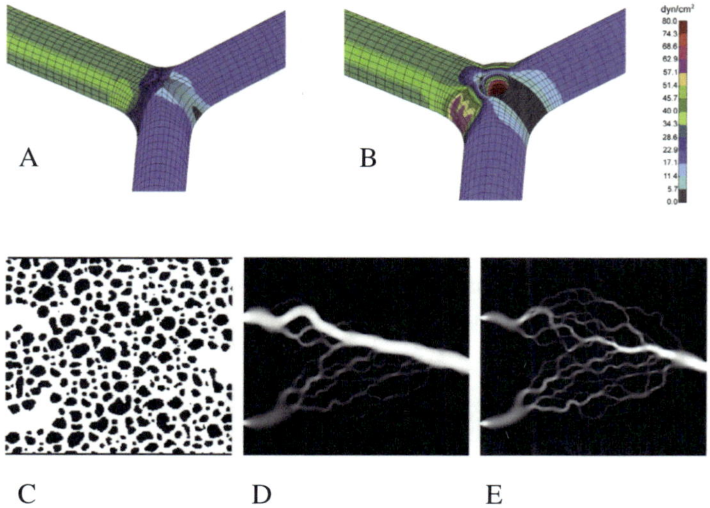

Fig. 5. Wall shear stress for a flow simulation of a Newtonian fluid in the geometry of a bifurcation (A) without pillar and (B) with a 10 μm diameter pillar. Figure from Filipovic et al. (2009) with permission of Elsevier B. V. Remodeling of an initial set of pillars (C) into a differentiated network. Flow pattern in the absence of any additional control: a large arterio-venous shunt forms (D). If, on the other hand, a steadily increasing concentration of strengthening fibers is considered, the arterio-venous anastomosis is avoided and numerous capillary vessels remain (E). Figure from Szczerba et al. (2009) with permission of Elsevier B. V.

these agents. However since the real dependence of the velocity on each one of these agents is not known experimentally, the authors consider the following simple form:

$$\mathbf{v} \sim (K - K_0) \frac{c_+}{c_+ + c_0} \mathbf{n} \,, \tag{4}$$

where K is the wall shear stress, K_0 the target shear stress, c_+ and c_- are respectively the concentration of pro- and anti-angiogenic factors, c_0 corresponds to the concentration of strengthening fibers and $\mathbf{n}$ is the normal vector pointing outwards.

First the authors simulate the model in three dimensions for the creation of a single pillar in the center of a vessel and its remodeling. They observe that the existence of the pillar increases the shear stresses in the walls near the pillar, leading to a force exerted on the pillar which leads to its elongation in the direction of the flow. This effect is verified experimentally (Hsiai et al., 2002). However the simulation in 3D is not feasible for a large system, and the authors opt for simulating a vascular network in 2D.

In Figure 5C the starting vascular network used in Szczerba et al. (2009) is presented. In this figure the black domains correspond to the spaces between vessels: the blood goes from left to right connecting the two arteries to the vein. When the system is remodeled with constant values of the factor concentrations, the authors observe non-functional network with a shunt connecting directly the artery and the vein (see Figure 5D). However when the concentration of strengthening fibrils or the concentration of anti-angiogenic factor increases progressively, the authors observe the creation of a hierarchical remodeled network (Figure 5E).

This model suggests new hypothesis about the mechanisms controlling intussusceptive angiogenesis and the creation of hierarchical vessel networks. In particular, it suggests that implementing mechanics is not enough to obtain a functional network. For the hierarchical network to be formed, something has to change progressively (concentrations of fibers or of angiogenic factors in this case), i.e. the system has to be driven.

As with vascular remodeling, many mechanisms present in intussusceptive angiogenesis are still unknown. Mathematical and computational modeling can definitely play an important role in understanding this process helping to determine what are the possible mechanisms present and what is the role of each one of them; how can the forces exerted by one cell on its neighbor be described; or what is the effect of the layering structure of the vessels in this process.

3.4 Sprouting angiogenesis

The process of sprouting angiogenesis is strikingly different form intussusceptive angiogenesis. It starts when endothelial cells of existing capillaries acquire the tip cell phenotype by the action of a protein cocktail produced typically by tissue cells in a hypoxic micro-environment. Tip cells lead the growth of new capillary sprouts formed by other endothelial cells which acquire the stalk cell phenotype. The migration of endothelial tip cells is directed towards increasing concentrations of relevant growth factors. The angiogenic role of VEGF is opposed by different anti-angiogenic factors in the tissue (Figg & Folkman, 2008). After the sprouting, further processes such as anastomosis (linkage of different branches on the network), and vessel remodeling by the blood flow and the intrinsic mechanical properties of the tissue, contribute to the formation of the new vessel network and are finely tuned to determine the final vascular patterning (Jones et al., 2006).

The tip cell migration is regulated in part by the production of extracellular MMPs (Matrix MetalloProteinases) that are responsible for the remodeling of nearby ECM. The movement of the sprout through the ECM is only possible through an accurate positioning of the regions where its cells exert traction forces on the matrix, and the zones where the ECM fibers are degraded by the action of MMPs (Ilina & Friedl, 2009). Forces and MMPs work as remodeling agents of the ECM: traction forces align the fibers in the ECM, while MMPs cleave the fibers and thus alter the mechanical properties of the ECM. Endothelial cells' traction forces are improved in stiffer gels (Discher et al, 2005; Pelham & Wang, 1997), and mobility and sprout development is improved in more compliant tissues (see review Shiu et al. (2005)). These complex mechanisms in sprout growing, result in a nontrivial dependence on the mechanical properties of the ECM (modeled in Painter (2009), for example).

In spite of the mathematical modeling of sprouting angiogenesis literature being very vast (Alarcón, 2009; Mantzaris et al., 2004; Peirce, 2008), most models, do not focus on the mechanical mechanisms of this process, except for modeling haptotaxis (Cai et al., 2009; Chaplain et al., 2006; Holmes & Sleeman, 2000), i.e. the influence of a non-uniform distribution of fibers in the migration of the sprouts. The hypothesis behind haptotaxis modeling is that an increase in fibronectin, or other similar protein, implies an increase in cellular traction forces, and so, the endothelial cells move along the gradient of fibronectin. Fibronectin in these models is produced and consumed by endothelial cells.

The choice for using a simplified description of mechanical processes, such as the one mentioned above, in most models of sprouting angiogenesis is understandable since the two main mechanisms driving sprouting angiogenesis are endothelial cell chemotaxis and proliferation. Nevertheless, there is nowadays an increasing need for models to provide quantitative predictions about vessel growth, and therefore the complex relations between the mechanical properties of the tissue and endothelial cell motility cannot keep being overlooked in this context.

Recently Bauer et al. (2009) implemented a two-dimensional cellular-Potts model of sprouting angiogenesis with the aim of investigating computationally the influence of matrix remodeling and fiber density orientation in vessel dynamics. In a cellular-Potts model each individual cell is a domain associated with an individual Potts ground-state (Graner & Glazier, 1992). The hamiltonian differs from the Potts hamiltonian since there are targets domain area and perimeter length, and an energy cost is associated to deviations from those targets. In other words, 2D cellular-Potts models create a tapestry of domains that during their dynamics maintain approximately their areas and perimeter lengths, akin to many real living cells.

In Bauer et al. (2009) the authors adapt the cellular-Potts model to sprouting angiogenesis, by including terms in the hamiltonian describing the chemotaxis and the adhesion to the matrix fibers (endothelial cells may grow filopodia and thus extend their perimeter, and so the perimeter constraint is not included in the model). The model also considers the different adhesions between an endothelial cell and the matrix fibers, the interstitial fluid and another endothelial cell. The authors explore carefully the parameter range of the model, comparing to experimental data, and thus obtaining its range of validity.

The authors observe a complex dependence of the sprout dynamics as a function of the matrix fiber fraction. At low fiber fractions the sprouts are thin, and ramified (since the matrix is sparse and in-homogeneous enough for some of the sprout cells to extend along directions not collinear with the leading VEGF gradient). As the fiber fraction increases it forms a scaffolding for the chemotaxis, and thus the number of branches decreases and the maximum sprout velocity is attained. For higher fiber density adhesion starts to dominate, the sprouting velocity becomes lower and the vessels thicker. Finally at very high fiber density, the sprouts are not able to form; though sprouting in these conditions is recovered by including in the model matrix degradation by the MMPs. These regimes have been recently observed in *in vitro* experiments (Shamloo & Heilshorn, 2010).

The model also predicts that matrix realignment does not influence in an appreciable manner the sprout velocity at low fiber densities, while at average densities variations in the fiber alignment can double the growth velocity. With respect to matrix degradation, it leads to an increase of sprout velocity (except for low matrix densities), and to more branching events.

While the cellular-Potts model is not a model suitable to study the effect of the elasticity or viscoelasticity of tissues in angiogenesis, since it does not include an unstressed reference frame, or a viscoelastic relaxation time, it is able to describe the adhesion properties of cells to the matrix fibers, thus putting forward relevant hypothesis about the complex dynamics of sprout formation that go well beyond the traditional haptotaxis formulation.

However, viscoelastic effects of the ECM in sprouting angiogenesis modeling have been included by some authors through coupling the endothelial cell movement to a spring-dashpot viscoelastic model of the ECM (Cai et al., 2009; Holmes & Sleeman, 2000) by incorporating a description used in vasculogenesis modeling (Murray & Oster, 1984) and in other models of cell locomotion (Moreo et al., 2010). The same spring-dashpot viscoelastic model has been used to model the elasticity of the endothelial cells themselves (Jackson & Zheng, 2010). Before concluding about the influence of the mechanical properties in angiogenesis, this type of modeling should be extended to other kinds of viscoelastic descriptions of the ECM, explored the coupling mechanisms of the ECM with the endothelial cells and compared to experimental results.

4. Conclusion

In this chapter we explored some of the most relevant mechanisms related to the mechanics of vessel growth and described the strategies used by several groups to model these mechanisms. Forces and the tissue mechanical properties are central to the different processes of vessel growth, nevertheless many of the details are not yet understood. While using non-linear elasticity to describe vessels and tissues permits the analysis of the stresses and strains in the system with great detail, the difficulty of implementing such models in a large system together with the lack of knowledge of how the different cells respond to the forces and interact with each other, lead to very different strategies in describing intussusceptive angiogenesis and vascular remodeling. Also, sprouting angiogenesis is controlled to great measure by the mechanical properties of endothelial cells and of the ECM, however very few models explore these features.

One of the possible strategies for the task of including mechanics in the sprouting angiogenesis modeling, is the use of the phase-field model. Originally developed by the physics community in the context of non-equilibrium systems, it achieved great success over the past decades in describing a whole range of Materials Science phenomena related to nucleation and growth. The phase-field permits an elegant and multifaceted numerical description of complex nonlinear problems with moving boundaries, being a tailorable method that can be easily adapted to describe quantitatively an extremely vast range of mechanical and dynamical properties of interfaces as a function of the bulk properties (Emmerich, 2008). In Materials Science, the various phase-field applications developed so far have matured sufficiently to allow their use in realistic applications with a high degree of accuracy. In tumor and angiogenesis modeling the use of phase-field simulations is currently in its early stages of development with promising results (Oden et al., 2010; Travasso et al., 2011a;b). Phase-field models are able to describe systems with different mechanical properties and are a great promise for exploring the influence of the tissue mechanics on vessel development.

We are left with the feeling that we are still starting to unveil the complexity of phenomena and interactions between the different cells, tissues and proteins related with vessel development. New mechanisms are being discovered that require to be understood in a quantitative way. For example, complete networks have been found to migrate *in vitro* in the presence stresses in the ECM (see Figure 6) (Kilarski et al., 2009). It is suggested that this mechanism could occur in cicatrization, explaining the fast growth of the vascularization in these emergencies. What are the forces that play an important role here? Can a vasculature be so easily affected by the action of stresses? How can we take advantage of this fact to help in the treatment of tumor growth, diabetic retinopathy, or heart ischemia? Mathematical modeling can obviously help in answering these questions, by providing testable hypothesis. Modeling can also determine

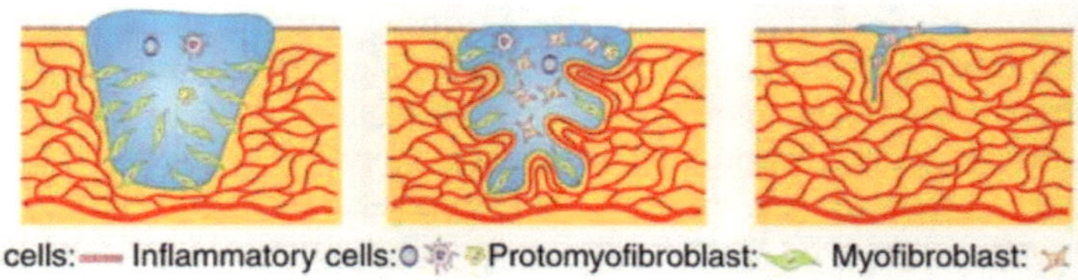

Fig. 6. Proposed model for dermal wound healing following the experiments on chick chorioallantoic membrane from Kilarski et al. (2009). Mechanical stresses provided by the fibroblasts pull the vasculature in the direction of closing the wound. Figure from Kilarski et al. (2009) with permission of Nature Publishing Group.

the mechanisms driving the process since it permits to test individually the effect of each one of them.
Much can be gained by following the research in the mechanical properties of vessel growth since it is pivotal in diverse pathological contexts, and this research can lead to definitive progresses in the therapeutics. However a stronger collaborative effort between Mathematics, Physics, computational simulations, together with advances in the understanding of the underlying biological processes has to be undertaken.

5. Acknowledgments

This work was supported by Fundos FEDER through Programa Operacional Factores de Competitividade - COMPETE and by Fundação para a Ciência e Tecnologia, through the project with reference number FCOMP-01-0124-FEDER-015708. It was also supported by Fundação Calouste Gulbenkian and Fundação para a Ciência e Tecnologia through the *Estímulo à Investigação* and *Ciência 2007* programs, respectively.

6. References

Adair T.H. & Montani, J.-P. (2010). *Angiogenesis*, Morgan & Claypool Life Sciences, San Rafael

Alarcón, T (2009). Modelling tumour-induced angiogenesis: A review of individual-based models and multiscale approaches, in *Mathematics, developmental biology and tumor growth*, 45-76, Herrero, M. A. & Giraldez, F. Eds., American Mathematical Society, Providence

Alberts, B. et al. (2002). *Molecular Biology of the Cell* (4th edn.), Garland, NewYork

Allen, R. J.; Bogle, I. D. L. & Ridley, A. J. (2011). A model of localised Rac1 activation in endothelial cells due to fluid flow, *J. Theor. Biol.*, Vol. 280, 34-42

Araújo, R.P. & McElwain, D.L.S. (2004). A history of the study of solid tumour growth: the contribution of mathematical modelling, *Bull. Math. Biol.*, Vol. 66, 1039-91

Bauer, A.L.; Jackson, T.L. & Jiang, Y. (2007). A cell-based model exhibiting branching and anastomosis during tumor-induced angiogenesis, *Biophys. J.*, Vol. 92, 3105-21

Bauer, A. L.; Jackson, T. L. & Jiang, Y. (2009). Topography of extracellular matrix mediates vascular morphogenesis and migration speeds in angiogenesis, *PLoS Comp. Biol.*, Vol. 5, e1000445

Bentley, K.; Gerhardt, H. & Bates, P.A. (2008). Agent-based simulation of Notch-mediated tip cell selection in angiogenic sprout initialisation. *J. Theo. Biol*, Vol. 250, 25-36

Bray, D. (2001). *Cell Movements* (2nd edn.), Garland, New York

Cai, Y. et al. (2009). Numerical simulation of tumor-induced angiogenesis influenced by the extra-cellular matrix mechanical environment, *Acta Mech. Sin.* Vol. 25, 889-95

Califano, J. P. & Reinhart-King, C. A. (2009). The effects of substrate elasticity on endothelial cell network formation and traction force generation, *31st Annual Inter. Conference of the IEEE EMBS*, 3343-45, Minneapolis

Chaplain, M.A.J.; McDougall, S.R. & Anderson, A.R.A. (2006). Mathematical modeling of tumor-induced angionenesis, *Annu. Rev. Biomed. Eng.*, Vol. 8, 233-57

Chlench, S. et al. (2007). Regulation of Foxo-1 and the angiopoietin-2/Tie2 system by shear stress, *FEBS Lett.*, Vol. 581, 673-80

Disher, D.E.; Janmey, P. & Wang, Y. (2005). Tissue cells feel and respond to the stiffness of their substrate, *Science*, Vol. 310, 1139-43

Djonov, V. G.; Kurz, H. & Burri, P. H. (2002). Optimality in the developing vascular system:branching remodeling by means of intussusception as an efficient adaptation mechanism, *Dev. Dyn.*, Vol. 224, 391-402

Emmerich, H. (2008). Advances of and by phase-field modelling in condensed-matter physics, *Adv. Phys.*, Vol. 57, 1-87

Figg, W.D. & Folkman, J. (2008). *Angiogenesis - an integrative approach from science to medicine*, Springer, New York; for example

Filipovic, N. et al. (2009). Computational flow dynamics in a geometric model of intussusceptive angiogenesis, *Microvasc. Res.*, Vol. 78, 286-93

Friedl, P. (2004). Prespecification and plasticity: shifting mechanisms of cell migration, *Curr. Opinion Cell Biol.* Vol. 16, 14-23

Friedl, P. & Wold, K. (2003). Tumor cell invasion and migration, *Nature Rev. Cancer*, Vol. 3, 362-74

Fung, Y. C. (1991). What are the residual stresses doing in our blood vessels?, *Ann Biomed Eng.*, Vol.19, 237-49

Gerhardt, H. et al. (2003). VEGF guides angiogenic sprouting using endothelial tip cell filopodia, *J. Cell. Biol.*, Vol. 161, 1163-77

Gerhardt, H. & Betsholtz, C. (2005). How do endothelial cells orientate?, in *Mechanisms of Angiogenesis*, 3-16, eds Clauss, M. & Breier, G., Birkhauser, Basel

Goriely, A. & Vandiver, R. (2010). On the mechanical stability of growing arteries, *IMA J. Appl. Math.*, Vol. 75, 549-70

Graner, F. & Glazier, J. A. (1992). Simulation of biological cell sorting using a two-dimensional extended Potts model". *Phys. Rev. Lett.*, Vol. 69, 2013-16

Hohberg, M. et al. (2010). Expression of ADAMTS1 in endothelial cells is induced by shear stress and suppressed in sprouting capillaries, *J. Cell. Physiol.*, Vol. 226, 350-61

Holmes, M. J. & Sleeman, B. D. (2000). A Mathematical Model of Tumour Angiogenesis Incorporating Cellular Traction and Viscoelastic Effects, *J. Theor. Biol.*, Vol. 202, 95-112

Holzapfel, G. A.; Gasser, T. C. & Ogden, R. W. (2000). A new constitutive framework for arterial wall mechanics and a compartive study of material models, *J. Elasticity*, Vol. 61, 1-48

Holzapfel, G. A. & Weizsäcker, H. W. (1998).Biomechanical behavior of the arterial wall and its numerical characterization, *Computers Biol. Med.*, Vol. 28, 377-92

Hsiai, T.K. et al. (2002). Endothelial cell dynamics under pulsating flows: significance of high versus low shear stress slew rates ($\partial\tau/\partial t$), *Ann. Biomed. Eng.*, Vol. 30, 646-56

Ilina, O. & Friedl, P. (2009). Mechanisms of collective cell migration at a glance, *J. Cell. Sci*, Vol. 122, 3203-08

Jain, RK (2005). Normalization of tumor vasculature: an emerging concept in antiangiogenic therapy, *Science*, Vol. 307, 58-62

Jacobsen, J. C.; Gustafsson, F. & Holstein-Rathlou, N.-H. (2009). A model of physical factors in the structural adaptation of microvascular networks in normotension and hypertension, *Physiol. Meas.*, Vol. 24, 891-912

Jacobsen, J. C. B.; Hornbech, M. S. & Holstein-Rathlou, N.-H. (2009). A tissue in the tissue: models of microvascular plasticity, *Eur. J. Pharm. Sci.*, Vol. 36, 51-61

Jakobsson, L. et al. (2010) Endothelial cells dynamically compete for the tip cell position during angiogenic sprouting, *Nature Cell Biol.* Vol.12, 943-53

Jackson, T. & Zheng, X. (2010). A cell-based model of endothelial cell migration, proliferation and maturation during corneal angiogenesis, *Bull. Math. Biol.*, Vol. 72, 830-68

Jones, E.A.V.; le Noble, F. & Eichmann, A. (2006). What determines blood vessel structure? Genetic prespecification vs. hemodynamics, *Physiology*, Vol. 21, 338Đ95

Kang, H.; Bayless, K. J. & Kaunas, R. (2008). Fluid shear stress modulates endothelial cell invasion into three-dimensional collagen matrices, *Am. J. Physiol. Heart Circ. Physiol.*, Vol. 295, H2087-97

Kilarski, W. W.; Samolov, B.; Petersson, L.; Kvanta, A. & Gerwins, P. (2009). Biomechanical regulation of blood vessel growth during tissue vascularization, *Nature Med.*, Vol. 15, 657-64

Korff, T. & Agustin, H. G. (1999). Tensional forces in fibrillar extracellular matrices control directional capillary sprouting, *J. Cell. Sci.*, Vol. 112, 3249-58

Kraning-Rush, C. M.; Carey, S. P.; Califano, J. P.; Smith, B. N. & Reinhart-King, C. A. (2011). The role of the cytoskeleton in cellular force generation in 2D and 3D environments, *Phys. Biol.*, Vol. 8, 015009

Learoyd, B. M. & Taylor, M. G. (1966). Alterations with age in the viscoelastic properties of human arterial walls, *Circul. Res.*, 18, 278-92

Maley, C.C. et al (2006). Genetic clonal diversity predicts progression to esophageal adenocarcinoma, *Nature Gen.*, Vol. 38, 468-73

Mammoto, A. et al. (2009). A mechanosensitive transcriptional mechanism that controls angiogenesis, *Nature*, Vol. 457, 1103-08

Mantzaris, N.; Webb, S. & Othmer, H. (2004). Mathematical modeling of tumor-induced angiogenesis, *J. Math. Biol.*, Vol. 49, 111-87

Markus, M.; Bohm, D. & Schmick, M. (1999). Simulation of vessel morphogenesis using cellular automata, *Math. Biosciences*, Vol. 156, 191-206

Mateus, A. R. et al. (2009). E-cadherin mutations and cell motility: a genotype-phenotype correlation, *Experimental Cell Res.*, Vol. 315, 1393-402

Mayer, R.J. (2004). Two Steps Forward in the Treatment of Colorectal Cancer, *N. Engl. J. Med.*, Vol. 350, 2406-08.

Merks, R. M. H.; Perry, E. D.; Shirinifard, A. & Glazier, J. A. (2008). Contact-inhibited chemotaxis in de novo and sprouting blood-vessel growth, *PLoS Comp. Biol.*, Vol. 4, e1000163

Milde, F.; Bergdorf, M. & Koumoutsakos, P. (2008) A hybrid model for three-dimensional simulations of sprouting angiogenesis, *Biophys. J.*, Vol. 95, 3146-60

Moreo, P.; Gaffney, E. A.; Garcìa-Aznar, J. M. & Doblaré, M. (2010). On the modelling of biological patterns with mechnochemical models: insights from analysis and computation, *Bull. Math. Biol.*, Vol. 72, 400-31

Mulvany, M. J. (1999). Vascular remodelling of resistance vessels: can we define this?, *Cardiovac. Res.*, Vol. 41, 9-13

Murray, J. D. (2003). *Mathematical Biology II: Spatial Models and Biomedical Applications*, (3rd edn.), Springer, Berlin

Murray, J. D. & Oster, G. F. (1984). Cell traction models for generation of pattern and form in morphogenesis, *J. Math. Biol.*, Vol. 19, 265-79

Nash, G. B. & Egginton, S. (2006). Modelling the effects of the haemodynamic environment on endothelial cell responses relevant to angiogenesis, in *Angiogenesis assays: a critical appraisal of current techniques*, 89-104, Staton, C. A.; Lewis, C. & Bicknell, R., Eds., John Wiley & Sons Ltd, Chichester

Nelson, C. M.; Pirone, D. M.; Tan, J. L. & Chen, C. S. (2004). Vascular endothelial-cadherin regulares cytoskeletal tension, cell spreading, and focal adhesions by stimulating RhoA, *Mol. Biol. Cell*, Vol. 15, 2943-53

Oden, J. T.; Hawkins, A. & Prudhomme, S. (2010). General diffuse-interface theories and an approach to predictive tumor growth modeling, *Math. Mod. Meth. Appl. Sci.*, Vol. 20, 477-517

Ogden, R. W. (2003). Nonlinear elasticity, anisotropy, material stability and residual stresses in soft tissue, in *Biomechanics of Soft Tissue in Cardiovascular Systems*, 65-108, Holzapfel, G. A. & Ogden, R. W. Eds., Springer, Vienna

Owen, M.R.; Alarcón, T; Maini, P.K. & Byrne, H.M. (2009). Angiogenesis and vascular remodelling in normal and cancerous tissues, *J. Math. Biol.*, Vol. 58, 689-721

Painter, K.J. (2009). Modelling cell migration strategies in the extracellular matrix, *J. Math. Biol.*, Vol. 58, 511-43

Peirce, S. M. (2008). Computational and mathematical modeling of angiogenesis, *Microcirculation*, Vol. 15, 739-51

Peirce, S. M.; Van Gieson, E. J. & Skalak, T. C. (2004). Multicallular cimulation predicts microvascular patterning and in silico tissue assembly, *FASEB J.*, Vol. 18, 731-33

Pelham, R. J. Jr & Wang, Y. (1997). Cell locomotion and focal adhesions are regulated by substrate flexibility, *Proc. Natl. Acad. Sci. USA*, Vol. 94, 13661-5

Perfahl, H. et al. (2011) Multiscale modelling of vascular tumour growth in 3D: the roles of domain size and boundary conditions, *PLoS ONE*, Vol. 6, e14790

Pries, A. R.; Reglin, B. & Secomb, T. W. (2005). Remodeling of blood vessels: responses of diameter an wall thickness to hemodynamic and metabolic stimuli, *Hypertension*, Vol. 46, 725-31

Pries, A. R. et al. (2009). Structural adaptation and heterogeneity of normal and tumor microvascular networks, *PLoS Comp. Biol.*, Vol 5, e1000394

Pries, A. R.; Höpfner, M.; le Noble, F.; Dewhirst, M. W. & Secomb, T. W. (2010). The shunt problem: control of functional shunting in normal and tumour vasculature, *Nature Rev. Cancer*, Vol. 10, 587-93

Pries, A. R. & Secomb, T. W. (2008). Modeling structural adaptation of microcirculation, *Microcirculation*, Vol. 15, 753-64

Rachev, A. & Hayashi, K. (1999). Theoretical study of the effects of vascular smooth muscle contraction on strain and stress distributions in arteries, *Ann. Biomed. Eng.*, Vol. 27, 459-68

Shamloo, A. & Heilshorn, S. C. (2010). Matrix density mediates polarization and lumen formation of endothelial sprouts in VEGF gradients, *Lab on a Chip*, Vol. 10, 3061-68

Shiu, Y.-T.; Weiss, J.A.; Hoying, J.B.; Iwamoto, M.N.; Joung, I.S. & Quam, C.T. (2005), The role of mechanical stresses in angiogenesis, *Critical Rev. Biomed. Eng.*, Vol. 33, 431-510

Styp-Rekowska, B.; Hlushchuk, R.; Pries, A. R. & Djonov, V. (2011). Intussusceptive angiogenesis: pillars against blood flow, *Acta Physiol.*, Vol. 202, 213-23

Szczerba, D.; Kurz, H. & Szekely, G. (2009). A computational model of intussusceptive microvascular growth and remodeling, *J. Theor. Biol.*, Vol. 261, 570-83

Travasso, R. D. M.; Corvera Poiré, E.; Castro, M.; Rodríguez-Manzaneque, J. C.; Hernández-Machado, A. (2011a). Tumor angiogenesis and vascular patterning: a mathematical model, *PLoS ONE*, Vol. 6, e19989

Travasso, R.D.M.; Castro, M. & Oliveira, J.C.R.E. (2011b). The phase-field model in tumor growth, *Phil. Mag.*, Vol. 91, 183-206

VanBavel, E.; Bakker, E. N.; Pistea, A.; Sorop, O. & Spaan, J. A. (2006). Mechanics of microvascular remodeling, *Clin. Hemorheol. Microcirc.*, Vol. 34, 35-41

Waters, S. L. et al. (2011). Theoretical models for coronary vascular biomechanics: progresses & challenges, *Prog. Biophys. Mol. Biol.*, Vol. 104, 49-76

Wood, L.D. et al. (2007). The genomic landscapes of human breast and colorectal cancers, *Science*, Vol. 318, 1108-13

10

A Novel Adult Marrow Stromal Stem Cell Based 3-D Postnatal De Novo Vasculogenesis for Vascular Tissue Engineering

Mani T. Valarmathi and John W. Fuseler
Department of Cell Biology and Anatomy,
School of Medicine, University of South Carolina
USA

1. Introduction

Vascular diseases are one of the leading causes of significant morbidity and mortality worldwide. Vascular diseases not only occur at all levels of vascular tree but also affect multiple organs and organ systems. Organ tissue engineering, including vascular tissue engineering, has been an area of intense investigation. The current major challenge to these approaches has been the inability to vascularize and perfuse in vitro engineered tissue constructs. Attempts to provide oxygen and nutrients to cells contained in biomaterial constructs have met with varying degrees of success. Engineering a tissue of clinically relevant magnitude requires the formation of extensive and stable microvascular networks within the tissue (Brey et al., 2005). Since most in vitro engineered tissue constructs do not contain the intricate microvascular structures of native tissue, the cells contained in scaffolds heavily rely on simple diffusion for oxygenation and nutritional delivery. The majority of cells need to be within 100-200 μm of a blood supply to receive adequate oxygen and nutrients for survival (Carmeliet & Jain, 2000). Otherwise, due to diffusion gradients, the cells in the interior regions of the artificial scaffold can experience hypoxia or anoxia and undergo cellular degeneration and necrosis. Hence, this necessitates the formation of appropriate in vitro three-dimensional (3-D) plexuses of new blood vessels within the pre-implanted biomaterial constructs through the process of in situ de novo vasculogenesis/angiogenesis for organ tissue engineering.

Development of postnatal new blood vessels occurs essentially by two temporally distinct but interrelated processes, vasculogenesis and angiogenesis. Vasculogenesis is the process of blood vessel formation occurring by a de novo production of endothelial cells in an embryo (primitive vascular network) or a formerly avascular area when endothelial precursor cells (angioblasts, hemangioblasts or stem cells) migrate and differentiate in response to local cues (such as growth factors and extracellular matrix) to form new intact blood vessels (Risau & Flamme, 1995). Angiogenesis refers principally to the sprouting of new blood vessels from the differentiated endothelium of pre-existing vessels. These vascular trees or plexuses are then pruned, remodeled and extended through angiogenesis to become larger caliber vessels (Carmeliet, 2000). In addition, there exists yet another unique mechanism of neovascularization, the postnatal vasculogenesis, where new blood vessels are formed by the process of fusion and differentiation of endothelial progenitors of bone marrow origin (Valarmathi et al., 2009). This indicates a potential role for bone marrow-derived progenitor cells in postnatal neovasculogenesis and/or neoangiogenesis. This implies that additional mechanisms besides angiogenesis can occur in the adult, and has opened up the possibility to investigate the embryonic origin and development of these putative progenitor cells.

The adult bone marrow contains two subsets of multipotential stem cells, hematopoietic stem cells (HSCs) and bone marrow stromal cells or mesenchymal stem cells (BMSCs/MSCs). BMSCs are a readily available heterogeneous population of cells that can be directed to differentiate into multiple mesenchymal and non-mesenchymal cells either in vitro or in vivo (Wakitani et al., 1995; Pittenger et al., 1999; Makino et al., 1999; Fukuda et al., 2001; Bianco et al., 2001; Valarmathi et al., 2009, 2010). Most noticeably BMSCs have been induced to undergo maturation and differentiation towards vascular endothelial and smooth muscle cell lineages. Previous reports indicate that BMSCs and bone marrow-derived multipotent adult progenitor cells (MAPCs) can be differentiated into endothelial-like cells in vitro and contribute to neoangiogenesis in vivo (Oswald et al., 2004; Reyes et al., 2002; Al-Khaldi et al., 2003). Additionally, it has been shown that BMSCs can augment collateral remodeling and perfusion in ischemic models through paracrine mechanisms rather than by cellular incorporation upon local delivery (Kinnaird et al., 2004). Therefore, the identification of bone-marrow-derived (hematopoietic and non-hematopoietic stem cells) and non-bone-marrow-derived (tissue-resident stem/progenitor cells - adipose, neural, heart, skeletal muscle; peripheral and cord blood-derived stem cells) endothelial progenitors cells (EPCs) has led to the realization of potential postnatal vasculogenesis (Urbich & Dimmeler, 2004).

For the above mentioned reasons, embryonic, fetal and postnatal stem cells as well as various types of progenitor cells, can be a potential cellular source for vascular tissue engineering (Levenberg, 2005). However, the source for the early-stage developmental cells is restricted. The utility of embryonic stem cells (ESCs) and induced pluripotent stem cells (iPSCs) in facilitating vascularized tissue/organ regeneration is still in its incipient stages. A number of issues, including a propensity for some implanted ESCs/iPSCs to form benign teratomas and/or malignant teratocarcinomas in the regenerating tissue/organ, remain to be addressed. In contrast to both ESCs/iPSCs, it has been well established that the adult stem cell, BMSCs exhibit multilineage differentiation potential in a well-controlled, predictable fashion. Moreover, unlike ESCs derivation, obtaining autologous or allogeneic BMSCs is feasible and can potentially be exploited to develop tissue-engineered blood vessel constructs for therapeutic purposes. Similarly, when compared to bone marrow-derived BMSCs, repeated isolation and rapid expansion of sufficient yield of autologous and/or allogeneic non-bone-marrow-derived resident stem cells/progenitors, especially from vital organs for routine therapeutic purposes are highly constrained. On the contrary, to certain extent autologous and/or allogeneic bone marrow-derived BMSCs are amenable for repeated isolation and reasonable in vitro expansion from the patients. In addition, the significant advantage of using these BMSCs is their low immunogenicity. And these autologous or allogeneic BMSCs have been reported to be immunomodulatory and immunotolerogenic both in vitro as well as in vivo. (Aggarwal & Pittenger, 2005). Taken together, these data strongly indicate that BMSCs can represent the potential cell of choice for adult autologous and/or allogeneic stem cell based vascularized tissue regeneration.

Extracellular molecules initiate biological signals and play a critical role in the control of cellular proliferation, differentiation, and morphogenesis. Many parameters, such as the presence and amount of soluble factors such as hormones, growth factors, and cytokines or the insoluble factors such as the physical configuration of the matrix which mediate the cell-cell interactions and cell-matrix interactions, exerts strong influence on the success of angiogenic processes in vitro and presumably in vivo (Even-Ram & Yamada, 2005; Carlson, 2007). The likelihood and ultimate success of in vitro cellular differentiation depends on how closer the cell-matrix interactions and relationships' mimic to those found during normal development or regeneration. In vascular tissue engineering, the application of these principles in vivo will be important to ensure that the matrix/scaffold to be implanted can support endothelial cell proliferation and migration resulting in endothelial tube formation (Ingber & Folkman, 1989). The vital issue for realistic clinical application is whether these scaffolds with preformed network of endothelial capillaries/microvessels can survive implantation into tissue defects and subsequently be able to anastomose to the host vasculature.

We therefore hypothesized that under appropriate in vitro physicochemical microenvironmental cues (combination of growth factors and extra cellular matrix, ECM) multipotent adult BMSCs could be differentiated into vascular endothelial and smooth muscle cell lineages. To test this hypothesis, we characterized the intrinsic vasculogenic differentiation potential of adult BMSCs when seeded onto a three-dimensional (3-D) tubular scaffold engineered from aligned type I collagen strands and cultured either in vasculogenic or non-vasculogenic growth medium. In these culture conditions, BMSCs differentiated and matured into both endothelial and smooth muscle/pericyte cell lineages and showed microvascular morphogenesis. We also explored the potential of the 3-D model system to undergo postnatal de novo vasculogenesis.

2. Experimental approach

The differentiation of rat BMSCs was carried out on a 3-D tubular scaffold made up of aligned type I collagen-gel fibers. Rat BMSCs were isolated from the tibial and femoral bone marrow of adult rats. The BMSCs isolated from the bone marrow were expanded, maintained and passaged to make sure that the attached marrow stromal cells were devoid of any non-adhering populations of cells. Phenotypic characterization of the BMSCs for cell surface markers was performed by confocal microscopy (qualitative evaluation) and single-color flow cytometry (quantitative analysis). This adherent population of cells were further purified and enriched by indirect magnetic cell sorting. The cells were subjected to CD90 positive selection. The resultant enriched $CD90^+/CD34^-/CD45^-$ fractions were expanded by subculturing and subjected to flow cytometric analysis to validate the proper phenotype. This population of purified BMSCs was used in all experiments. For vasculogenic differentiation of BMSCs, the expanded and purified population of $CD90^+$ BMSCs was seeded into the collagen-gel tubular scaffold and cultured either in vasculogenic or non-vasculogenic culture medium for 28 days. At regular intervals of 7, 14, 21 and 28 days the tube cultures were assayed by RT-qPCR, immunofluorescence, ultrastructural and biochemical analyses for various endothelial and smooth muscle cell differentiation markers as shown in table 1 and 2. These times were chosen for the following reasons: these time points cover the range of both vasculogenic and angiogenic processes seen in vivo and/or in vitro and mimic the progression of microvascular development.

3. Research methods

3.1 Fabrication of tubular scaffold

Briefly, a 25 mg/ml solution of bovine collagen type I was extruded with a device that contained two counter-rotating cones. The liquid collagen was fed between the two cones and forced through a circular annulus in the presence of an NH_3-air (50-50 vol/vol) chamber. This process results in a hollow cylindrical tube of aligned collagen fibrils with an inner central lumen. The dimensions of tubes produced for this set of experiments had a length of 30 mm with a luminal diameter of 4 mm and an external diameter of 5 mm, leaving a wall thickness of 1 mm. The collagen tubes had a defined fiber angle of 18° relative to the central axis of the tube and had pores ranging from 1 to 10 μm. The tubes were sterilized using gamma radiation 1200 Gy followed by Stratalinker UV crosslinker 1800 (Stratagene) and then placed in Mosconas's solution (in mM: 136.8 NaCl, 28.6 KCl, 11.9 $NaHCO_3$, 9.4 glucose, 0.08 NaH_2PO_4, pH 7.4) (Sigma-Aldrich) containing 1 μl/ml gentamicin (Sigma-Aldrich) and incubated in 5% CO_2 at 37°C until cellular seeding (Valarmathi et al., 2010). The rationale for the particular orientation of collagen fiber was based on our previous work on cardiovascular tissue engineering (Yost et al., 2004). When proepicardial organ cells (PECs) were seeded onto this scaffold, they underwent maturation and differentiation and produced elongated vessel-like structures reminiscent of in vivo-like phenotype (Valarmathi et al., 2008).

3.2 BMSCs isolation, expansion and maintenance

The initial step is to isolate the mononuclear cells from the bone marrow by aspiration and centrifugation followed by plating and isolation of the cells based on differential adherence capacity to tissue culture dishes (passage 0 cells). Rat BMSCs were isolated from the bone marrow of adult 300g Sprague Dawley®™ SD®™ rats (Harlan Sprague Dawley, Inc.). Briefly, after deep anesthesia, the femoral and tibial bones were removed aseptically and cleaned extensively to remove associated soft connective tissues. The marrow cavities of these bones were flushed with Dulbecco's Modified Eagle Medium (DMEM; Invitrogen) and combined. The isolated marrow plugs were triturated, and passed through needles of decreasing gauge (from 18 gauge to 22 gauge) to break up clumps and cellular aggregates. The resulting single-cell suspensions were centrifuged at 200g for 5 minutes. Nucleated cells were counted using a Neubauer chamber. Cells were plated at a density of $5 \times 10^6 - 2 \times 10^7$ cells per T75 cm^2 flasks in basal medium composed of DMEM supplemented with 10% fetal bovine serum (FBS, lot-selected; Atlanta Biologicals, Inc.), gentamicin (50 μg/ml) and amphotericin B (250 ng/ml) and incubated in a humidified atmosphere of 5% CO_2 at 37°C for 7 days. The medium was replaced, and changed three times per week until the cultures become ~70% confluent (between 12 and 14 days). Cells were trypsinized using 0.05% trypsin-0.1% EDTA and re-plated at a density of 1×10^6 cells per T75 cm^2 flasks. After three passages, attached marrow stromal cells were devoid of any non-adhering population of cells. These passaged BMSCs were cryopreserved and stored in liquid nitrogen until further use (Valarmathi et al., 2011).

3.3 Immunophenotyping of BMSCs by flow cytometry and confocal microscopy

BMSCs are a heterogeneous population of cells with varying degrees of cell shapes and sizes. Stringent characterization of BMSCs used in experimental procedures is required for various cell surface markers; this is to ensure that the employed population of cells contains solely stem/progenitor cells. This will obviate the possible contaminating marrow-derived endothelial cells and macrophages that are part of the adherent population of cultured cells. Therefore, characterization of BMSCs included qualitative evaluation for various cell surface markers and was performed on cells grown in the Lab-tek™ chamber slide system™ (Nunc) using a Zeiss LSM 510 Meta confocal scanning laser microscope (Carl Zeiss, Inc.), and quantitative analysis of the same set of markers was performed by single-color flow cytometry using a Coulter® EPICS® XL™ Flow Cytometer (Beckman Coulter, Inc.) as previously described (Valarmathi et al., 2009).

Immunophenotyping of undifferentiated BMSCs for various cell surface markers by flow cytometry revealed that the fluorescent intensity and distribution of the cells stained for CD11b, CD31 and CD45 were not significantly different from the intensity and distribution of cells stained with isotype controls (Figure 1E-G), indicating that these cultures were devoid of any possible hematopoietic stem and/or progenitor cells as well as differentiated bone-marrow-derived endothelial cells. In contrast, BMSCs exhibited high expression of CD90 surface antigens (Figure 1H), which is a consistent characteristic of undifferentiated BMSCs. Phenotypic characterization using the same set of markers on BMSCs by confocal microscopy also revealed that these cells were negative for CD11b, CD31 and CD45 (Figure 1A-C) and, strongly positive for CD90 (Figure 1D). The expression profiles of these surface molecules were consistent with previous reports and the minimal criteria for defining multipotent mesenchymal stromal cells, enunciated by the international society for cellular therapy (ISCT) position statement (Dominici et al., 2006; Valarmathi et al., 2009; Reyes et al., 2002).

3.4 Purification and enrichment of CD90$^+$ BMSCs by magnetic-activated cell sorting (MACS)

Purification and enrichment of input BMSCs (such as CD45$^-$, CD34$^-$, CD90$^+$/CD105$^+$) are mandatory either using MACS (magnetic activated cell sorter) or FACS (fluorescent activated cell sorter). Since the unpurified fraction may contain sizable number of contaminating adherent macrophages and bone marrow-derived endothelial progenitors and differentiated endothelial cells. The adherent populations of BMSCs were further purified by indirect magnetic cell labeling method using an autoMACS™ Pro Separator (Miltenyi Biotech). Thus, these cells were subjected to CD90 positive selection by incubating the cells with FITC- labeled anti-CD90 antibodies (BD Pharmingen), followed by incubation with anti-FITC magnetic microbeads (Miltenyi Biotech), and passed through the magnetic columns as per the manufacturer's instructions. The resultant enriched CD90$^+$/CD34$^-$/CD45$^-$ fractions were expanded by subcultivation and subjected to flow cytometric analysis as described previously (Valarmathi et al., 2010).

3.5 BMSCs vasculogenic differentiation

For vasculogenic differentiation of BMSCs, the purified population of CD90$^+$ BMSCs were seeded into the collagen-gel tubes at a density of 0.5 x 10^6 cells/30 mm tube length and cultured either in mesenchymal stem cell growth medium supplemented with 10% FBS, penicillin and streptomycin (Poietics® MSCGM™ BulletKit®; Lonza Ltd.) or microvascular endothelial cell growth medium (Clonetics® EGM®-MV Bullet Kit®; Lonza Ltd.) supplemented with 5% FBS, bovine brain extract, human epidermal growth factor (hEGF), hydrocortisone, amphotericin B and gentamicin for 28 days. These BMSCs seeded tubes were cultured either in vasculogenic or non-vasculogenic medium for the defined time periods of 7, 14, 21 or 28 days. In addition, BMSCs were seeded in 65-mm Petri dishes at a density of 3 x 10^3 cells/cm^2 and cultured either in non-vasculogenic (MSCGM) or vasculogenic (EGMMV) medium for 7, 14, 21 or 28 days.

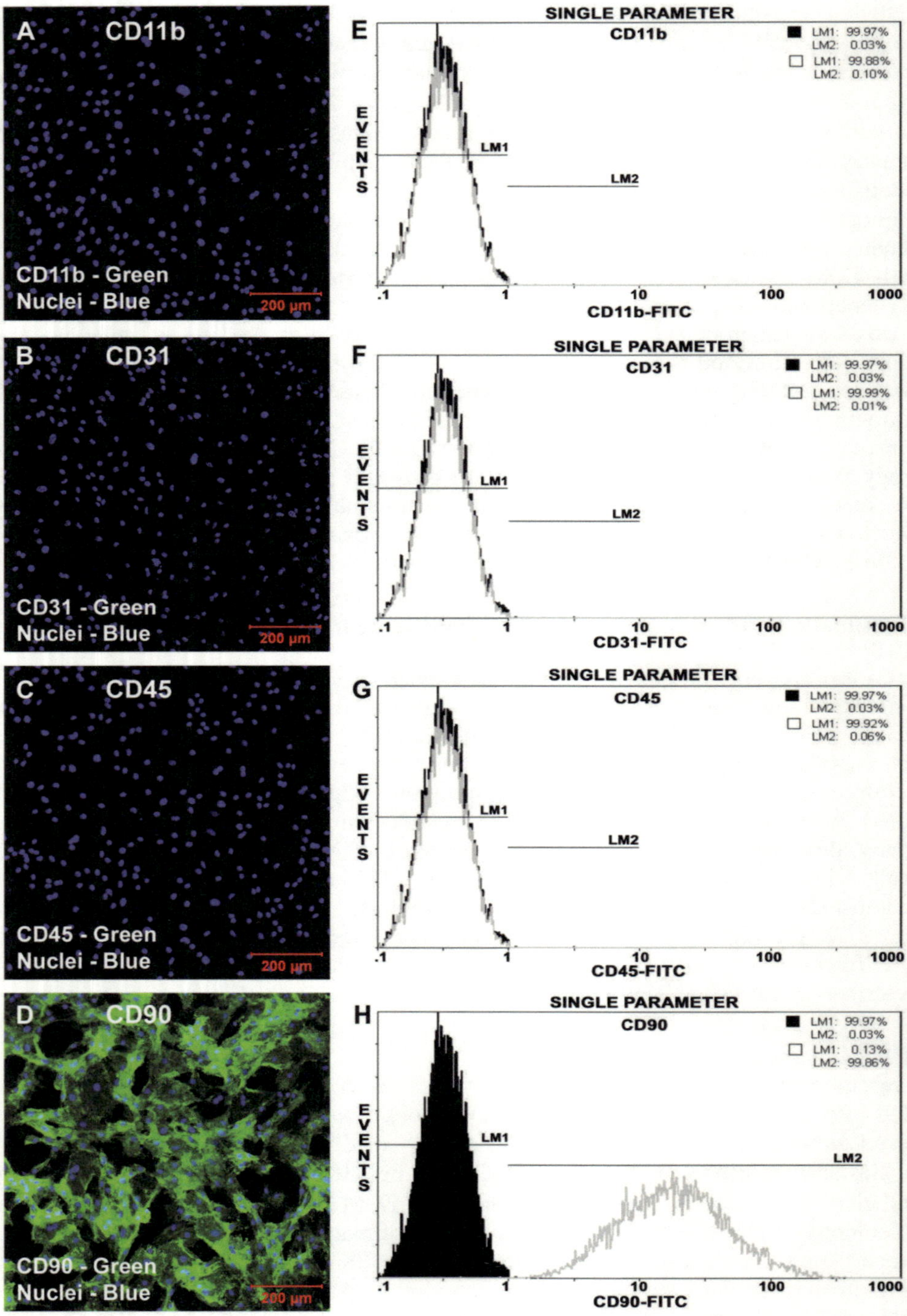

Fig. 1. Immunophenotyping of undifferentiated rat BMSCs by confocal microscopy and flow cytometry. Immunostaining and confocal microscopy revealed that BMSCs were

negative for CD11b (A), CD 31 (B) and CD45 (C) and; were uniformly positive for CD90 surface antigen (D), consistent with their undifferentiated state. Isotype and/or negative controls were included in each experiment to identify the level of background staining. Cells were also stained for nuclei (blue - DAPI). Additionally, the same population of BMSCs was subjected to flow cytometric analysis. Single parameter histograms showing the relative fluorescence intensity of staining (abscissa) and the number of cells analyzed, events (ordinate). Isotype controls were included in each experiment to identify the level of background fluorescence (black, shaded peaks). The intensity and distribution of cells stained for hematopoietic and endothelial markers; CD11b, CD31 and CD45 (grey, open peaks) were not significantly different from those of isotype control (black, shaded peaks) (E-G), indicating that these cultures were devoid of any potential contaminating hematopoietic and/or endothelial cells of bone marrow origin. The fluorescent intensity was greater (shifted to right) when BMSCs were stained with CD90 (grey) compared to isotype control (black) (H). The predominant population of BMSCs consistently expressed CD90 surface molecule, a property of rat bone marrow-derived mesenchymal/stromal stem cells. (DAPI - 4′,6-diamidino-2-phenylindole).
Merged images A-D (A-D, scale bar 200 μm).

4. BMSCs based postnatal de novo vasculogenesis and in situ vascular regeneration

The 3-D collagen-gel tubular scaffold has previously been used to create vascularized bone elements (Valarmathi et al., 2008 a, b). Here we report the utility of a 3-D tubular construct for its ability to support the vasculogenic differentiation of BMSCs culminating into microvascular structures, which are similar to those structures resulting from postnatal de novo vasculogenesis and angiogenesis (Valarmathi et al., 2008 a, b).

In the developing vertebrate embryo, the initial event of blood vessel formation is the differentiation of vascular endothelial cells, which subsequently cover the entire interior surface of all blood vessels. Angioblasts are a subpopulation of primitive mesodermal cells that are committed to differentiate into endothelial cells and later on form the primitive vascular labyrinth (Risau & Flamme, 2000). In addition, endothelial cells can also arise from hemangioblasts, a common precursor for both hematopoietic and endothelial cells (His et al., 1900).

In adults, endothelial precursor cells have been identified in bone marrow, peripheral blood and blood vessels (Prater et al., 2007). Two subsets of multipotential stem cells, HSCs and BMSCs/MSCs are resident in the postnatal bone marrow. Of these cells, BMSCs can be differentiated into osteoblasts, chondrocytes, adipocytes, smooth muscle cells and hematopoietic supportive stroma either in vitro or in vivo (Bianco et al., 2001). Previous studies have provided substantial evidence that bone-marrow-derived stem and/or progenitor cells can be differentiated into either endothelial or smooth muscle cells in vitro and in pathological situations are capable of contributing to neoangiogenesis in vivo by cellular integration (Carmeliet & Luttun, 2001).

Although there are a plethora of studies focused on developing viable scaffolds for osteogenic, chondrogenic, adipogenic and musculogenic differentiation of BMSCs (Lanza et al., 2000), the optimal scaffolds that are capable of inducing and supporting the growth and differentiation of BMSCs into vascular cell lineages are yet to be identified and characterized. Despite the much known vasculogenic potential and transgermal plasticity of BMSCs; none of these studies explicitly demonstrated the postnatal de novo vasculogenic potential of BMSCs in vitro (Reyes et al., 2002; Oswald et al., 2004).

When compared to 2-D planar cultures, the potential 3-D models of vasculogenesis allow us to understand the role of specific factors under more physiological and spatial conditions with respect to dimensionality, architecture and cell polarity. Nevertheless, the molecular composition and the natural complexity and diversity of in vivo extra cellular matrix (ECM) organization cannot be easily mimicked or reproduced in vitro (Vailhe et al., 2001). In addition, even though quite a few in vitro 3-D models of vasculogenesis based on fibrin and collagen gels are in vogue (Folkman & Haudenschild, 1980); none have explored the behavior of BMSCs and their intrinsic vasculogenic differentiation potential on a topographically structured 3-D tubular scaffold made of uniformly aligned type I collagen fibers.

Previous studies demonstrated that the formation of endothelial tubes in vitro was largely influenced by the nature of the substrate (Kleinman et al., 1982). The formation of endothelium lined tubular structures was enhanced when the substrate was rich in laminin (Madri et al., 1988), whereas a matrix rich in type I collagen would not promote rapid tubulogenesis (Montesano et al., 1983; Ingber & Folkman, 1989). Similarly, Ingber & Folkman (1989) documented that under a given cocktail of growth factors, the local physical nature of the interaction between endothelial cells and the underlying matrix/substrate ultimately determined the tubular morphogenesis. Substrates containing abundant fibronectin promoted adhesion, spreading and growth of endothelial cells. In contrast, less adhesive substrate or matrix materials that were arranged three-dimensionally permitted the endothelial cells to retract and form tubes (Ingber & Folkman, 1989).

In general, successful in vitro differentiation of cells depends on cell-cell as well as cell-matrix interactions. Therefore, we hypothesized that under appropriate in vitro local environmental cues (combination of growth factors and ECM) multipotent postnatal BMSCs could be induced to undergo microvascular development. Hence, we developed a 3-D culture system in which a pure population of $CD90^+$ rat BMSCs was seeded and cultured on a highly aligned, porous, biocompatible collagen-fiber tubular scaffold for differentiation purposes. Here, we utilized two types of growth media for vasculogenic differentiation purpose, MSCGM (non-vasculogenic) as control and EGMMV (vasculogenic) preferentially for microvascular differentiation. Both of these culture media consistently promoted the vasculogenic differentiation of BMSCs and also supported the formation of endothelium lined vessel-like structures within the constructs.

A number of early and late stage markers associated with rodent vascular development in vivo were used in this study to characterize the rat BMSCs derived microvascular structures at mRNA and protein levels, which included: CD31/Pecam1, Flt1 (Vegfr1), Flk1 (Vegfr2/Kdr), VE-cadherin (CD144), CD34, Tie1, Tek (Tie2), and Von Willibrand factor (Vwf). Platelet/endothelial cell adhesion molecule, also known as CD31, is a transmembrane protein expressed abundantly early in vascular development that may mediate leukocyte adhesion and migration, angiogenesis, and thrombosis (Albelda et al., 1991). The other early stage differentiation markers Flk1 and Flt1, which are receptors for the vascular endothelial cell growth factor-A (Vegf) essentially, play a vital role in embryonic vascular and hematopoietic development (Shalaby et al., 1997). Similarly, VE-

cadherin, a member of the cadherin family of adhesion receptors, is a specific and constitutive marker of endothelial cell plays an important role in early vascular assembly. Vascular markers that are expressed at a later stage include CD34 and Tie-2 (Bautch et al., 2000). CD34 is a transmembrane surface glycoprotein that is expressed in endothelial cells and hematopoietic stem cells. Tie1 and Tek are receptor kinases on endothelial cells that are essential for vascular development and remodeling in the embryo and may also mediate maintenance and repair of the adult vascular system. In late phases of vasculogenesis, the mature endothelial cells will synthesize and secrete Vwf homolog, a plasma protein that mediates platelet adhesion to damaged blood vessels and stabilizes blood coagulation factor VIII.
In any type of in vitro cellular differentiation, the cytodifferentiated cells need to be critically evaluated for their maturation and differentiation at transcriptional, translational and functional levels. Therefore, to study the expression pattern of key vasculogenic gene transcripts in the 3-D tube constructs; we examined the time-dependent expression pattern of Pecam1, Kdr, Tie1, Tek and Vwf at mRNA level in the tube constructs by real-time PCR (Table 1, Figure 2A-D).

Genes	Forward primer	Reverse primer	Product length (bp)	Annealing temperature (°C)	GenBank accession No
Pecam1	5′-CGAAATCTAGGCCTCAGCAC-3′	5′-CTTTTTGTCCACGGTCACCT-3′	227	56	NM_03159.1
Kdr	5′-TAGCGGGATGAAATCTTTGG-3′	5′-TTGGTGAGGATGACCGTGTA-3′	207	56	NM_013062.1
Tie1	5′-AAGGTCACACACACGGTGAA-3′	5′-TGGTGGCTGTACATTTTGGA-3′	174	56	XM_233462.4
Tek	5′-CCGTGCTGCTGAACAACTTA-3′	5′-AATAGCCGTCCACGATTGTC-3′	201	56	NM_001105737.1
Vwf	5′-GCTCCAGCAAGTTGAAGACC-3′	5′-GCAAGTCACTGTGTGGCACT-3′	163	56	XM_342759.3
Gapdh	5′-TTCAATGGCACAGTCAAGGC-3′	5′-TCACCCCATTTGATGTTAGCG-3′	101	56	XR_007416.1

Table 1. RT-qPCR primer sequences used in this study (Valarmathi et al., 2009; Rozen and Skaletsky, 2000).

Constitutive expressions of these markers were detected at low to very low levels in undifferentiated BMSCs. RT-qPCR results showed that differentiation of BMSCs under vasculogenic tube culture conditions for 28 days resulted in increased expression of transcripts coding for various endothelial cell associated proteins such as Pecam1, Kdr, Tek and Vwf. The peak expression of Vwf, the endothelial specific protein occurred around day 21 (over 400 fold) indicating that the differentiating cells acquired a distinctive phenotype and biosynthetic activity of differentiated and matured endothelial cells (Figure 2D). The upregulation of Tek during this period may represent the continual development and remodeling of the developing microvessels within the tubular constructs. Whereas differentiation of BMSCs under non-vasculogenic tube culture conditions for 14 days showed signs of early and rapid induction of transcripts coding for both early and late stage endothelial cell markers such as Kdr, Tie1, Tek and Vwf. The peak expression of Vwf occurred during day 14 (over 20 fold) (Figure 2B) (Valarmathi et al., 2009).

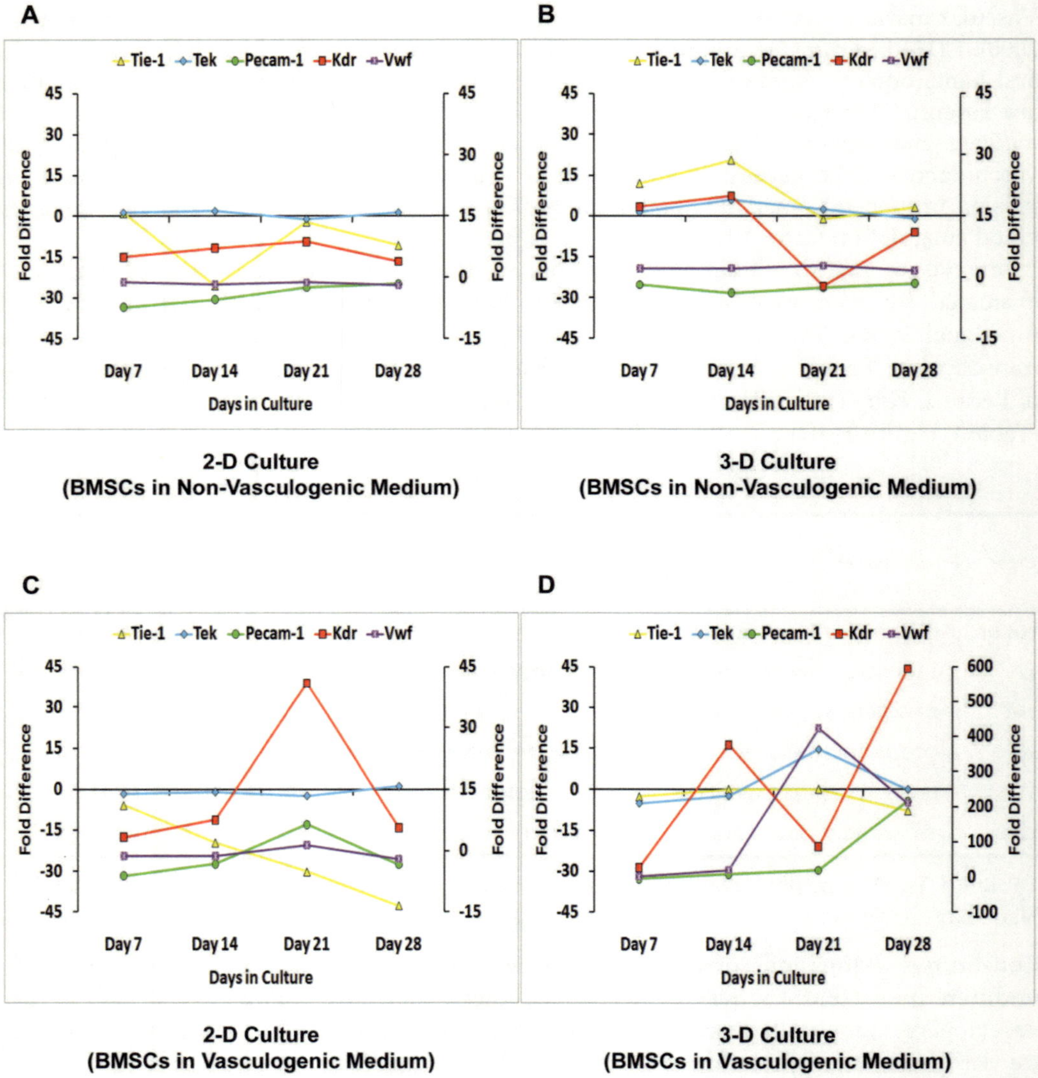

Fig. 2. Real-time reverse transcriptase quantitative polymerase chain reaction (RT-qPCR) analysis of various key vasculogenic markers. RT-qPCR analysis of various key vasculogenic markers such as tyrosine kinase with immunoglobulin-like and EGF-like domains 1 (Tie1), endothelial-specific receptor tyrosine kinase (Tek/Tie2), platelet/endothelial cell adhesion molecule 1 (Pecam1), kinase insert domain protein receptor (Kdr/Flk1/Vegfr-2), and Von Willebrand factor homology (Vwf) as a function of time (abscissa). BMSCs cultured in Petri dishes (2-D culture) in mesenchymal stem cell growth medium (A) and, in microvascular growth medium (C). BMSCs cultured in

collagen-gel tubular scaffolds (3-D culture) in mesenchymal stem cell growth medium (B) and, in microvascular growth medium (D). The calibrator control included BMSCs day 0 sample and; the target gene expression was normalized by a non-regulated reference gene expression, Gapdh. The expression ratio (ordinate) was calculated using the REST-XL version 2 software. The values are means ± standard errors for three independent cultures (n=3). (Tie-1 and Tek - plotted with respect to 1° Y-axis; Pecam-1, Kdr and Vwf - plotted with respect to 2° Y-axis) (Pfaffl, 2001, 2002; Valarmathi et al., 2008 a).

As revealed by immunostaining for various vasculogenic markers, day 21 vasculogenic and non-vasculogenic tube cultures showed that BMSCs were able to adhere, proliferate, migrate and, undergo complete maturation and differentiation into microvascular structures (Figure 3A-C). BMSCs derived microvessel formation is a combination of de novo vasculogenesis i.e., in situ endothelial cell differentiation and endothelium-lined tube formation, and angiogenesis, endothelial sprouting from existing endothelial tubes. In addition, these microvessels are stabilized by association with BMSCs derived smooth muscle cells and/or pericytes.

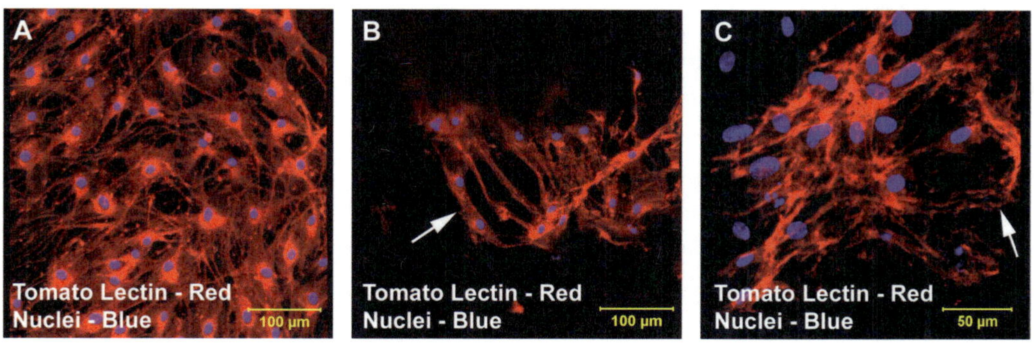

Fig. 3. Localization of BMSC-derived endothelial cells by Texas Red labeled Lycopersicon Esculentum lectin/Tomato Lectin (LEL/TL) staining. BMSCs cultured in collagen-gel tubular scaffolds under vasculogenic or non-vasculogenic culture conditions were incubated with tomato lectin (1:50 in 10 mM N-2-hydroxyethylpiperazine-N'-2-ethanesulfonic acid, pH 7.5; 0.15 M NaCl) to identify endothelial cells. Confocal laser scanning microscopic analysis of day 14 tubular scaffolds in these media conditions demonstrated the typical cobblestone appearance of differentiating endothelial cells (A), fusion and self-assembly (B), and evolving primitive capillary plexus with attempted lumen formation (B-C, white arrows). Cells were also stained for nuclei (blue, DAPI). Image (A) shows a projection representing 19 sections collected at 5.05 µm intervals (90.90 µm). Image (B) shows a projection representing 13 sections collected at 4.05 µm intervals (48.60 µm). Image (C) shows a projection representing 15 sections collected at 6 µm intervals (84.00 µm). Merged images (A-C). (A-B, scale bar 100 µm; C, scale bar 50 µm).

To validate the findings of mRNA expression pattern of important vasculogenic markers in these tube cultures and to determine whether these messages were in fact translated into proteins, immunostaining of the BMSC tube culture was carried out (Table 2; Figure 4A-L; Figure 5A-L).

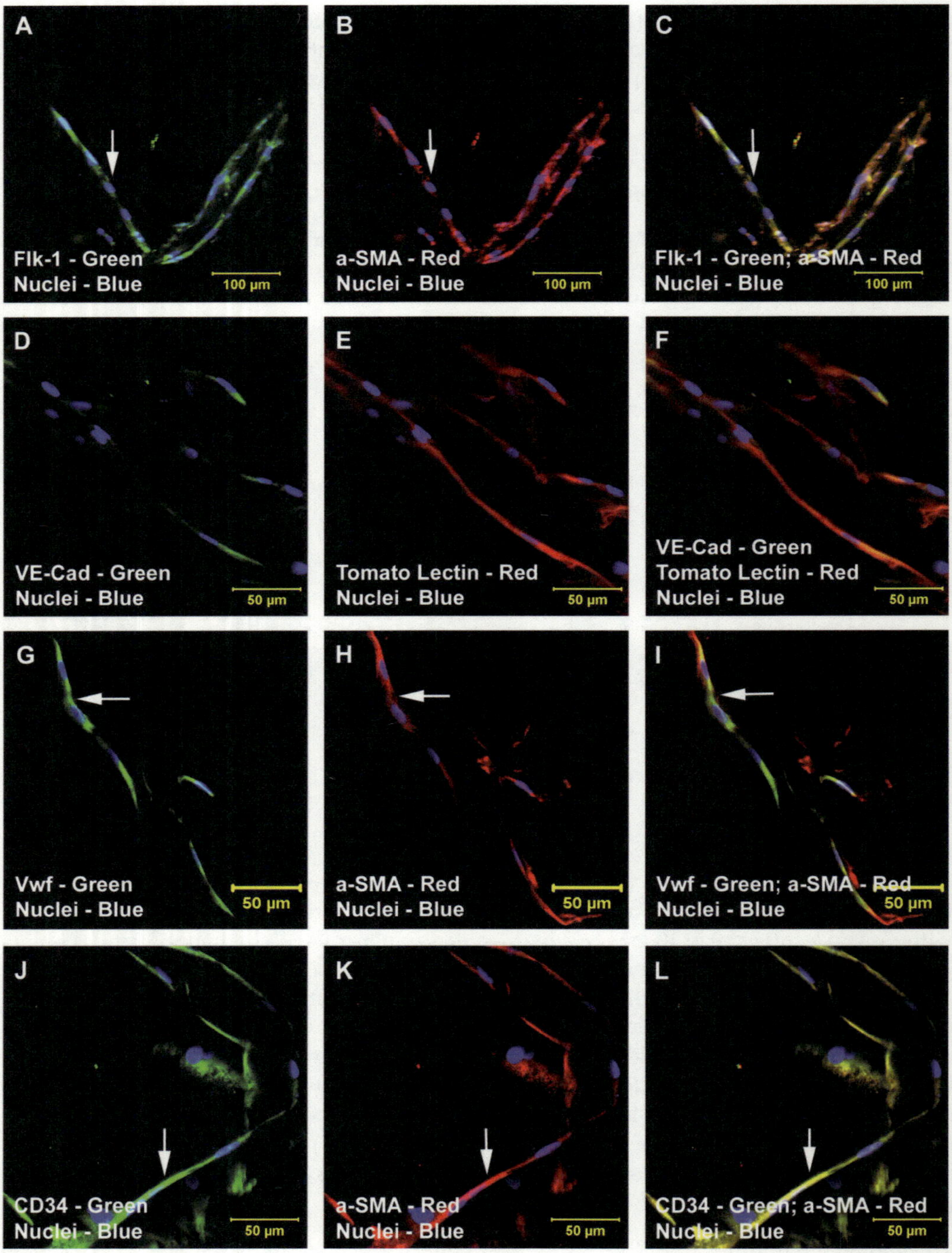

Fig. 4. Expression pattern of various vasculogenic markers in tubular scaffold by confocal microscopy. Localization of key endothelial and smooth muscle cell phenotypic markers of day 21 vasculogenic and non-vasculogenic tube cultures demonstrated the expression of

Flk1 (A, C), VE-cadherin (D, F), Vwf (G, I), CD34 (J, L), tomato lectin (E, F) and α-SMA (B-C, H-I, K-L). Dual immunostainings of these tube cultures (mesenchymal stem cell growth media, MSCGM or microvascular endothelial growth medium, EGMMV) revealed areas of elongated and flattened cells composed of varying degrees of mature endothelial and smooth muscle cells (A-L). These cells were organized into a loose delicate monomer network of nascent capillary-like structures composed of mature endothelial and smooth muscle cells. In addition, tube-like structures were emanating from the mixed population of differentiating vasculogenic cells represented by their distinct morphology and phenotypic expression (white arrows, A-C; white arrows, G-L). Cells were also stained for nuclei (blue, DAPI). Images (A-C) show a projection representing 15 sections collected at 3.05 μm intervals (42.70 μm). Images (J-L) show a projection representing 15 sections collected at 5.05 μm intervals (70.70 μm). Merged images (A-L). (A-C, scale bar 100 μm; D-L, scale bar 50 μm). Adapted from Valarmathi et al., 2009.

Primary antibodies	Dilutions	Source	Cell target
BMSCs characterization markers			
CD11b	1:50	BD Pharmingen	Leukocytes
CD31	1:10	Abcam	Endothelial
CD45	1:50	BD Pharmingen	Hematopoietic
CD90	1:50	BD Pharmingen	BMSCs
Endothelial cell differentiation markers			
CD34	1:100	Santa Cruz Biotechnology	Endothelial
Flk-1	1:100	Santa Cruz Biotechnology	Endothelial
VE- cadherin	1:100	Santa Cruz Biotechnology	Endothelial
Pecam1	1:100	Santa Cruz Biotechnology	Endothelial
Vwf	1:100	Santa Cruz Biotechnology	Endothelial
Tomato lectin	1:50	Vector Laboratories	Endothelial
Smooth muscle cell differentiation markers			
α-SMA	1:100	Sigma-Aldrich	Smooth muscle

Table 2. Primary antibodies used in this study (Valarmathi et al., 2009).

It is well known that endothelial cells share a large majority of their characteristic antigenic markers with other types of hematopoietic and mesenchymal cells (Bertolini et al., 2006). Therefore, antigens such as CD31, CD34, CD144 (VE-cadherin), CD146, Vwf or CD105 are not only expressed by endothelial cells but also expressed by hematopoietic cells (specifically HSCs), platelets and certain subpopulations of fibroblasts. Hence to identify the differentiated and matured endothelial cells in the tubular scaffold a battery of various early and late stage vasculogenic markers such as Pecam1, CD34, Flt1, Flk1, VE-cadherin and Vwf were employed. In addition, tomato lectin, another marker specific for rat vascular endothelial cells, was found closely associated with Flk1 and Vwf staining. These endothelial associated markers localized to endothelial cell clusters and capillary-like structures that were present throughout the tubular construct. This suggests that BMSC-derived endothelial cells assembled into endothelium-lined tube-like structures and initiated the process of vasculogenesis, consistent with our previous report (Valarmathi et al., 2008). In addition, the BMSC-derived cells and the microvessel-like structures expressed the smooth muscle antigens, α-SMA. These α-SMA positive cells were recruited in juxtaposition to the tandemly arranged endothelial cells and, were attached and wrapped around in such a way that is reminiscent of in vivo microvessel morphogenesis.

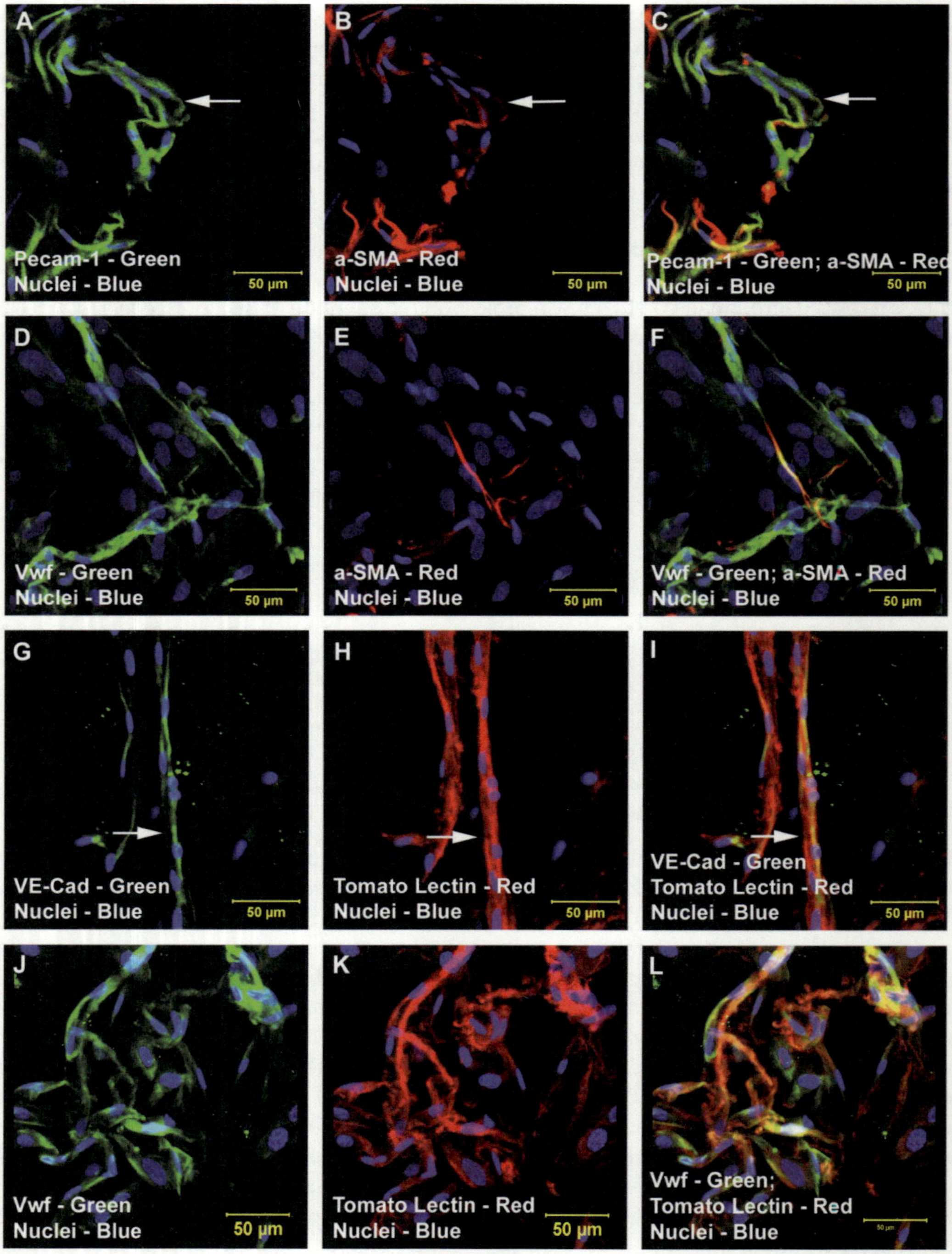

Fig. 5. Expression pattern of various vasculogenic markers in tubular scaffold by confocal microscopy. Localization of key endothelial and smooth muscle cell phenotypic markers of day 21 vasculogenic and non-vasculogenic tube cultures demonstrated the expression

of Pecam1 (A, C), Vwf (D, F; J, L), VE-cadherin (G, I), tomato lectin (H-I; K-L) and α-SMA (B-C, E-F). Dual immunostainings of these tube cultures (mesenchymal stem cell growth media, MSCGM or microvascular endothelial growth medium, EGMMV) revealed areas of elongated cells composed of both mature endothelial and smooth muscle cells (A-L). These cells were organized into a loose delicate network of nascent capillary-like structures composed of mature endothelial and smooth muscle cells and showed evidence of central lumen formation (white arrows, A-C, G-I). These cells formed developing microvessel-like structures (D-L). The linear nascent capillary-like structures showed translucent central lumen (white arrows, G-I). In addition, the cells were organized into a loose network of vascular cells and were in a ribbon-like configuration (D-F). These aligned vascular cells transformed into thin tube-like structures reminiscent of in vivo microvessel morphogenesis (D-L). Cells were also stained for nuclei (blue, DAPI). Images (A-C) show a projection representing 19 sections collected at 5.05 μm intervals (90.90 μm). Images (D-F) show a projection representing 16 sections collected at 4.05 μm intervals (60.75 μm). Images (G-I) show a projection representing 13 sections collected at 3.05 μm intervals (36.60 μm). Images (J-L) show a projection representing 23 sections collected at 4.05 μm intervals (89.10 μm). Merged images (A-L). (A-L scale bar 50 μm). Adapted from Valarmathi et al., 2009.

Similarly, it is critically important to characterize the ultrastructural morphology of any stem cells that are directed to differentiate into vascular lineage cells. Scanning electron microscopic (SEM) analysis of the tubular constructs depicted the pattern of microvessel morphogenesis and maturity. These formed nascent capillary-like structures and elongated tube-like structures revealed patent lumen-like structures, elucidating the vessel-maturation (Figure 6A-H). Besides, transmission electron microscopic (TEM) analysis revealed elongated capillary-like structures lined by differentiating endothelial cells (Figure 7A-F). These cells showed electron dense bodies as well as numerous small pinocytotic vesicles adjacent to the endothelial cell membranes as well as in their cytoplasm (Figure 7B, black arrows). In addition these cells exhibited variously sized cell-cell junctions, which have the appearance of typical in vivo endothelial tight junctions (Figure 7C-F).

Furthermore, the ability to identify endothelial cells based on their increased metabolism of Ac-LDL was examined using Ac-LDL tagged with the fluorescent probe, Dil-Ac-LDL. BMSC-derived endothelial cells and the nascent capillary-like structures were brilliantly fluorescent whereas the fluorescent intensity of smooth muscle cells/pericytes was barely detectable as reported previously (Valarmathi et al., 2009). This suggests that the formed endothelial cells were not only fully differentiated but also functionally competent and matured (Figure 8A-C).

This behavior of BMSCs and their exhibition of vasculogenic differentiation potential can be attributed to the nature of microenvironmental factors in this culture conditions. The preconditioned factors in the growth microenvironment rendered by the aligned type I collagen fibers of the tubular scaffold and the soluble differentiating factors provided by the vasculogenic or non-vasculogenic medium may be behind the BMSC fate determination. Further work is ongoing to determine whether our prevascularised tubular scaffolds can survive implantation into a tissue defect and is able to anastomose promptly with vascular sprouts emanating from the host. Finally, our morphological, molecular, immunological and biochemical data reveal the intrinsic vasculogenic differentiation potential of BMSCs under appropriate 3-D environmental conditions.

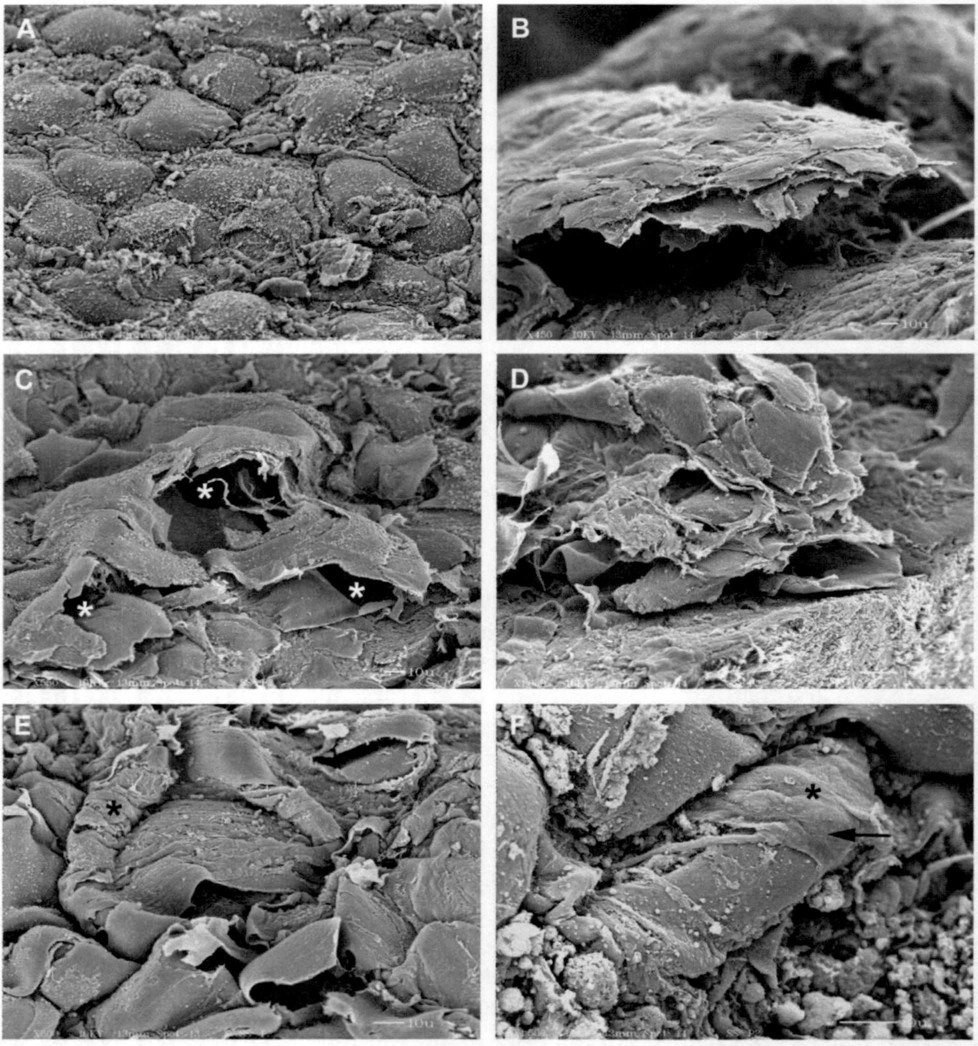

Fig. 6. Scanning electron microscopic (SEM) analysis of tubular constructs. SEM analysis of day 28 tubular constructs under vasculogenic or non-vasculogenic culture conditions

showed the typical cobblestone appearance of differentiating endothelial cells (A), stratification and networking (B-D), and the presence of smooth-walled tube-like structures with its attached smooth muscle cells and/or pericytes (black arrows, F-H). Multiple smooth muscle-like cells were wrapping around these tube-like structures (black asterisks, Figure E-H). These cylindrical structures revealed the presence of evolving patent lumens (white asterisks, C, G, H). (A-H, scale bar 10 μm). Adapted from Valarmathi et al., 2009.

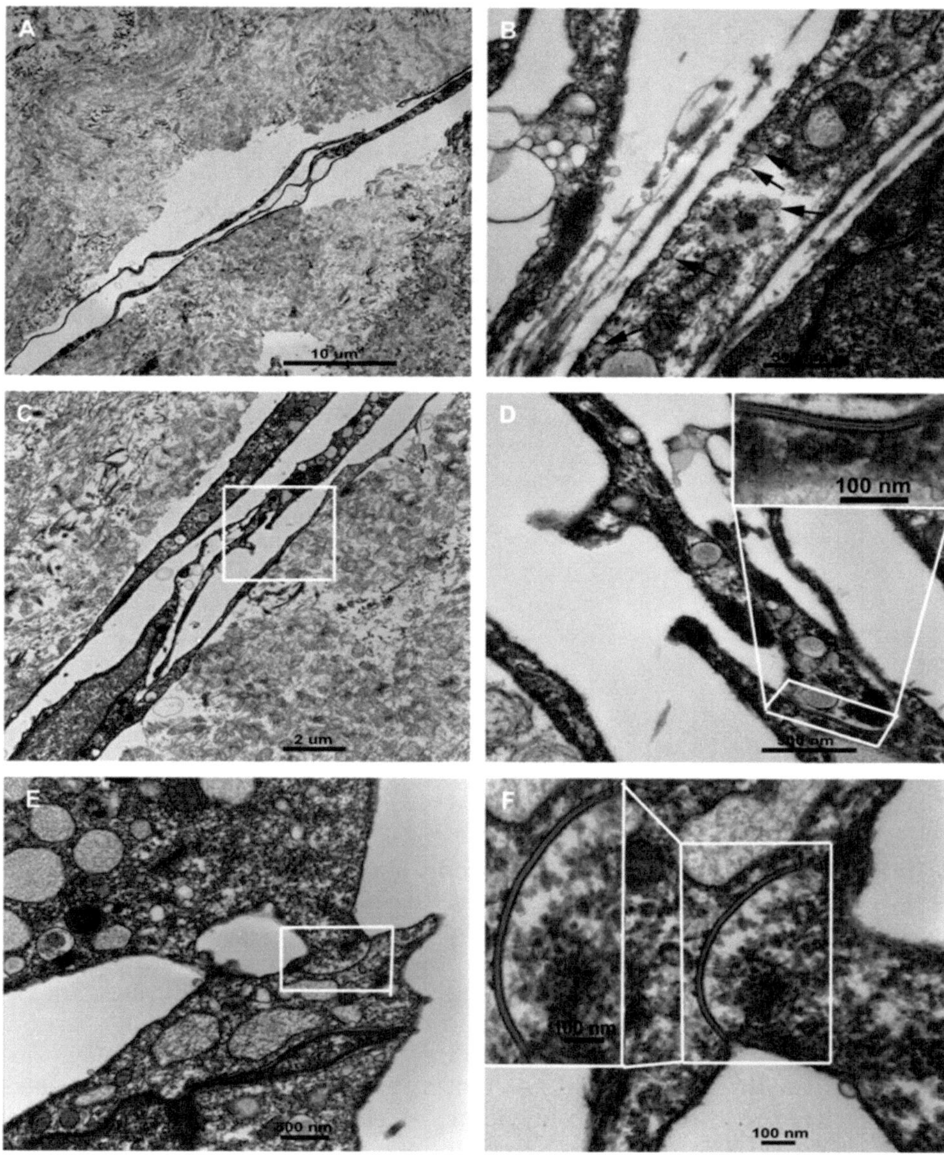

Fig. 7. Transmission electron microscopic (TEM) analysis of tubular constructs. TEM analysis of day 28 tubular constructs under vasculogenic or non-vasculogenic culture conditions showed a

vessel-like structure containing many small dense bodies within endothelial cells on either side of the lumen (A). Note the most obvious feature of endothelial cells, the concentration of small vesicles (pinocytotic vesicles) adjacent to the endothelial cell membranes and cytoplasm (B, black arrows). The interdigitating endothelial cells showing junctional regions (C, E, inserts, lower magnification). The typical adherent junction could be visualized between two overlapping endothelial cell processes (D, F, inserts, higher magnification). (Hanaichi et al., 1986).

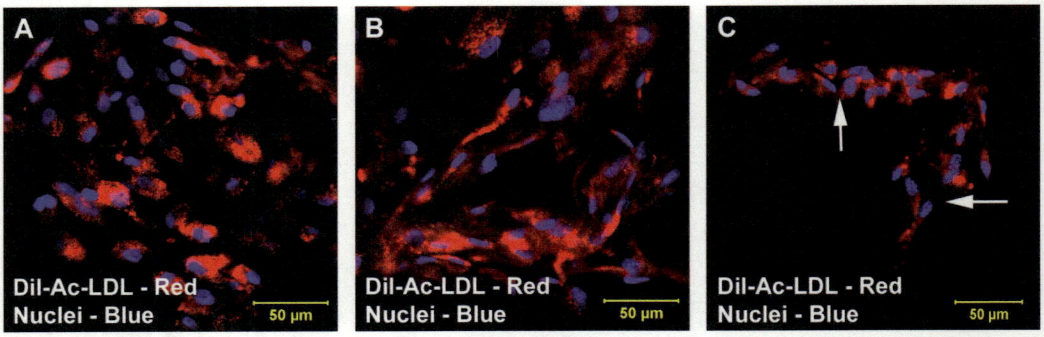

Fig. 8. Characterization of BMSC-derived endothelial cells by Dil-Ac-LDL uptake. BMSCs cultured in collagen-gel tubular scaffolds in vasculogenic or non-vasculogenic culture conditions were incubated with 10 µg/ml of Dil-Ac-LDL for 4 to 6 hours. Confocal laser scanning microscopic analysis of day 21 tubular scaffolds in microvascular endothelial cell growth medium (EGMMV) revealed typical abundant punctate perinuclear bright red fluorescence of the differentiated and matured endothelial cells (A). These labeled vascular cells were self-organized into tangled nascent linear capillary-like structures (B), assembled into solid cord of cells and, transformed into tube-like structure with attempted lumen formation (C, white arrows). Cells were also stained for nuclei (blue, DAPI). Image (C) shows a projection representing 22 sections collected at 5 µm intervals (105.00 µm). Merged images (A-C). (A-C, scale bar 50 µm). (Voyta et a., 1984) (Adapted from Valarmathi et al., 2009)

Previously, it has been shown that mature vascular endothelium can give rise to smooth muscle cell (SMC) via endothelial-mesenchymal transdifferentiation, coexpressing both endothelial and SMC-specific phenotypic markers (Frid et al., 2002). Recently, it has been show that Flk1-expressing blast cells derived from embryonic stem cells can act as precursors that can differentiate into both endothelial and mural cell populations of the vasculature (Yamashita et al., 2000). In this study, clonal analyses revealed the bi-lineage potential of BMSCs, suggesting that both endothelial and smooth muscle/pericytes could be derived from single colonies. However, in general, BMSCs-derived colonies are clonal or nearly clonal. The colonies of BMSCs resultant from a number of cells may represent co-existence of several subclones, each capable of differentiating into specific lineages. Hence, single cell-derived colonies that are stably transfected with lineage specific markers are needed to gain more meaningful insights and address the origin of both lineages.

Our results indicate that the 3-D tubular scaffold with its unique characteristics provides a favorable microenvironment that permits the development of in situ microvascular structures. Moreover, this is the first ever documentation that explicitly demonstrates that adult BMSCs under appropriate in vitro environmental cues can be induced to undergo vasculogenic differentiation culminating in microvessel morphogenesis (Valarmathi et al.,

2009). Our model recapitulates many aspects of in vivo de novo vasculogenesis. Thus, this unique culture system provides an in vitro model to investigate the maturation and differentiation of BMSC-derived vascular endothelial and smooth muscle cells in the context of postnatal vasculogenesis. In addition, it allows us to elucidate various molecular mechanisms underlying the origin of both endothelial and smooth muscle cells and especially to gain a deeper insight and validate the emerging concept of 'one cell and two fates' hypothesis of vascular development (Yamashita et al., 2000).

5. Conclusions

Here we report a unique 3-D culture system that recapitulates many aspects of postnatal de novo vasculogenesis. This is the first comprehensive report that evidently demonstrates that BMSCs under appropriate in vitro environmental conditions can be induced to undergo vasculogenic differentiation culminating in microvessels. Since BMSCs differentiated into both endothelial and smooth muscle cell lineages, this in vitro model system provides a tool for investigating the cellular and molecular origin of both vascular endothelial cells and smooth muscle cells. In addition, this system can potentially be harnessed to develop in vitro engineering of microvascular trees, especially using autologous bone-marrow-derived BMSCs for therapeutic purposes in regenerative medicine.

6. Acknowledgements

"This material is based upon work supported by the National Science Foundation/EPSCoR under Grant No. (EPS - 0903795)." - The South Carolina Project for Organ Biofabrication, as well "This work was supported by an award from the American Heart Association." - National Scientist Development Grant (11SDG5280022) for Valarmathi Thiruvanamalai.

7. References

Aggarwal, S. & Pittenger, M. F. (2005). Human mesenchymal stem cells modulate allogeneic immune cell responses. *Blood,* 105, 1815-1822.

Albelda, S. M.; Muller, W. A.; Buck, C. A. & Newman, P. J. (1991). Molecular and cellular properties of PECAM-1 (endoCAM/CD31): a novel vascular cell-cell adhesion molecule. *J Cell Biol,* 114, 1059-68.

Al-Khaldi, A.; Eliopoulos, N.; Martineau, D.; Lejeune, L.; Lachapelle, K. & Galipeau, J. (2003). Postnatal bone marrow stromal cells elicit a potent VEGF-dependent neoangiogenic response in vivo. *Gene Ther,* 10, 621-29.

Anokhina, E.B. & Buravkova, L. B. (2007). Heterogenecity of stromal cell precursers isolated from rat bone marrow. *Cell and Tissue Biology,* 1, 1-7. (Original article in Russian - Tsitologiya 2007;49:40-47.)

Bautch, V. L.; Redick, S. D.; Scalaia, A.; Harmaty, M.; Carmeliet, P. & Rapoport, R. (2000). Characterization of the vasculogenic block in the absence of vascular endothelial growth factor-A. *Blood,* 95, 1979-87.

Bertolini, F.; Shaked, Y.; Mancuso, P. & Kerbel, R. S. (2006). The multifaceted circulating endothelial cell in cancer: towards marker and target identification. *Nat Rev Cancer,* 6, 835-45.

Bianco, P.; Riminucci, M.; Gronthos, S. & Robey, P. G. (2001). Bone marrow stromal stem cells: nature, biology, and potential applications. *Stem Cells,* 19, 180-92.

Brey, E. M.; Uriel, S.; Greisler, H. P.; Patrick Jr., C. W. & McIntire, L. V. (2005). Therapeutic neovascularization: contributions from bioengineering. *Tissue Eng,* 11, 567-84.

Carlson, B. M. (2007). Tissue engineering and regeneration In: ed. *Principles of regenerative biology*, Amsterdam: Elsevier, pp. 259-278.

Carmeliet, P. & Jain, R. K. (2000). Angiogenesis in cancer and other diseases. *Nature,* 407, 249-257.

Carmeliet, P. & Luttun, A. (2001). The emerging role of the bone marrow-derived stem cells in (therapeutic) angiogenesis. *Thromb Haemost,* 86, 289-97.

Carmeliet, P. (2000). Mechanisms of angiogenesis and arteriogenesis. *Nat Med,* 6, 389-95.

Dominici, M.; Le Blanc, K.; Mueller, I.; Slaper-Cortenback, I.; Marini, F. & Krause, D. et al. (2006). Minimal criteria for defining multipotent mesenchymal stromal cells. The International Society For Cellular Therapy position statement. *Cytotherapy,* 8, 315-7.

Even-Ram, S. & Yamada, K. M. (2005). Cell migration in 3D matrix. *Curr Opin Cell Biol,* 17, 524-32.

Folkman, J. & Haudenschild, C. (1980). Angiogenesis in vitro. *Nature,* 288, 551-56.

Frid, M. G.; Kale, V. A. & Stenmark, K. R. (2002). Mature vascular endothelium can give rise to smooth muscle cells via endothelial-mesenchymal transdifferentiation: in vitro analysis. *Circ Res,* 90, 1189-96.

Fukuda, K. (2001). Development of regenerative cardiomyocytes from mesenchymal stem cells for cardiovascular tissue engineering. *Artif Organs,* 25, 187-193.

Hanaichi, T.; Sato, T.; Iwamoto, T.; Malavasi-Yamashiro, J.; Hoshino, M. & Mizuno N. (1986). A stable lead by modification of Sato's method. *J Electron Microsc (Tokyo),* 35, 304-06.

His, W. (1900). Lecithoblast und Angioblast der Wirbeltiere. *Abhandl Math-Phys Ges Wiss,* 26, 171-328.

Ingber, D. E. & Folkman, J. (1989). How does extracellular matrix control capillary morphogenesis? *Cell,* 58, 803-05.

Ingber, D. E. & Folkman, J. (1989). Mechanochemical switching between growth and differentiation during fibroblast growth factor-stimulated angiogenesis in vitro: Role of extracellular matrix. *J Cell Biol,* 109, 317-30.

Kinnaird, T.; Stabile, E.; Burnett, M. S.; Shou, M.; Lee, C. W. & Barr, S. et al. (2004). Local delivery of marrow-derived stromal cells augments collateral perfusion through paracrine mechanisms. *Circulation,* 109, 1543-49.

Kleinman, H. K.; McGarvey, M. L.; Liotta, L. A.; Robey, P. G.; Tryggvason, K. & Martin, G. R. (1982). Isolation and characterization of type IV procollagen, laminin, and heparan sulfate proteoglycan from the EHS sarcoma. *Biochemistry,* 21, 6188-93.

Lanza, R. P.; Langer, R. & Vacanti, J. (2000). *Principles of tissue engineering*, San Diego, CA: Academic Press.

Levenberg, S. (2005). Engineering blood vessels from stem cells: recent advances and applications. *Curr Opin Biotechnol,* 16, 516-23.

Madri, J. A.; Pratt, B. M. & Tucker, A. M. (1988). Phenotypic modulation of endothelial cells by transforming growth factor-β depends upon the composition and organization of the extracellular matrix. *J Cell Biol,* 106, 1375-84.

Makino, S.; Fukuda, K.; Miyoshi, S.; Konishi, F.; Kodama, H. & Pan, J. et al. (1999). Cardiomyocytes can be generated from marrow stromal cells in vitro. *J Clin Invest,* 103, 697-705.

Montesano, R.; Orci, L. & Vassalli, J. D. (1983). In vitro rapid organization of endothelial cells into capillary-like network is promoted by collagen matrices. *J Cell Biol,* 97:1648-52.

Oswald, J.; Boxberger, S.; Jorgensen, B.; Feldmann, S.; Ehninger, G. & Bornhauser, M. et al. (2004). Mesenchymal stem cells can be differentiated into endothelial cells in vitro. *Stem Cells,* 22, 377-84.

Pfaffl, M. W. (2001). A new mathematical model for relative quantification in real-time RT-PCR. *Nucleic Acids Res* 29, e45.

Pfaffl, M. W.; Horgan, G. W. & Dempfle, L. (2002). Relative expression software tool (REST) for group-wise comparison and statistical analysis of relative expression results in real-time PCR. *Nucleic Acids Res,* 30, e36.

Pittenger, M. F.; Mackay, A. M.; Beck, S. C.; Jaiswal, R. K.; Douglas, R. & Mosca, J. D. et al. (1999). Multilineage potential of adult human mesenchymal stem cells. *Science,* 284, 143-147.

Prater, D. N.; Case, J.; Ingram, D. A. & Yoder, M. C. (2007). Working hypothesis to redefine endothelial progenitor cells. *Leukemia,* 21, 1141-49.

Reyes, M.; Dudek, A.; Jahagirdar, B.; Koodie, L.; Marker, P. H. & Verfaillie, C. M. (2002). Origin of endothelial progenitors in human postnatal bone marrow. *J Clin Invest,* 109, 337-46.

Risau, W. & Flamme, I. (1995). Vasculogenesis. *Annu Rev Cell Dev Biol,* 11, 73-91.

Rozen, S. & Skaletsky, H. J. (2000). Primer3 on the WWW for general users and for biologist programmers. In: Krawetz S, Misener S (eds) Bioinformatics Methods and Protocols: *Methods in Molecular Biology,* Humana Press, Totowa, NJ, pp. 365-386.

Shalaby, F.; Ho, J.; Stanford, W. L.; Fischer, K-D.; Schuh, A. C. & Schwartz, L. et al. (1997). A requirement for Flk-1 in primitive and definitive hematopoiesis and vasculogenesis. *Cell,* 89, 981-90.

Urbich, C. & Dimmeler, S. (2004). Endothelial progenitor cells functional characterization. *Trends Cardiovasc Med,* 14, 318-22.

Vailhe, B.; Vittet, D. & Feige, J. J. (2001). In vitro models of vasculogenesis and angiogenesis. *Lab Invest,* 81, 439-52.

Valarmathi, M. T.; Goodwin, R. L.; Fuseler, J. W.; Davis, J. M.; Yost, M. J. & Potts, J. D. (2010). A 3-D cardiac muscle construct for exploring adult marrow stem cell based myocardial regeneration. *Biomaterials,* 31, 3185-200.

Valarmathi, M. T.; Davis, J. M.; Yost, M. J.; Goodwin, R. L. & Potts, J. D. (2009). A three-dimensional model of vasculogenesis. *Biomaterials,* 30, 1098-112.

Valarmathi, M. T.; Fuseler, J. W.; Goodwin, R. L.; Davis, J. M. & Potts, J. D. (2011). The mechanical coupling of adult marrow stromal stem cells during cardiac regeneration assessed in a 2-D co-culture model. *Biomaterials,* 32, 2834-50.

Valarmathi, M. T.; Yost, M. J.; Goodwin, R. L. & Potts, J. D. (2008a). A three-dimensional tubular scaffold that modulates the osteogenic and vasculogenic differentiation of rat bone marrow stromal cells. *Tissue Eng,* 14, 491-504.

Valarmathi, M. T.; Yost, M. J.; Goodwin, R. L. & Potts, J. D. (2008b). The influence of proepicardial cells on the osteogenic potential of marrow stromal cells in a three-dimensional tubular scaffold. *Biomaterials,* 29, 2203-16.

Voyta, J. C.; Via, D. P.; Butterfield, C. E. & Zetter, B. R. (1984). Identification and isolation of endothelial cells based on their increased uptake of acetylated-low density lipoprotein. *J Cell Biol,* 6, 2034-40.

Wakitani, S.; Saito, T. & Caplan, A. I. (1995). Myogenic cells derived from rat bone marrow mesenchymal stem cells exposed to 5-azacytidine. *Muscle Nerve,* 18, 1417-26.

Yamashita, J.; Itoh, H.; Hirashima, M.; Ogawa, M.; Nishikawa, S. & Yurugi, T. et al. (2000). Flk1-positive cells derived from embryonic stem cells serve as vascular progenitors. *Nature,* 408, 92-96.

Yost, M. J.; Baicu, C. F.; Stonerock, C. E.; Goodwin, R. L.; Price, R. L. & Davis, M. et al. (2004). A novel tubular scaffold for cardiovascular tissue engineering. *Tissue Eng,* 10, 273-84.